Creole Remedies of Trinidad and Tobago

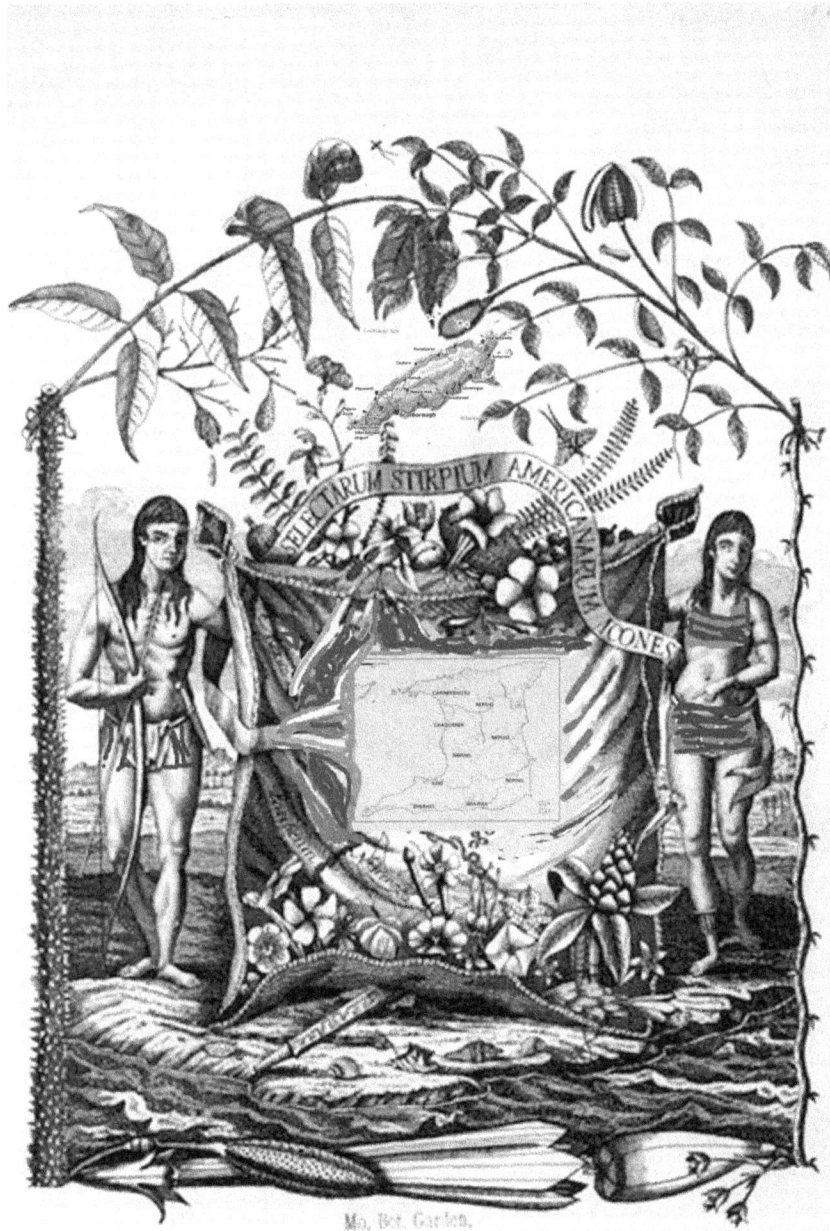

Mo. Bot. Garden.

Cheryl Lans, PhD

Creole Remedies of Trinidad and Tobago

ISBN: 978-0-9880852-0-6

Publication Date: 2012-05-10
Original publication lulu.com
Publisher: Lans, Cheryl

All of the plant pictures are used with the permission of the Missouri Botanical Garden Rare Book collection. This edition has black and white pictures.
Disclaimer: this book is not a replacement for qualified medical or veterinary advice.

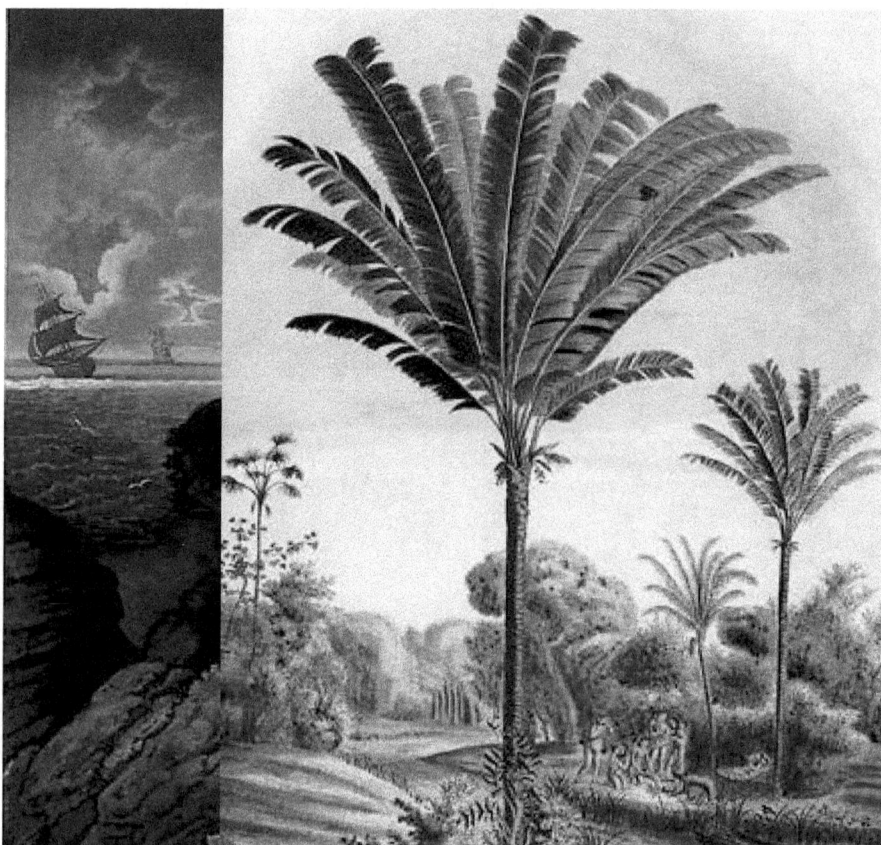

Cover illustration: Selectarum stirpium Americanarum historia (Kew): in qua ad Linnaeanum systema determinatae descriptaeque sistuntur plantae illae, quas in insulis Martinica, Jamaica, Domingo aliisque et in vicinae continentis parte, observavit rariores; adjectis iconibus ad autoris archetypa pictis. Author:Jacquin, Nikolaus Joseph, Freiherr von. Amerindian ethnic groups in Trinidad, ca. 1600. Legend: (1) 100-m contourline; (2) swamps and marshes. Source: Boomert, 2006.

Figure 2. Compiled images representing the coming of the Europeans to the Caribbean
Sources: New illustration of the sexual system of Carolus von Linnaeus: and the temple of Flora, or garden of nature, Historia naturalis palmarum: opus tripartium / Carol. Frid. Phil. de Martius.

Preface

This book describes research done in the spirit of the pledge initiated by the Student Pugwash Group in the United States as quoted by Rotblat (1999).

I promise to work for a better world, where science and technology are used in socially responsible ways. I will not use my education for any purpose intended to harm human beings or the environment. Throughout my career, I will consider the ethical implications of my work before I take action. While the demands placed upon me may be great, I sign this declaration because I recognise that individual responsibility is the first step on the path to peace.

The research documents ethnoveterinary practices used in Trinidad and Tobago, which are based on ethno- or folk medicine. It does not include the thesis chapters that have been already published in a variety of journals.

History of the research proposal

The Caribbean Agricultural Research and Development Institute (CARDI) was the implementing agency for a Sheep Production and Marketing Project (CSP/M) funded by the Canadian International Development Agency (CIDA). The project worked with low-resource farmers in Barbados, Guyana and Tobago. Farmer-participants in Tobago used folk medicines as anthelmintics. Edward Evans the Production Economist attached to the CSP/M concluded that improved technologies [including purchased drugs] could not be justified under the socio-economic and cultural framework in which these farmers operated (Evans, 1992). A research topic was then born.

The research process was an attempt to reshape (bio) technological knowledge of ethnoveterinary medicine by bringing ethnoveterinary knowledge into western science. This necessitated a process of negotiation with veterinarians, Animal Science and Medicinal Plant journal editors and reviewers, in order to validate ethnoveterinary practices and to classify the practices into recommended versus non-recommended for further research.

Some of the knowledge claims on which ethnoveterinary practices are based are open to debate. Yet there is still the need to reach compromise, consensus or accommodation, so that a process of validation satisfactory to all parties can be achieved. The research is thus an attempt to facilitate joint action on ethnoveterinary remedies, since the market will not provide tropical plant-based medicines in the short term.

One idea that shaped the research came from Foucault (1980) who talks about an: 'insurrection of subjugated [non-scientific] knowledges' and 'render[ing] these knowledges capable of opposition and of struggle against the coercion of a theoretical, unitary, formal and scientific discourse.' A second idea shaping the research was that: 'Knowledge is effective action in the domain of existence.' Maturana and Varela (1992: 244) as quoted by (Röling, N., Jiggins, J., and Coehoorn, C., 1999).

Validated ethnoveterinary knowledge can help all interested farmers become better at the performance of farming (Richards, 1989; Nitsch, 1991). Farm [performance] is not a matter of doing everything correctly, but of making a totality run in a satisfactory way using a pattern of continuous observation and adjustment (Richards, 1989; Nitsch, 1991). What western thought has long seen as magical beliefs and practices are the real challenge posed by indigenous knowledge (Marglin, 1990b; Giarelli, 1996). The challenge for scientists is to reconsider not only the nature of medicine, but also the nature of science and scientific knowledge itself (Giarelli, 1996).

Acknowledgements

Wageningen UR funded the research on which the present book is based under the sandwich program. Wageningen UR also provided a fellowship for the first phase of the research and the M.Sc. training. I am indebted to the Department of Ecological Agriculture for the first phase of the research. The Tobago sheep farmers provided me with the research question and their prayers helped me through the first phase. The Department of Communication and Innovation Studies and the Working Group Technology and Agrarian Development supported the second phase of the research. My gratitude extends to them also.

During the fieldwork friendship and support was offered by many staff members of the School of Veterinary Medicine, Faculty of Medical Science, University of the West Indies, Trinidad and Tobago. Some of the staff members participated in the fieldwork, some were co-authors of the published case studies and three had many roles. Dr. Gabriel Brown, (one of the co-promotors, co-authors and long-term friends), Dr. Gustave Borde (co-author), Dr. Elmo Bridgewater (co-author), Professor C.D. Ezeokoli (supporter), Dr. Tisha Harper (friend and co-author), Dr. Karla Georges (friend and co-author), Dr. Veronica Offiah (co-author). Others who were helpful in various ways were Dr. Webb, Dr. Reece, Mrs. Turner, Ashley and Rambo.

I owe much to my promotors Professor Paul Richards of the Working Group Technology and Agrarian Development and Professor Niels Röling of the Chair Group Communication and Innovation Studies. Professor Niels Röling co-supervised the first phase of the research with Dr. Jan Diek van Mansvelt of the Department of Ecological Agriculture and encouraged me to continue to do the doctorate.

Both Professor Paul Richards and Professor Niels Röling kept in constant touch during the fieldwork for the second phase despite their busy schedules and despite the uncertainty of the outcome. My co-promotor Dr. A. J.J. van den Berg of the Department of Medicinal Chemistry at the University of Utrecht, worked very hard in sorting through the chemical compounds and asked for changes in the text that would make it acceptable to the pharmacological audience.

My co-promotor Dr. Gabriel Brown was the day-to-day supervisor for the fieldwork period and always cleared a space for me to work in his crowded office. He acted as a sounding board for many of my ideas and theories and provided much needed support and guidance. Dr. Lionel Robineau, formerly of *enda-caribe* in the Dominican Republic provided friendly support and information on the under-researched plants.

The co-operation from the respondents was tremendous. The hospitality of all was wonderful. The *demi tasse* of local coffee that was always provided in Paramin was very much appreciated as was the 'bake and buljol / smoked herring' breakfasts provided on the hunting trips by Dr. Bridgewater.

Thanks especially to my family. Lastly this book is dedicated to Iris, Violet, Julia, Emily and Lucia.

Cheryl Lans

June 1, 2006

Contents

List of Figures

ADB	Agricultural Development Bank
CACAM	Caribbean Association of Complementary and Alternative Medicine
CARAPA	Caribbean Association of Researchers and Herbal Practitioners
CARDI	Caribbean Agricultural Research and Development Institute
CARICOM	Caribbean Community and Common Market
CARIRI	Caribbean Research Institute
CGIAR	Consultative Group on International Agricultural Research
CIDA	Canadian International Development Agency
CPDC	Caribbean Policy Development Centre
CSP/M	Caribbean Sheep Production and Marketing Project
EBUTROP	Economic Biology of Under-Utilised Tropical Plants
FAO	Food and Agriculture Organisation of the United Nations
GDP	Gross Domestic Product
IADB	Inter-American Development Bank
IICA	Inter-American Institute for Co-operation in Agriculture
IIRR	International Institute of Rural Reconstruction
IMF	International Monetary Fund
IPGRI	International Plant Genetic Resources Institute
IPR	Intellectual Property Rights
MALMR	Ministry of Agriculture, Land and Marine Resources, formerly Ministry of Food Production and Marine Exploitation
OAS	Organisation of American States
PAHO	Pan American Health Organisation
PBR	Plant Breeders' Rights
PGR	The Commission on Plant Genetic Resources
PSU	Poultry Surveillance Unit
THA	Tobago House of Assembly
TRAMIL	Traditional Medicine in the Islands
TRIPS	Trade-related aspects of Intellectual Property Rights
TTAIHP	Trinidad and Tobago Association of Integrative Healthcare Practitioners
UNCTAD	United Nations Conference on Trade and Development
UNEP	United Nations Environment Programme
UNESCO	United Nations Educational, Scientific and Cultural Organisation
UVI	University of the Virgin Islands
UWI	University of the West Indies
WIPO	World Intellectual Property Organisation

Introduction

As Trinidad is an English colony, one's first idea is that the people speak English; and one's second idea, when that other one as to the English has fallen to the ground, is that they should speak Spanish, seeing that the name of the place is Spanish. But the fact is that they all speak French (Trollope, 1859).

1. Background and motivations for the study

Introduction

The first chapter of this book outlines the context and justification of the research and gives a brief overview of the potential for ethnobotanical research and the relevance of medicinal plants to human and animal health in the Caribbean.

Background

Herbal remedies are one of the world's primary therapeutic arsenals to fight disease (Croom, 1983). In November 1998 the *Archives of Internal Medicine*, the *Journal of American Medicine* and eight other speciality medical journals devoted whole issues to alternative medicines (Dalen, 1998).

One of the Caribbean region's major problems is access to timely and cost effective medical and veterinary services. Some human health concerns in the Caribbean region are Measles, Neonatal tetanus, Foot and Mouth, Leprosy, Rubella, Chagas' Disease, Tuberculosis, Onchocerciasis, Dengue, HIV, HBV, HCV, Malaria, Cholera, Hepatitis, Diabetes, Cancer, Heart Disease, Asthma, *Treponema pallidum* and Yellow fever (PAHO, 1996). Many Caribbean rural people are involved in the production, marketing and processing of medicinal and culinary herbs. Regional policy makers have recognised that many problems in primary health care are due to lack of knowledge and sensitivity to local health practices, and to the economic and cultural factors associated with these practices (Bentley *et al.*, 1988). There is potential for locally available herbal medicines to be used in primary health care and agricultural development. However available herbal products, have no clear statement of content or medically related information on the package labels, and have not been validated or certified by any recognised body. This concerns consumers (potential and actual) and medical practitioners who may unknowingly counter-prescribe these herbal products (Maurice and Cream, 1989). Not all of the plants reported to be useful are harmless (Oubré *et al.*, 1997; MacGregor *et al.*, 1989).

Ethnoveterinary medicine in this thesis is the local, mainly plant-based medicines used for animals. As defined by McCorkle (1989), veterinary anthropology is folk management of animal health in the context of the whole farming system, with consideration for other socio-economic and political realities. The study of ethnoveterinary medicine is typically undertaken to assess its usefulness, but the majority of the studies are descriptive. It has been a named and recognised area of academic interest since the mid-1970s. Biodiversity, ethnomedicine and ethnoveterinary knowledge are greatly influenced by cultural beliefs, religion, societal norms and trends and by the materia medica available in terms of local flora, fauna and minerals (Mathias-Mundy and McCorkle, 1997; Guyer and Richards, 1996). Multi-disciplinary fieldwork is necessary to understand all the aspects of its complexity. In Trinidad and Tobago ethnoveterinary knowledge is based on folk medicine, a phenomenon which has been documented in other cultures (McCorkle and Green, 1998). This study has documented the ethnoveterinary and ethnomedicinal knowledge in Trinidad and Tobago.

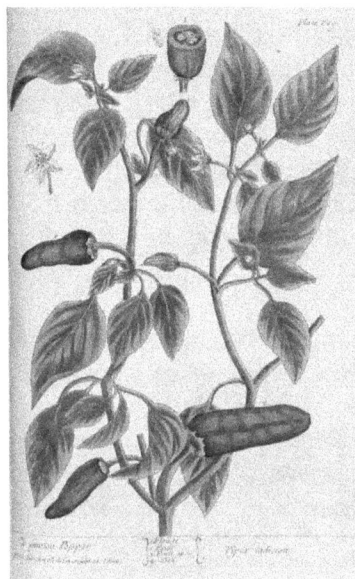

Figure 3. *Piper indicum*
Figure 4. *Coccoloba uvifera*
Figure 5. *Justicia lithospermifolia*

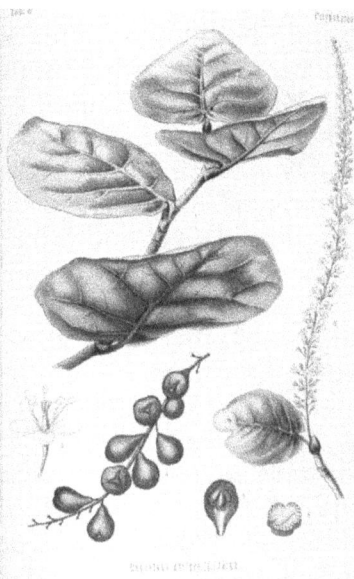

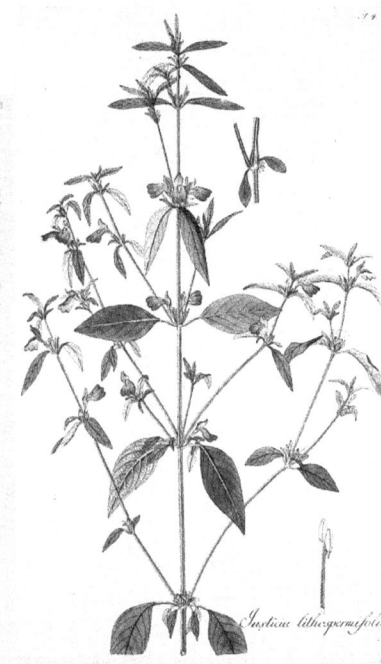

Creolization

The word Creole comes from the Spanish and means native to the settlement though not ancestrally indigenous to it (*criar*: to create, imagine, establish, found, settle and *colono*: a colonist, founder settler) (Brathwaite, 1971). In linguistics the word means a pidgin or reduced language that has become a native language to the local born population (Brathwaite, 1971). Glissant defines Creolization in the Caribbean as the cultural construct that distils the main constituents of Caribbean history. These are slavery, colonialism, and racism and the dehumanising experiences of transportation or migration (from Africa, Asia and Europe). Creolization processes integrate colonial historical experiences into a self-consciously de-centered, subversive and transformative creative Caribbean identity (Richards, 1996; Balutansky, 1997). Immigrants in their new Caribbean space use locally adapted technology which was obtained by matching the knowledge of their origins to the locally available plants for emergent health needs. Some of these plants might have been botanically related to previously known plants while others would have been seen for the first time. Creolized folk medicine then developed from the exploitation of synergy between the local knowledge of the Amerindian population and the external knowledge of the immigrants (Richards, 1996). Creolized folk medicine would not have been judged on the origins of its ideas and practices, but only on the standpoint that the plants used alleviated health problems (Richards, 1996).

Caribbean folk medicine is based on this synergy between European folk medicine; scientific medicine; African-based practices; Amerindian medicine and Indian-

11

based medicine with inclusions from other sources. It is a product of inter-group borrowing or medical syncretism or 'the pattern of social institutions and cultural traditions that evolve from deliberate behaviour to enhance health' (Laguerre, 1987). Folk medicine as a system includes: home remedies; folk aetiologies of disease; preventative medicine; reproductive techniques; medicinal properties of plants; anatomical knowledge, and healers. This ethnoveterinary medicinal study looks at some aspects of these different traditions. During preliminary research conducted in 1995, hunters were found to be using plants from the forests for snakebites and for their dogs, while medicinal plants from different sources were being used by livestock and poultry farmers as anthelmintics, for reproductive purposes and as antidiarrhoeal agents (Lans, 1996). Very little information was found on ethnoveterinary medicines for pigs. These core traditions of ethnoveterinary medicine were recently documented and published for the first time (Lans and Brown, 1998 a & b). Herskovits and Herskovits (1947) and Mischel (1959) have also documented folk medicine. Simpson (1962), Mahabir (1991), Littlewood (1988), Laguerre (1987) and Wong (1976) focus on either one community or one ethnic group.

Scientific validation of the effects and side effects of medicinal plants is needed before they can be recommended (or not) for use (Farnsworth, 1993). Research is also needed to establish whether medicinal plants have fewer long term adverse complications, such as antibiotic resistance, than commercial drugs. This is important since a 1997 study has shown that seven species of bacteria from animals in Trinidad are showing increasing resistance to five antimicrobial/antibacterial drugs: gentamicin, trivetrin, penicillin, amoxicillin and erythromycin (Suepaul, 1997). Lambie *et al.*, (2000) found that 50% of all *Escherichia coli* isolates from diseased broilers submitted to postmortem examination from 1990 to 1997 in Trinidad were resistant to several antimicrobial drugs. More than 85% of the isolates were resistant to streptomycin, tetracycline, and triple sulfa. Almost 50% of the isolates were resistant to amoxicillin, ampicillin, apramycin, gentamicin, neomycin and sulfamethoxazole-trimethoprim. Additionally the routine use of acaricides in the Third World is counterproductive due to loss of animals' natural resistance to illness, the acaricides high cost and the resulting tendency for farmers to underdose (Fielding, 2000). The ethnoveterinary medicinal research fits the call by the World Bank (and the Pan American Health Organisation (PAHO)) for public health research where public benefits exceed the economic returns that traditional investors typically seek (PAHO, 1997). PAHO (1997) has called for a science and technology system that dovetails with socio-economic realities. This entails linking the scientists who are dedicated to the production of knowledge and those dedicated to its utilisation.

The focus and main purpose of this study

This research stands at the interface of Beta/Gamma, where Beta stands for the Natural Sciences and Gamma for the Social Sciences. Together, Beta and Gamma sciences are becoming increasingly involved in the 'interactive design' of technology, knowledge systems, natural resource use and other forms of 'land use negotiation' (Röling, 2000). The research stands at the interface because it is not content with the pure anthropological approach of focussing on connected systems of local knowledge (Ellen, 1996a); it is also concerned with transforming local knowledge into information. The research also addresses the question of how institutions can organise to realise technological solutions based on indigenous knowledge / information for those in need of low-cost, low-tech solutions to common agricultural problems, while protecting the integrity and credibility of extension as an information source.

Traditionally, veterinarians have tried to discourage traditional medicines in favour of the modern medicine in which they were trained (Fielding, 2000; Lans, 1996; Mischel, 1959). However in financial crises 'modern' medicines are economically unrealistic to those in the low income groups, those living in remote areas and sometimes to government ministries (Niehoff, 1959; Guèye, 1999; Lans, 1996). Ethnoveterinary remedies on the other hand are often freely available, or have a cost in proportion to the value of the animal, or are already part of the culture, often work and are relatively easy to administer (Fielding, 2000). Previous research (Lans, 1996) has indicated that there are minor illness that farmers can treat with medicinal plants if it can be established that these plants are safe and effective. Schillhorn van Veen and de Haan (1995) predict a new era of cost effectiveness in which disease control is mandated, financed and executed by the farmer or lay personnel. Shifting minor health concerns to farmers can then free the Veterinarians to concentrate on health problems that may be getting inadequate attention and resources (Lans, 1996). The provision of and availability of a local pharmacopoeia supported by scientific data could impact positively on the health status of animals whose owners have inadequate access to or resources for the use of modern drugs and on the livestock industry.

Documentation and preliminary evaluation of medicinal plants is a necessary first step in establishing whether these ethnoveterinary remedies can provide affordable options for farmers' veterinary health needs. Indications that this would indeed be the case was provided in the first phase of the research when it was discovered that farmers in the 'modern' and commercially viable poultry industry were successfully using ethnoveterinary medicines to meet the health needs of the poultry sector (Lans, 1996). The first and second phases of the research were designed to codify and record collective memory of medicinal plants and thus provide a broad picture of the ethnoveterinary knowledge base of livestock farmers, pet owners and hunters in both Trinidad and Tobago. Ethnomedicinal knowledge was also recorded because there are many interconnections between ethnomedicinal and ethnoveterinary knowledge. Documenting the ethnomedicinal knowledge is an important first step in tracing the origins of the ethnoveterinary knowledge in Trinidad and Tobago. The origin of the knowledge is important in the verification process, why things are done in certain ways, and if there are any theories behind the practice. In addition to documenting and presenting the medicinal plants used in species-specific case studies, the medicinal plants listed in this thesis were also subjected to a non-experimental validation process. Experts in ethnoveterinary medicine consider that validation is still a weak point in the discipline (Schillhorn van Veen, 1997). This validation process is seen as a preliminary step to establish which plants should have priority in future clinical trials or research projects.

Written, public knowledge is revised, tested and challenged by others and is not lost to future generations, it becomes 'universalised and immortalised, oral knowledge does not (Laguerre 1987). Creolization-based technologies are not judged on the basis of their origins, only that they work in the local context. Western science has become the main means of establishing whether a technology works and how (Nelkin, 1996; Watson-Verran and Turnbull, 1995). The non-experimental validation of the ethnoveterinary medicines was undertaken in recognition of this fact. Analysis requires that all knowledge claims be subjected to a minimalist standard of rationality that requires that belief be apportioned to evidence and that no assertion about folk medicine or 'theory' (even the Doctrine of Signatures) be immune from or rejected without critical assessment (Hawkesworth, 1989).

Anthropologists like Posey (1998) and Hastrup and Elsass (1990) claim that anthropologists should not decide whether indigenous beliefs and practices are or are not scientific as this has colonial overtones. Other anthropologists claim that indigenous knowledge systems represent the cultural dimension of development and cannot be reduced to the empirical knowledge that they contain (Warren, Slikkerveer and Brokensha, 1995)[1]. These anthropological reservations have some value; however validation of ethnoveterinary medicines is important since most scientists will not use local medicines without some form of validation. For example during the second research phase one unbiased local veterinarian decided to research the effect of Neem (*Azadirachta indica*) on ticks, because the insecticidal properties of Neem were already published. An equivalent local plant (*Cordia curassavica*) existed, and its use to control ectoparasites had been published by a colleague (Lans and Brown, 1998a&b). However in contrast to Neem, little research work had been done on the insecticidal properties of *Cordia curassavica*.

The evaluation of the ethnoveterinarymedicinal plants was conducted using a non-experimental method (Browner *et al.*, 1988; Heinrich *et al.*, 1992), which consisted of:
1. botanical identification
2. reframing the folk medicinal data in terms of bioscientific concepts and methods
3. searching the chemical / pharmaceutical literature for the plant's known chemical constituents
4. searching the pharmacological literature to determine the known physiological effects of either the plant, related species, or isolated chemical compounds that the plant is known to contain; and
5. assessing whether the plant use is based on empirically verifiable principles; or, whether symbolic aspects of healing are of greater relevance (Heinrich *et al.*, 1992; Browner *et al.*, 1988).

The evidence gathered and the critical reflection / validation process which occurred during the documentation and preliminary validation of the medicinal plants can provide a 'developed, tested and critically-examined rationale' for locally used ethnomedicines and ethnoveterinary medicines (Hatten *et al.*, 2000).

Research objectives and Research questions
The objective of this thesis was to document ethnoveterinarymedicinal knowledge in Trinidad and Tobago and to explore whether it can usefully complement formal veterinary and medicinal knowledge; and if so, how?

The main research questions
- Which practices can be identified as ethnoveterinary practices in Trinidad and Tobago and is ethnoveterinary medicine a separate field from human folk medicine?
- How are ethnoveterinary medicinal practices being used for livestock, sport animals and pets? And what kind of socio-cultural environment does this folk knowledge exist in?
- Are the ethnoveterinary practices based on culture, religion, or on the indigenous knowledge of different subsets of the population? Can these practices be traced to the original continents of Trinidad and Tobago's current population?
- Are there positive things to say about this Creole legacy and does this folk medicinal knowledge fit a theory of [ethnomedicinal] agrarian creolization?
- Are the folk/ethnoveterinary medicinal practices derived from a body of knowledge that is ancient, coherent and global in nature? Do the different traditional medical systems that exist in Caribbean folk medicine share a common explanatory model?
- Does the ethnomedical literature support the claimed uses of the medicinal plants?

In the thesis there was no radical dis-identification with conventional biomedicine (Scheper-Hughes, 1990), and no 'flight from reason after the death of God' (Latour, 1998), but an attempt to create the necessary space for the folk medicinal paradigm to co-exist with

---

[1] These viewpoints are examined in more detail in Chapter 3.

western medicine. A framework of indigenous / ethnoveterinary knowledge that can interface with science and technology is more likely to influence scientific research agendas and development work (Sillitoe, 1998). This research can contribute to a systematic and comparative understanding of different ways of conceiving and treating human and veterinary medical problems which will add useful data to medicinal and pharmaceutical science (Tarbes, 1989). A methodology for the systematic cross-cultural study of traditional medical systems and their diagnostic and therapeutic efficiency could provide an important contribution to the medical anthropological literature (Tarbes, 1989).

Traditional medicine is a health care system and both the botanical and cultural aspects of this system need to be studied (Croom, 1983). A holistic approach is necessary to properly document ethnoveterinary practices due to the strong influence that religion and culture and the environment have on this oral knowledge (Mintz, 1983; Ingold, 1996; Rappaport, 1993). A holistic approach will ensure that future scientific validation is not wasted on plants that are used only as cultural artefacts (Elisabetsky and de Moraes, 1990; Eigner and Scholz, 1999). This is important not only because of the waste of time, money and energy, but because negative results can lead to the discrediting of further effort (Eigner and Scholz, 1999). Drawing parallels between ethnomedical systems and the biochemical system is difficult because sickness and health are not only biological states, but also social, cultural and psychological phenomena (Weniger, 1991). The so-called objective sciences - chemistry and pharmacology – are therefore not the only valid parameters to evaluate ethnomedicines (Weniger, 1991).

Documentation of both the ethnoscientific empirical material, and also the non-empirical dimension of this knowledge is necessary since the local symbolic system is an integral part of traditional knowledge (Giarelli, 1996). Knowing is a practical, embodied, situated activity, constituted by a past, but reconstituted and changing in current use of the practices (Escobar, 1999). Decontextualised models alter the relationship between person and environment by subordinating or obscuring the local details which generate meanings (Hornborg, 1996). It is in this context that Etkin (1993) cautions that cultural connotations and preparatory details need to be considered in the assessment of the 'efficacy' of medicinal plants. For instance how the knowledge of phytochemical potential translates to the circumstances of actual plant use during illness (Etkin, 1993). If culture influences the use of the plant-based medicine this is not sufficient reason to dismiss the use as 'non-scientific' since medico-religious or magical understandings of disease aetiology can at times lead to effective therapeutic or management action. For practical scientific reasons, therefore supernaturally motivated practices cannot truly be separated from other aspects of ethnoveterinarymedicine (McCorkle and Mathias-Mundy, 1992). This last point will be elaborated on in subsequent chapters.

Medical Anthropological research recognises that illness and healing are lived events (Scheper-Hughes, 1990). All popular clinical discourse[2], western or non-western, utilises familiar and tangible referents, either through personalisation (e.g. Obeah) or naturalisation (interaction of natural elements) (Littlewood, 1988; Tan, 1989). An anthropological study needs to deal with (non) biological forms of healing in terms of their own meaning-centred and emic[3] frames of reference (Scheper-Hughes, 1990).
Baer (1996, 1997) sets out four premises for a Critical Medical Anthropology.
   o First, the recognition that local events can be influenced by external forces.

---

[2] Discourses are historically, socially, and institutionally specific structures of statements, terms, categories, and beliefs or bodies of knowledge. As texts, they assert truths and claims for authority and legitimisation (Foucault, 1980).
[3] Emic - categories which are drawn from the way local people perceive things (Martin, 1995).

- o Second, a holistic understanding of sickness and an examination of the power relationships that exist in medicine.
- o Third, the realisation that all theories have a cultural basis, including the anthropological theories of sickness and healing.
- o Fourth, the acceptance of research and theorising as social acts that can be made into ethical acts.

An analytical framework combining the emic perspective of ethnomedicine with the etic[4] measures of bioscience can generate new interpretations for cross-cultural, comparative studies of ethnomedicine (Browner *et al.*, 1988). The research fits into the framework of applied anthropology, which is a complex of related, research-based, instrumental methods which produce change or stability in specific cultural systems through the provision of data, initiation of direct action and/or the formation of policy (Peterson, 1988). Applied anthropology has been described as a process rather than a field (Warry, 1992). In this process the relevant stages are discovery/planning, intervention and evaluation. A dialectical relationship exists between theory and praxis in applied anthropology since applied anthropology seeks to use the insights offered by ethnography as a basis for intervention and planned change, advocacy and information dissemination as well as theory development (Johannsen, 1992; Giarelli, 1996; Rappaport, 1993).

Fieldwork was conducted from September 1996 to September 2000. Semi-structured interviews and participant observation were used to collect the data. The approach was partly anthropological using the definition of anthropology as a specialism of non-specialism (Rapport and Overing, 2000). Research methodologies based on knowledge-based action provided the framework used to collect the ethnoveterinary and ethnomedicinal data. These are non-traditional methodologies. This type of research can lead to stronger linkages between organisations and research centres and to organisational knowledge development and improvement (Nereu *et al.*, 1997).

An overview of the book's contents and the structure of the book

An introductory chapter gives the overview and background. Chapter 2 gives details on agriculture in Trinidad and Tobago with a focus on livestock and poultry production. Chapter 3 outlines the methodological approach taken. The approach compares 'hard' and 'soft' science, and gives a brief overview of social constructivism and knowledge-based action. Chapter 4 examines the concepts and theories embedded in folk medicine and the origins of the folk medicine in the Caribbean. Chapter 5 provides details on the methods used to collect the data. Chapter 6 outlines the folk medicinal terms used. Chapter 7 contains case study 1 on backyard animals. Chapter 8 comprises case study 2 on horses. Chapter 9 contains case study 3 on [human] ethnomedicine. Chapter 10 looks at the actor networks involved in science and folk medicine, pointing out some of the processes by which knowledge is accepted into or excluded from science. Chapter 11 examines the cultural factors that shape ethnomedicinal creolization. Chapter 12 contains the conclusions.

---

[4] Etic - categories taken from the way the researcher perceives and classifies the world (Martin, 1995).

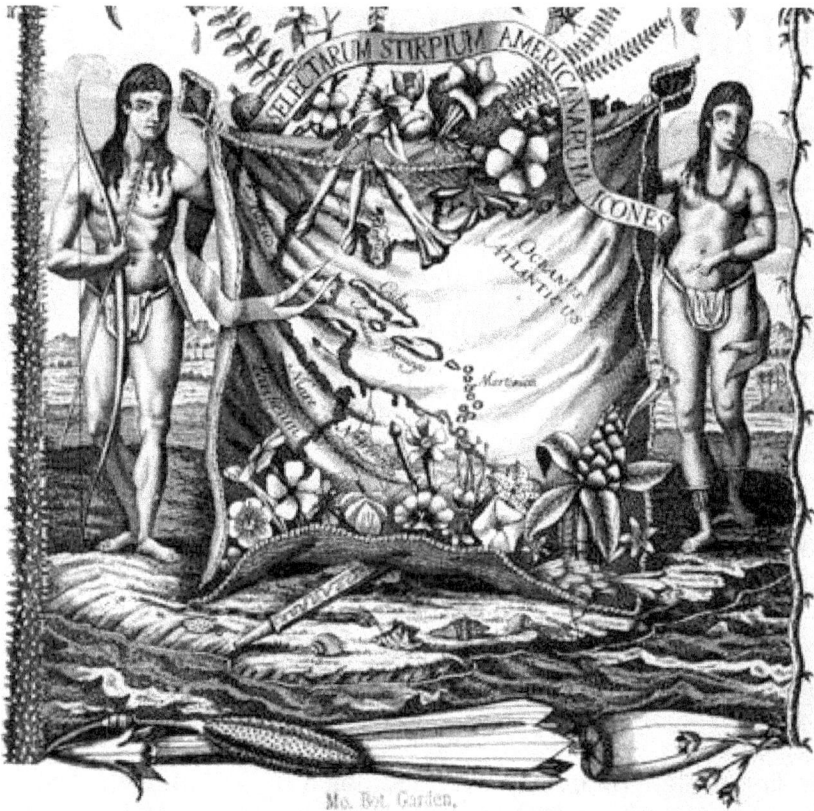

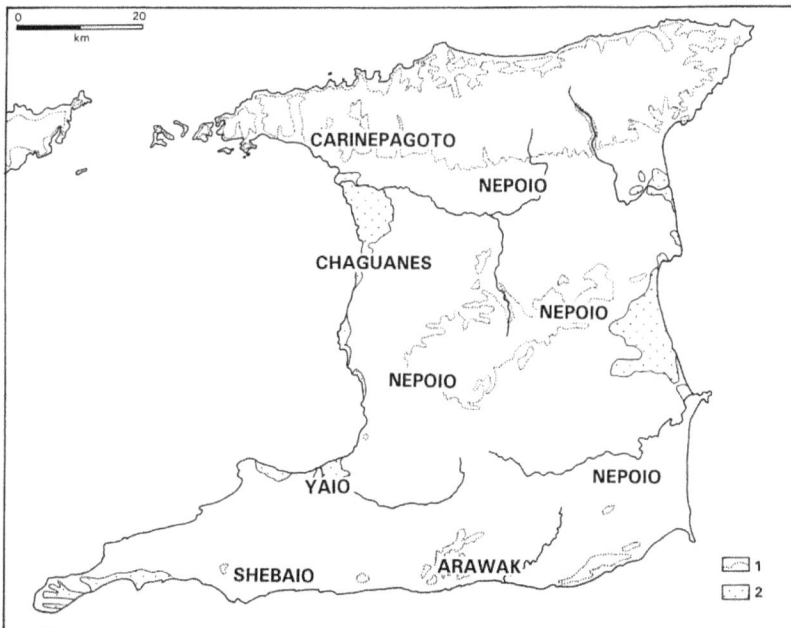

Figure 6a. Frontispiece.
Selectarum stirpium Americanarum historia (Kew): in qua ad Linnaeanum systema determinatae descriptaeque sistuntur plantae illae, quas in insulis Martinica, Jamaica, Domingo aliisque et in vicinae continentis parte, observavit rariores; adjectis iconibus ad autoris archetypa pictis. Author:Jacquin, Nikolaus Joseph, Freiherr von

Figure 6b. Amerindian ethnic groups in Trinidad, ca. 1600.
Legend: (1) 100-m contourline; (2) swamps and marshes. Source: Boomert, 2006.

Agriculture in Trinidad and Tobago

2. Agriculture in Trinidad and Tobago

Trinidad and Tobago is one country consisting of two adjacent islands located just northeast of the Venezuelan coast. Trinidad was first Spanish then a British colony. Tobago's cigar-like shape gave it its Spanish name (*cabaco, tavaco, tabaco*) and possibly its Amerindian names of *Aloubaéra* (black conch) and *Urupaina* (big snail) (Boomert, 2000). Historian E.L. Joseph claimed that Trinidad's Amerindian name was *Iere* derived from the Amerindian name for hummingbird *ierèttê* or *yerettê*. However Boomert claims that *Cairi* or *Caeri* does not mean hummingbird and *tukusi* or *tucuchi* does (Boomert, 2000)[5]. Both islands became independent of Britain in 1962 and attained the status of a republic in 1976. The republic is located between latitudes 10 ° and 11 ° north and spans longitude 61 ° west. The republic has a combined area of 5070 km^2. Geologically, Trinidad is an outlier of the South American continent. It lies 18 km north-east of Venezuela, and has an area of 4769 km^2. Tobago lies 35 km north of Trinidad and has an area of 301 km^2. The wet season lasts from June to December. The human population of 1.25 million is multi-ethnic, religious and cultural. The population increases at 1% annually. In Trinidad, the major population centres are concentrated along the west coast and along an east-west transportation corridor in the north of the island.

Antonio de Sedeño first settled Trinidad in the 1530s as a means of controlling the Orinoco and subduing the *Warao* (Whitehead, 1997). Cacique *Wannawanare* (*Guanaguanare*) granted the St Joseph area to Domingo de Vera e Ibargüen in 1592 and then withdrew to another part of the island (Boomert, 2000). San José de Oruña (St. Joseph) was established by Antonio de Berrío on this land. Ralegh arrived in *Trinedado* on March 22 1595 casting anchor at Curiapan/Punta de Gallos and described the pitch lake (*Piche* or Tierra de Brea) and the *Annaperima* hill. This hill was known to the *Warao* as the home of the sea god *Na'barima* (Whitehead, 1997; 131). Ralegh soon attacked San José and captured and interrogated de Berrío obtaining much information from him and from the cacique *Topiawari* (Whitehead, 1997). In the 1700s, Trinidad belonged as an island province to the vice royalty of New Spain along with modern Mexico and Central America (Besson, 2000). The Dutch and the Courlanders had established themselves in Tobago in the 16th and 17th centuries and produced tobacco and cotton. However Trinidad in this period was still mostly forest, populated by a few Spaniards with their handful of slaves and a few thousand Amerindians (Besson, 2000). Spanish colonisation in Trinidad remained tenuous. In 1762, after three hundred years of Spanish rule San José de Oruña and Puerto España (Port of Spain) were hamlets rather than towns. Because Trinidad was considered underpopulated, Roume de St. Laurent, a Frenchman living in Grenada, was able to obtain a Cédula de Población from the Spanish King Charles III on the 4th November, 1783. This Cédula de Población was more generous than the first of 1776 and granted free lands to Roman Catholic foreign settlers and their slaves in Trinidad willing to swear allegiance to the Spanish king. The land grant was thirty two acres for each man, woman and child and half of that for each slave brought. As a result, Scots, Irish, German, Italian and English families arrived. The Protestants among them profited from Governor Don José Maria Chacon's generous interpretation of the law. The French Revolution (1789) also had an impact on Trinidad's culture since it resulted in the emigration of Martiniquan planters and their slaves to Trinidad who established an agriculture-based economy (sugar and cocoa) for the island (Besson, 2000).

---

[5] Boomert (2000) claims that *Warao* identify *Nibo-yuni* (without-men), the *Matininó* of the Taino as Trinidad

The population of Puerto de España (Port of Spain) increased from under 3,000 to 10,422 in five years and the inhabitants in 1797 consisted of mixed-races, Spaniards, Africans, French republican soldiers, retired pirates and French nobility (Besson, 2000). The total population of Trinidad in 1797 was 17718; 2,151 of which were "white", 4,476 were "free blacks and people of colour", 10,009 were slaves and 1,082 Amerindians. In 1797, General Sir Ralph Abercromby and his squadron sailed through the Bocas and anchored off the coast of Chaguaramas. The Spanish Governor Chacon decided to capitulate without fighting. Trinidad became a British crown colony, with a French-speaking population and Spanish laws (Besson, 2000). The conquest and formal ceding of Trinidad in 1802 led to an influx of settlers from England or the British colonies of the Eastern Caribbean. After the abolition of slavery and the collapse of the French planters' cane economy, the 'French Creole' planters and the peasant population of mixed Spanish-Amerindians turned to cocoa cultivation. By the 1950s cocoa had become a staple in Trinidad's export market and was responsible for a growing middle-class. Early Caribbean settlers helped tie the Caribbean into international markets as suppliers of sugar cane, spices, bananas and arrowroot. Arrowroot starch is used to thicken soups and other culinary dishes. The starch is also used industrially in paper, board, glues, soaps and powders (Sanderson, 2005). These crops have not provided sustainable incomes to small scale growers, and have resulted in environmental degradation.

The history of sugar cane and cocoa meant that livestock production was always marginalised. This is clearly seen in the figures presented by the Minister of Agriculture in the 1999 Budget Speech. The export earnings for agriculture were TT$553.0 million, which represented 24% of non-oil exports and 8.1% of total exports. The contribution of sugar to this figure was $217 million or 38.3%, fruit and vegetables contributed 9.6% or $52.9 million, fish and fish preparations contributed $41.1 million or 7.4% and cocoa and coffee contributed $38.1 million or 6.9%. The contribution of livestock was not reported. The only initiatives reported for livestock in this budget were the establishment of a Livestock and Livestock Producers Board comprised of stakeholders to assist in the promotion and development of the sub-sector, and a new subsidy of TT$2000.00 for pasture establishment. The 2005-2006 Budget Speech represented the government's objective for agriculture as food security in rice, root crops, small ruminants, aquaculture dairy and rice, however at the beginning of 2005 the national rice mill was shut down.

Trinidad and Tobago is heavily dependent on imported food because of the historical legacy of sugar monoculture. At the small farm level, a wide variety of fruits, vegetables, root crops, legumes and livestock were produced for subsistence and/or sale on the local market. However plantation owners were reluctant to diversify from sugar and thus lose the social and political privileges that were linked to sugar monoculture (Pemberton, 1990). They firmly believed it made greater economic sense to export sugar and import everything else. According to Bennett (1986) 'forty years ago it was the general consensus of opinion among the plantocracy of Trinidad, that any poultry or livestock project would be doomed to failure, due to our tropical environment, in particular the wet and humid season, which created a haven for internal parasites. In addition to the fact that our grasses were not nutritious enough and that no cereal grains were grown in the tropics to provide concentrate feed supplements'. These attitudes are the basis for the current marginality of the livestock sector. The agriculture sector is also weak because historically peasant farmers were considered poor credit risks by the Canadian, American and British interests that controlled the banking system until the mid-1960s. This attitude towards small farmers was reinforced by the colonial education system which taught disdain for manual labour in general and agriculture in particular. In addition, because farming is still associated with slavery, it has never been, and is still not, a first-choice occupation for the ex-slaves and their descendants. To this day it is still considered something 'to escape from'. Of those involved in agriculture in 1990, squatters were approximated at 25,000, and legal landholders at 35-40,000, 79% of the farming population was over 40 years old, of which 56% was over 50, and only 2% were less than 25. Pemberton (1990) traces the downward trend in agricultural employment from 23.4% in 1970 to 9.4% in 1986. The 2004 Census recorded 19,143 holders, with 974 of these in Tobago. Crop farmers comprised 72.4% and livestock farmers 9.6% of the total. The majority of the holdings (96%) were under 10 ha. There was a greater percentage of livestock farmers in Tobago (28.5%) and a greater proportion of mixed farmers (30.6%) than in Trinidad (17.9%).

Centralised government employment and the high wage industrial and construction sectors escalated the exodus from agriculture (McElroy and de Albuquerque, 1990). The Public Works program (a form of social support for low income workers) was characterised by higher wages and also by the fact that the number of hours worked per day was negligible in contrast to agriculture which involved long hours with higher risks and smaller financial returns (Harrison, 1994). In the 1960s the Government attempted to restructure the agriculture sector, and to break the dichotomy between plantation and small scale farming by the implementation of the State Lands Development Project (Pemberton, 1990). In this project five-acre plots with the infrastructure for beef, dairy or pig production were leased out to farmers. The Agricultural Development Bank (ADB) gave credit to farmers, based on this project and on private farmer initiatives, but this credit was often given for political rather than economic reasons - contributing to the poor performance of the agriculture sector. Government also subsidised fertilisers and animal feeds to encourage farming. In the post-World War II era of 'progress by unlimited growth', 'industrialisation by invitation' was seen as the way to 'develop' the Caribbean. Western corporations set-up 'screwdriver' assembly industries and light manufacturing plants when local Governments promised them cheap labour, tax holidays and tax laws on profit remittances. The emphasis given to import substitution in manufacturing led to shoddy manufactured goods and worsened the agricultural terms of trade. Consumption and intermediate goods were obtained by the agricultural sector at inflated prices, and this raised costs of agricultural production and affected competitiveness. These factors were compounded by a formerly over-valued currency (Bishnodat, 1988).

Oil is the major source of export earnings in Trinidad and Tobago, as high as 90% for some years of the boom of 1974-81 (Harrison, 1994). The share of petroleum in the total output at current market prices moved from 25% of GDP (Gross Domestic Product) (1966-73) to 40.5% (1974-87) and 24.5% in 1988-90 (U.S. Department of Commerce, Bureau of Economic Analysis, 1999). It currently contributes 40% of GDP, 80% of exports and 50% of government revenue (IMF, 2005). Also important are the petroleum-based industries (natural gas, fertilisers, methanol, iron and steel). In 1988, agriculture was considered the second largest industry providing 2% of the country's foreign exchange earnings and occupying a third of the cultivated land. However, the sugar-producing State enterprise CARONI accounted for most of this. The contribution of sugar to agricultural GDP in 1998 was 44% (1999 MALMR Budget Speech). Exports of sugar in 1997 were 109.3 ('000 tons) and declined to 59.5 ('000 tons) in 2001 (TT Parliament, 2004).

In the 1980s the public sector accounted for 25% of employment compared to a combined employment of 20% in agriculture, mining, and manufacturing. In June 1998 employment in agriculture was 42,300 (1999 MALMR Budget Speech). Agriculture's contribution to GDP declined from 6.6% in 1966-73 to 3.7% in 1988-90. Trinidad and Tobago used the high oil prices in the 1970s to expand public sector employment and to develop its economic and social infrastructure, including the natural gas sector. The fall in the price of oil in the mid-1980s made these strategies unsustainable; the economy retracted and was pushed into structural reform by the IMF and World Bank. Between 1983 and 1993, per capita income fell by four percent per year, unemployment soared, and there was a significant out-migration of relatively skilled labour (U.S. Department of Commerce, Bureau of Economic Analysis, 1999). A severe recession ensued until 1994. Since 1994, the economy has stabilised and grown at an average rate of three percent a year, mostly as a result of high foreign investment in natural gas-related industries and growth in the services sector. The capital-intensive energy sector and the narrow economic base curtailed job creation in the 1990s. However 28,000 jobs were created in 2004 and the unemployment rate was 7.8% in the last quarter of 2004 (Budget Speech 2005-2006). From 1992 the T&T government followed IMF/World Bank mandates and partially or fully privatised the majority of state-owned companies and dismantled most trade barriers. In April 1993 the government removed exchange controls and floated the TT Dollar (U.S. Department of Commerce, Bureau of Economic Analysis). Trinidad and Tobago is highly import-dependent; the food import bill from January to June 1997 was $743.5 million (1999 MALMR Budget Speech).

In the 1980s there were 512,000 ha. of arable land (Dindial, 1991) and 6000ha in Tobago (IMA, 2006). Since the 1980s there has been some loss of agricultural land to more profitable and speculative uses like tourist resorts and tourism-related infrastructure (McElroy and de Albuquerque, 1990). The positive links between tourism and local farming were unrealised at first but have improved slightly. There was a decline in agriculture's contribution to GDP between 1960 and 1980. From 1985 to 1989, the average annual contribution of domestic agriculture, excluding sugar, to the GDP increased from 1.5 - 2.1%. In the period 1988 to 1996 Trinidad and Tobago had the smallest variability in agriculture (2.5%) as a percentage of GDP in Latin America and the Caribbean (Tavernier, 1999). The arable land under tree crops increased by 5000 ha with fresh fruit exports increasing from 31 (1000 MT) to 36 (1000 MT), but a decline in cocoa exports from 1453.5 ('000 kg) in 1997 to 718.5 ('000 kg) in 2001. The agricultural labour force declined from 11% to 8% of the total labour force (ESSA, 2005). Agriculture's contribution to the GDP varied from 1.1% to 1.4% from 2003 to 2005 (First Citizens Bank, 2004).

The recent modernisation of the sector (Agricultural Sector Reform Programme (ASRP) was funded by a loan from the Inter-American Development Bank (IADB) (IADB, 1995). The program was expected to generate foreign exchange through increased exports and more rational land utilisation, and it was supposed to foster economic diversification and increased sectoral employment. The US $65 million loan was tied to a series of reforms including trade and price policy, land use policy and administration, restructuring and divestment of state-owned enterprises like CARONI and public policy reform to improve agricultural support services and sector policy, programming, and budget functions. There was an additional IADB loan of US$9 million to finance technical co-operation / private sector participation. CARONI was restructured with the loss of 9,000 jobs since it was producing sugar in 2002 at a cost 2.7 times higher than the average cost of the ten lowest cost world producers and 1.4 times higher than the cost of other Caribbean countries (TT Parliament, 2004). CARONI's shut down is reflected in the decline of citrus exports in 2001. CARONI's land was disbursed - 7247 former workers received 1 ha plots and 6755 are promised residential plots (First Citizens Bank, 2004; 2005-2006 Budget Speech). However the 2005-2006 Budget Speech claims that an inflation rate > 4% is linked to the high price of imported food. While claiming that the high price of oil had also boosted the country's external reserves to US $3.8 billion it was revealed that this was the equivalent to only 7 months of imports. The agricural trade balance of exports to imports has improved from US$ -255.3 MLN (1979) to US $ –140.3 MLN (2003) (ESSA, 2005).

Livestock Production

There are some feedlot systems but more commonly farmers tether or graze animals on the roadside verges, communal pastures, family land, or unused land. A number of farmers cut fodder on the roadside verges or [in Tobago] collect it after the authorities have cut the verges. Some farmers have no real 'farms', but they have animals on houselots. The domestic market in Trinidad and Tobago is limited, agriculture is low-input, and marketable surplus is small. Most farmers are part-time and input costs in Tobago are higher due to shipping costs from Trinidad. There are also transport costs to ship goods from Tobago to Trinidad. Poultry and pigs are usually raised in intensive modern systems. There are some large and small ruminant feedlot systems, on deep litter and on slatted floors, but by and large, ruminants are still traditionally raised as a low-input, low operating cost investment. Small ruminant farmers in the Caribbean are not solely profit-maximisers (Evans and Ganteaume-Farrell, 1993). These farmers keep sheep for social security reasons since they have high reproductive rates and lower economic risk of loss and are readily converted into cash (Craig and Lans, 1993). The niche market for fresh, local meat is very small, since the average householder and their political representatives are interested in cheap imported food. Livestock are traditionally sold on an ad-hoc basis to hucksters, but that pricing is random and often bears no relevance to the weight or quality of the animal. Sometimes animals are sold for "next-to-nothing" if the farmer is in desperate need for cash. Farmers accept orders for festive occasions like the Muslim festival of Eid (Craig and Lans, 1993).

Trinidad and Tobago is considered to be 100% self-sufficient with respect to pigs, poultry meat and eggs. Poultry farming is one of two productive, intensive and efficient forms of meat production in Trinidad and Tobago (Ministry of Food Production and Marine Exploitation, 1989). Government subsidies were removed, and most of the inputs for poultry production (hatching eggs, feed ingredients, equipment and drugs) are imported. In 2005 the population of broilers was 5 million birds, layers 50,000 birds, ducks 100,000, common fowl 10,000 and the number of turkeys was estimated at 2000 (Thomas, 2005). Poultry production typically fluctuates to match consumption.

Ninety-percent of dairy farms have less than 25 head of cattle. The estimated annual milk production was 16.9 million kg of fresh milk of which 10.2 million kgs are processed by Nestlé (Trinidad Guardian 16th October 1997, pg. 5). The domestic market size is estimated at 110 m kg. The Trinidad and Tobago Holstein Breeders Association and Dairy Farmers Association represent 569 dairy farmers who supply fresh milk to Nestlé at $2.55 / kg (Trinidad Guardian 16th October 1997, pg. 5). The Government milk subsidy was $1.00 / kg, and Nestlé's contribution was $1.55. This price is a 25% increase instituted on September 29, 1997 from $2.00. The previous Government subsidy of $0.90 was established in 1972. Nestlé has milk collection centres at Orange Field, Las Lomas, Turure and Wallerfield (Trinidad Guardian 16th October 1997, pg. 5). The production of milk increased by 5% in 1998. Under the current trade regime, small-scale production of sheep is unprofitable (Evans and Ganteaume-Farrell, 1993), although the ruminant sub-sector is still being targeted by the government of Trinidad and Tobago as an essential component of a revitalised agricultural sector (2005-2006 Budget Speech).

Pig production is dealt with in the case study on pigs in Chapter 6.

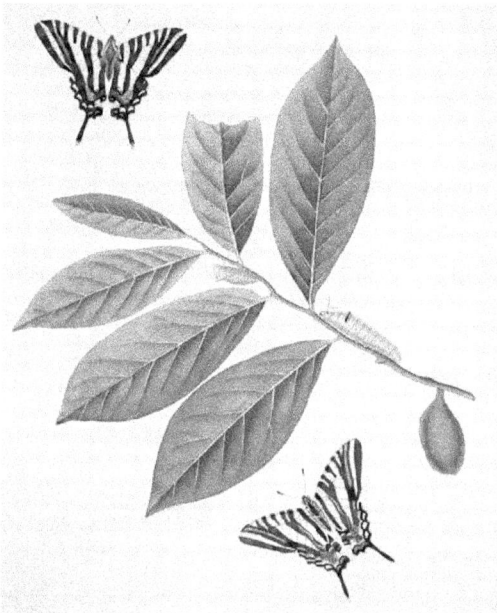

Figure 7. Papilio ajax/Annona glabra
Figure 8.Eclipta prostata

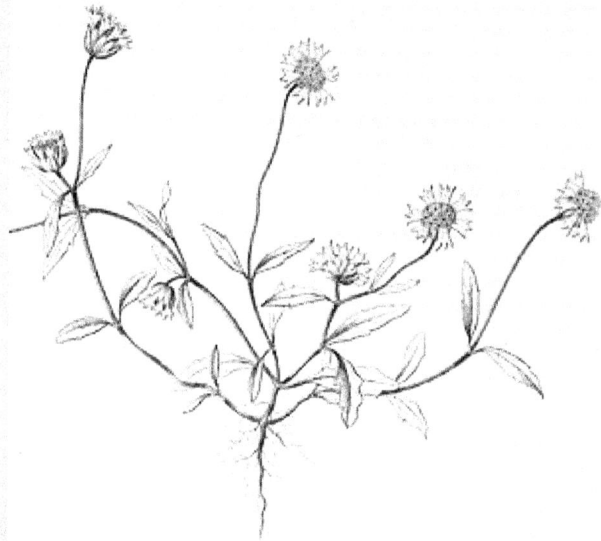

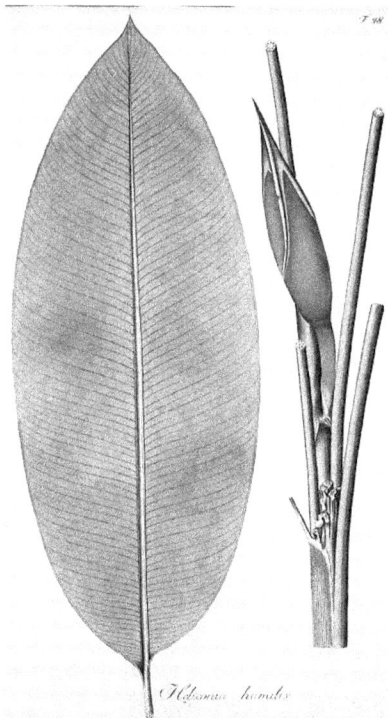

Figure 9. Heliconia bihai
Figure 10. Centropogon cornutus
Figure 11. Lantana camara

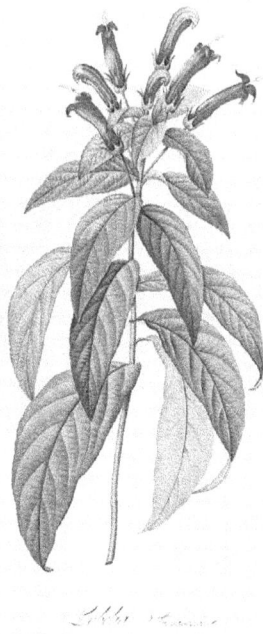

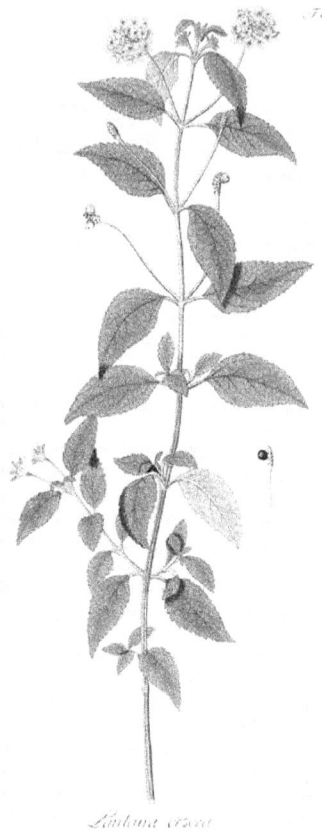

Contriving my own fable, as I grow stiff and uncited, before the necrologists get at me (Geertz, C. 2000, cited by Nigel Rapport, 2001).

Soft science, hard science, mirror images

Theory is certainly not to be treated as sacrosanct and enshrined in 'texts' to be endlessly pored over like chicken entrails (Stanley and Wise, 1990)

3. Soft science, hard science, mirror images

Methodology

Methodology provides both theory and analysis of the research process while Epistemology is concerned with providing a philosophical grounding for deciding what kinds of knowledge are possible and how we can ensure that they are both adequate and legitimate (Maynard, 1994). Epistemology includes questions about what is defined as knowledge, and under what circumstances, what differentiates knowledge from beliefs, who is seen as a legitimate knower and how competing knowledge claims are adjudicated (Maynard, 1994). Epistemology is important because the way that research questions are framed shapes the questions that can be asked and provides clues and directions as to where answers can be sought (Ferguson, 1997). Different ways of knowing can be categorised into four characteristics: epistemology, transmission, innovation and power (Röling, 1988; Marglin, 1990c).

Soft science

As an interdisciplinary discipline anthropology has sometimes claimed an 'intellectual poaching licence and an amateurish use of all manner of information which enables the examination of complex systems' (Rapport and Overing, 2000). Applied anthropology typically means analyses of particular human problems, situations, or processes for the purposes of understanding their causes, dynamics, and consequences; and, in some instances, for developing courses of action designed to influence those situations or processes so that they are brought into agreement with [the researcher's] goals or values (Rappaport, 1993). Sillitoe (1998) considers that harnessing anthropology to technical knowledge in order to facilitate development will put the discipline at the centre of the development process before others "steal Anthropology's disciplinary clothes" (Ferradás 1998).

In the past anthropologists have tended to select research projects that could at worst do little harm and that might occasionally serve some good purpose (Kielstra, 1979). These researchers tried to exercise as little influence as possible on the social phenomena they studied and left the active intervention in the situation to other agencies (Kielstra, 1979). Positivistic approaches in anthropology are based on three deeply embedded views of its objectives: 1. Knowledge accumulation is an end in itself, 2. Studies are preferably done on tribal and peasant societies to which anthropologists have easy access. These more or less autonomous, traditional communities do not change while contemporary society, which does change, is a less suitable subject of study. Unchanging societies provide the theoretical basis for the evolutionist, diffusionist or functionalist anthropologists who assume the existence of more or less closed and finite social systems in order to demonstrate their theories of social equilibrium (Kielstra, 1979), 3. Long-term studies are preferable to short-term analyses of cultural systems (Kielstra, 1979; Weaver, 1985; Shore and Wright, 1996).

While still existing, these traditional attitudes have been joined by the more contemporary views of Posey (1998) and Hastrup and Elsass (1990) who do not support the idea that the anthropologist should use his/ her knowledge for a particular cause by deciding for example whether indigenous beliefs and practices are or are not scientific as this would be a modified form of colonialism. Some anthropologists also claim that local knowledge should not be treated as a marketable category and encoded in Intellectual Property Rights regimes since that would reinforce Cartesian dualisms (Pálsson, 1996; Posey, 1998). If indigenous knowledge systems represent the cultural dimension of development (Warren, Slikkerveer and Brokensha, 1995), these anthropologists say, then they cannot be reduced to the empirical knowledge that they contain. If a culture is a system as some anthropologists maintain, then when a cultural item is removed this removal disrupts the set of relationships into which it is locked, and the cultural item cannot be imported into another culture without bringing with it some of the trappings of those former relationships and disturbing its new surroundings, therefore cultural change is problematic (Milton, 1996). While macro issues such as communication across cultural boundaries have been happening for millennia, this continues to befuddle the culture/system anthropologists who wonder how such a thing is possible (Milton, 1996). There are constraints to taking a critical approach in anthropology, for example some clinical anthropologists are asked to function solely as cultural interpreters and their critiques of health care arrangements and their political-economic environments are not welcomed (Baer, 1993). Nereu *et al. (*1997) state that society is the victim of the distancing of science from social change since research outcomes often end up forgotten on some dusty shelf without any practical application other than support for further theoretical research.

Hard science

Western science has often been used as the standard by which other knowledges should be evaluated (Watson-Verran and Turnbull, 1995). Combatants over socially controversial issues enlist scientific experts to support their causes resulting in science serving conflicting agendas (Nelkin, 1996). Science is frequently portrayed as being of unequivocal social benefit, which if properly funded (and given unrestricted freedom to conduct curiosity-driven research unencumbered by excessive public or government control) would eventually solve all problems (Middendorf and Busch, 1997; Rotblat, 1999).

The failure of centrally planned systems and their scientific products is often cited as a justification for the continuation of a production and profit based approach to agricultural research (Zimdahl, 1998). Positivistic scientists assume that there is a radical separation between science and politics, and science and society. The scientific 'citadel' is a 'culture of no culture' (Franklin, 1995). Science need not be done in the public interest nor should democratic principles guide science, since the lay public would bring un-informed subjectivity (values, beliefs, attitudes and politics) to the scientific decision making process (Middendorf and Busch, 1997). These 'subjectivities' are labelled as 'externalities' to science that have little bearing on the practice of science and are seldom integrated into decision making (Zimdahl, 1998). The scientists' only obligation is to operate from within the existing paradigm and make the research results known to the public (Rotblat, 1999). The increasing corporate involvement and funding of science is not seen as involvement in politics and the external society but as a way of conducting research in the public's interest which is conveniently funded by the commercial organisation (Zimdahl, 1998).

When research is funded by corporate entities to serve their short-term needs only one set of production-related questions are asked and only one type of research (technological tinkering at the margin of science) is conducted (Zimdhal, 1998). Since externalities are excluded and evidence that dominant paradigms are flawed is treated as an externality for long periods; science proceeds along non-neutral paths determined by the short-term production goals. Every new technological step gives rise to new steps and new directions and closes off others (Zimdhal, 1998). Information that can be quantified assumes importance beyond its true value while the alternative approaches are shelved and the hypotheses that are not recognised drop out of sight. According to Dolby (1979) if a problem is not resolvable by immediate empirical test most scientists abandon the issue as non-science. Science is then only what can be derived by the rules of logic (Marglin, 1990c; 234). Editors in the top science journals are full-time professionals who are very sensitive to the latest scientific trends and very cautious about publishing new work where the level of rigour cannot be as high as work in familiar territory (Lawrence, 1999).

There are other reasons why alternative theories find it hard to maintain themselves in a world of 'normal science'. Scientists' reputations hinge on the validity of their research conclusions (Ikerd, 1993). To ignore the existence of something real means a scientist fails to make a discovery -disappointing but not harmful to the reputation, so scientists are more willing to do this than take conclusion risks. What counts for the scientist is replication and comparison, but controlled-experiments are 'out of time' (Richards, 1989). Farmers' sequential performances are always 'in time' and embedded within their particular context. What counts for the farmer is fitting available resources to changing circumstances so that they make it through the season (Richards, 1989). Farmers take decision risks, the risks of wrong choices among alternatives (Ikerd, 1993). The scientists' risk is often smaller than the farmers' risk of a wrong decision based on the scientists' conclusion.

Scientific knowledge bases its claim to superiority on the basis of universal validity while local knowledge is assumed to be bound by time and space (Raedeke and Rikoon, 1997). Some ecological science has been recognised as 'local' and situational so that what is learned about one population or one conservation strategy in one place at one time is not readily transferable (Hinrichsen, 2000). While Elisabetsky and de Moraes (1990) caution that culturally specific practices are not universally applicable, Kloppenburg (1991) calls local knowledge 'mutable immobiles', with little utility outside of particular places. It is then the role of scientific disciplines like Agroforestry to identify which aspects can be translated and adapted to fit into other situations. However before the advance of science ordinary people were responsible for carrying local knowledge to new regions, where, if relevant, it was quickly adopted (McClure, 1982). Busch and Lacy (1983) and Wittrock (1985) have stated that 'the vested political interests that guide some science diverts attention from questions of ends; what is the good society? To questions of means; how can productivity be increased? When society as a whole feels some negative effects from this approach to science and agriculture, these deleterious consequences are dismissed by some scientists and farmers, or are redefined as adjustment problems, or tolerated as the price of scientific progress' or claims are made that scientists are not responsible for the misapplication of science (Banuri, 1990; Rotblat, 1999). The technological disasters of the late twentieth century like Bhopal, Chernobyl, the Challenger and environmental degradation suggest that expert assessments need to be tempered by broader visions in the same way that the common-law system has promoted the integration of expert knowledge with layman's values, ethics and perceptions (Nandy and Visvanathan, 1990; Jasanoff, 1999).

There are scientists who have claimed that scientific positivism and detached observation are no longer considered necessary conditions in the search for scientific truth (Barrett,

1997; Autumn, 1996; Rappaport, 1993; Krumeich, 1994). Polanyi (1967) claims that if tacit thought forms an indispensable part of all knowledge it is impossible to establish a strictly detached, objective knowledge. Jiggins and Röling (2000) among others are calling for a new social contract for science (Lubchenco, 1998; Latour, 1998; Zimdhal, 1998; Gibbons, 1999; Rotblat, 1999). For them, science is not only part of the problem but very much a source of solutions since it is difficult to opt out of science (James Lovelock).

Post-normal science goes beyond 'normal' (in the Kuhnian sense) (Funtowicz and Ravetz, 1993; Jiggins and Röling, 2000). It would include widespread involvement in, if not a total democratisation of, science. This type of science produces 'socially robust knowledge' with three aspects: it is valid inside and outside the laboratory; its validity is achieved through involving an extended group of experts, including 'lay' experts; and thirdly this participatory-generated knowledge is likely to be less contested (Funtowicz and Ravetz, 1993; Gibbons, 1999). Externalities such as health and safety of living things, resource and energy use and other societal goals would be internalised in this type of science (Zimdahl, 1998). Research would become a co-learning activity that develops mutual accountability (Jiggins and Gibbon, 1997). Co-learning develops ways of understanding the world that re-enter society and affect action in society (Jiggins and Gibbon, 1997). In other words science as knowledge-based action or a form of reflective activity underlying rational action: action is then concerned with change; is present and future oriented; and requires the anticipation of the effects of action, rather than the interpretation of prior event (Vasquez, 1977).

Cernea (1995) claims that: 'Science becomes applicable and theory becomes practical when it first allows us a definite grip of empirical reality'. The reality is that ethnoveterinary knowledge in Trinidad and Tobago exists in a politically charged environment. The project of validating ethnoveterinary medicine cannot come into existence if the range of interests gathered around the project do not intersect (Latour, 1993). It is thus necessary to show what the scientific interests are in Trinidad and Tobago. There are some local extension agents, animal health assistants, agricultural chemical agents, scientists and veterinarians who undervalue ethnoveterinary knowledge in favour of the scientific principles in which they were trained. There are others who are actively promoting the use of this knowledge. The reasons for both attitudes towards ethnoveterinary knowledge will be examined using the constructivist perspective that all knowledge is socially constructed, with both strengths and weaknesses.

The Social Construction of Scientific Knowledge

Foundationalism or naïve idealism is the idea that truth exists independently of the knower (Maynard, 1994). The social shaping of theory is not commonly known because scientific knowledge hides its labour process through a series of textual means (Stanley, 1990). Social constructivism is the treatment of scientific knowledge and other knowledge as social constructions. Using this viewpoint, fact making becomes a social enterprise, and 'truth' becomes relative and contextual (Pinch and Bijker, 1987; Hubbard, 1988; Foucault, 1980). The principle of epistemic relativity states that all beliefs are socially produced, so that all knowledge is transient, and neither truth-values nor criteria of rationality exist outside historical time (Baber, 1992). The social production of knowledge comes from the social life of scientists, their shared goals and understandings, codes of conduct, definitions of time and space and created self-identities (Franklin, 1995). The [scientific] epistemological stance can be described as [scientists] power to create the world from their own point of view, which then becomes the truth to be described (Maynard, 1994). Epistemic relativity means rejection of the doctrine of judgmental relativism which means that all beliefs are equally valid, in the sense that there can be no rational grounds for preferring one to another, for it allows each group to disqualify the criticism of others by claiming that there are no common grounds for argument (Baber, 1992; Scheyvens and Leslie, 2000).

Pinch and Bijker (1987) talk about three stages of the social construction of scientific knowledge. In the first stage there is some interpretative flexibility in the findings, so scientific controversies are present in this stage. The level of confidence in the scientific model by the scientific community increases with the level of scientific confirmation (i.e. scientific activities that cumulatively corroborates the theory's hypotheses or the fraud's claims) (Deichmann and Müller-Hill, 1998; Bradshaw and Borchers, 2000). In the second stage scientific flexibility reduces as papers, findings and models are published, disseminated, debated and cited giving rise to new funding and new research. A scientific consensus builds as to what the 'truth' is. Typically younger scientists defer to the judgement of eminent scientists and don't express contrasting opinions. This process of creating scientific orthodoxy is called 'closure' (Pinch and Bijker, 1987). Or in other words 'research creates controversies while science puts an end to the vagaries of human disputes' (Latour, 1998). In the third stage Pinch and Bijker (1987) propose that the closure mechanisms can be related to the 'wider social-cultural milieu'. Latour (1993) criticises both the theory and the application of social constructivism to science. Part of the difficulty is how to have an account of the historical contingency of all knowledge claims, a commitment to valid accounts of an existing reality, and also retain the capacity the subject all knowledge claims to critical scrutiny (Hawkesworth, 1989; Kerr, 1998).

Mainstream scientists criticise social constructivism because they are reluctant to reveal the ambiguities and uncertainties built into science for fear of diminishing their public credibility (Dolby, 1979; Bradshaw and Borchers, 2000). Franklin (1995) points out that the epithet 'antiscience' used to describe any critical studies of science suggests that scientists accept only internal-disciplinary criticism dedicated to improving results or preventing fraud. The sense of threat felt by scientists (as evidenced in the 'science wars') when their disciplines are questioned as foundational belief systems reveals the importance of science as a source of deeply-felt cultural values (Franklin, 1995). Scientific entities like genes can assume cultural meanings and lay people 'hijack' scientific symbols. Conversely scientists like sociobiologists draw moral and philosophical lessons from science and other scientists 'hijack' religious imagery such as the 'bible' or 'book of man' used to describe the human genome (Nelkin, 1996).

Scientific knowledge is hierarchical internally, and even more hierarchical externally, (i.e. it disenfranchises those outside the knowledge network) (Dolby, 1979; Marglin, 1990c). Eminent scientists are deferred to and lesser scientists are constrained from expressing contrary views (Dolby, 1979).The élitism in science and technology is not seen as problematic since the scientific élite see themselves as the only appropriate group to make scientific, technological and policy decisions based on authoritative knowledge, given an increasingly complex world which requires highly technical and specialised expertise (Middendorf and Busch, 1997; Jasanoff, 1999).

The social construction of scientific knowledge becomes important when scientific bodies like the International Council for Science (ICSU) are asked to carry out a study on the concept of 'traditional knowledge' (Dickson, 1999). This took place in the context of the signing of the Declaration on Science and the Framework for Action at the 1999 World Conference on Science in Budapest, and the 26th General Assembly of the ICSU in Cairo, Egypt (Nakashima and Guchteneire, 1999).

Prior to the signing debate took place on whether indigenous knowledge (IK) was scientific or not and scientists expressed surprise at seeing the issue on the agenda. Scientists suggested that including indigenous and traditional knowledge on the agenda might lend ill-deserved credibility to IK or open the door to anti- and pseudoscientific[6] approaches like creationism and astrology. Nakashima and Guchteneire (1999) wondered whether the discomfort of the scientists might be related to their unwillingness to view science as one knowledge system among many. The debate led to a discussion on the nature of scientific knowledge itself; for example what makes the theory of natural evolution 'scientific' and thus distinguishable from astrology when neither can be replicated or reproduced? (Anon, 1999).

The ICSU's critical study on traditional knowledge' and other publications on indigenous knowledge inscribe a formerly subjugated knowledge in the hierarchical order of power associated with science (Foucault, 1980). These scientific 'inscriptions'.... 'can be recombined in various ways, communicated across space and time and they thus become very important and significant' (Latour, 1986). However the original oral knowledge and its holders are not so important and need 'scientific validation' by the ICSU (O'Brien and Butler Flora, 1992). Validation 'acts to reaffirm the order of development, the stamp of approval or denial rests at the top of the development or scientific hierarchy' (O'Brien and Butler Flora, 1992). Scientific objectivity is a 'translation' that scientists use to deny other people access to decision or fact making power (Hubbard, 1988).

Hubbard (1988) claims that: 'science is made by a self-perpetuating, self-reflective group, by the chosen for the chosen', not for the poor and marginal. These latter, left out of the Science network, continue to use 'non-empirical belief systems' or cultural rationality which is then both a means to survive and also 'attempts to achieve certainty' (Brown and Mikkelson, 1990; Krimsky and Plough, 1988). Cultural rationality is based on folk wisdom, peer groups, and traditions. This type of rationality asks non-technical questions like why do we need this product? It also looks at direct and personal effects of social, technical and environmental risks.

The dichotomy between science and traditional knowledge has increasingly been questioned and the overlaps and disjunctures between them have been outlined (Franklin, 1995). The phrase 'knowledge communities' emphasises the dynamic networks of actors, processes of negotiation and the diverse ways in which knowledge is constructed and performed (Richards, 1993; Raeder and Rikoon, 1997). The phrase 'communities' implies that individuals may participate in and utilise multiple knowledge communities. Finally the word 'community' also reflects the idea that the boundaries between knowledge groups are not closed and that there may be considerable overlap between knowledge communities. Knowledge communities influence and reflect the organisation of science and folk medicine. What scientists and lay people perceive as potential management options and constraints and where lay people and farmers look for potential alternatives depends on the individual's participation in different knowledge communities. The social construction of knowledge is revisited in Chapter 12.

The definition of indigenous knowledge based on that developed by Ellen (1996a) is local, orally transmitted, a consequence of practical experimentation reinforced by experience, not easily recognised as theoretical, repetitive, fluid and negotiable, shared but asymmetrically

---

[6] The American National Institutes of Health has a new National Center for Complementary and Alternative Medicine (NCCAM) which replaces the predecessor, the Office of Alternative Medicine (OAM). The OAM was called a 'child of politics, that gained a reputation as a counterculture enclave for pseudoscience'....and it was condemned for sponsoring inconclusive research and bestowing prestige on practices that resembled "witchcraft" (Stokstad, 2000).

distributed, largely functional, and embedded in cultural matrices. Questions related to the terms indigenous and traditional are where a particular body of knowledge has to be to be called indigenous and when it can be called traditional (Pálsson,1996). A distinction between empirical/ordinary knowledge and non-empirical/non-ordinary knowledge is preferable (Giarelli, 1996). The latter category would include witchcraft, magic and spirits (Giarelli, 1996).

The popular pharmacopoeia of Trinidad and Tobago is the result of a Creole pan-Caribbean culture, closely linked to history, and the result of a South American Indian, African, European and Asian heritage (Lans, 1996; Moodie-Kublalsingh, 1994; Littlewood, 1988; Simpson, 1962; Niehoff, 1959). Cultural knowledge is the contextual glue that binds the use of tacit and explicit knowledge and gives it meaning (Bontis and Choo, 2002). Tacit knowledge is embedded in people and difficult to access, communicate or share with others because it is the noncodifiable accumulation of skills that results from learning by doing (Porac et al., 2002). There are four aspects of tacit knowledge according to Polanyi (1967): functional, phenomenal, semantic and ontological. Learning the technical skills related to indigenous knowledge depends on technology acquisition support systems (Ingold, 1996). These are systems of apprenticeship or relationships between more and less experienced mentors or practitioners in hands-on contexts of activity. There is no blueprint, only instructions or rules of thumb that take on meaning in the context of the engagement with the environment and in a socio-cultural and historical background (Maturana and Varela, 1987; Escobar, 1999). This does not mean that there is always a systematic body of cultural representations (Ingold, 1996; Maturana and Varela, 1987). The continuity of the apprenticeship relationships is essential for the continuity of a technical tradition (Ingold, 1996). The death of knowledgeable individuals; lack of verbal transfers to the next generation, and acculturation, all impact negatively on culturally encoded indigenous knowledge (Longuefosse and Nossin, 1996; Douglas, 1995).

Knowledge-based action in [Veterinary] Medical Anthropology

Science is increasingly seen as a social process of making narratives where meanings are contested and stabilised for a time through the productive relations of power (Morawski, 1988). This means that the epistomological paradox of using political enterprises like feminism or knowledge-based action research to achieve a more accurate, coherent and less masculinist science can be resolved through the reconsideration and alteration of existing social relations of power (Morawski, 1988). Objective, value-free science is being replaced by a science in which social conditions, ethical conduct, and identification with the research subjects are integral components (Barrett, 1997; Autumn, 1996; Pálsson, 1996). Rappaport (1993) calls for an engaged anthropology that would comprehend contemporary problems in anthropologically derived terms, but would resemble applied anthropology in trying to develop programs that would correct these problems. Anthropology's traditional tools—such as ethnographic interviews and participant observation—are thus employed within the framework of a more general research action methodology (Giarelli, 1996).

Informed, directed and committed action is often referred to as 'praxis' (Hatten et al., 2000). Praxis research questions the validity of 'etic' interpretations[7]. The truly 'reflective practitioner' actively participates in the moulding of the social order through 'praxis' (Hatten et al., 2000). Praxis or knowledge-based action can be defined as a property of individuals that emerges from the interactions of the theories (beliefs) that they hold, the actions that they practice, the values that they assume, and the contexts that they interpret of the 'world around them'

---

[7] Etic intepretations are those which at some level cannot be judged by the actors (Warry, 1992).

(Bawden, 2000). The Community-centred praxis approach recognises that all action, even the casual observation characteristic of positivistic research affects a system and that inaction is consequential and thus ultimately partisan (Warry, 1992; Singer, 1994). Action/praxis research takes this insight within its approach (Nereu et al., 1997). Each researcher is an actor in the research process. Each researcher brings particular values, self-identities and experiences to the research; however we do not know how these stances affect the research (Holland and Ramazanoglu, 1994).

Non-experimental validation

Phyto-therapeutic products are usually compared with allopathic drugs based on their unproven effectiveness, their variability, impurity and the potential health hazards they might cause. In comparison pure compound formulations are assumed to be effective, standardised, pure and safe (Elisabetsky and de Moraes, 1990). However until recent times there were 607 drug products used in the USA market for at least 18 years with no officially recognised substantial evidence of effectiveness in well-controlled studies (Elisabetsky and de Moraes, 1990). These non-evidence based drugs were not described as unconventional or snake oil because they were introduced from within the mainstream of western medicine[8] (Dalen, 1998). In this sense western science-derived technologies are different from Creolization-derived technologies. As stated before, Creolization-based technologies are not judged on the basis of their origins; only that they work in the local context.

Western science has become the main means of establishing whether a technology works and how. The non-experimental validation of the ethnoveterinary medicines was undertaken in recognition of that fact. In this research farmer's knowledge is taken and validated scientifically and in the future there are plans to return this validated knowledge to farmers. This approach can be justified in engaged anthropology, one of whose aims is to identify indigenous institutions or processes that could be strengthened and to support processes that could lead to culturally appropriate or effective corrective programs (Rappaport, 1993). There are precedents to this type of engagement. The staff of the Leiden Ethnosystems and Development Programme (LEAD) are involved in collaborative multi-country projects on indigenous knowledge and practice in agriculture and food production (Slikkerveer, 1995).

Role of the researcher in the research

It cannot be argued that theory emerges from research since most researchers start from a theoretical perspective. Rigour in research involves being clear about one's theoretical assumptions, the nature of the research process, the criteria against which 'good' knowledge can be judged and the strategies used for interpretation and analysis (Mascia-Lees et al., 1989; Maynard, 1994). There is a difference between personal and theoretical reflexivity, the former being seen as the unique thoughts, feelings and experiences of the researcher while the latter is a theoretical understanding of the site from which one is working (Kelly et al., 1992). There are few canons about the practical role of the anthropologist apart from the old one of remaining objective and staying away from the native women (Hastrup and Elsass, 1990). By taking the place of the researched into account we can raise questions about what the research is for (Holland and Ramazanoglu, 1994).

Cox (1997) claims that choosing applied research may bring conflict with community power groups and brokers and also a loss of professional peer support. Anthropological advocacy has been called a contradiction in terms and advocacy has been said to be incompatible with

---

[8] More of this discussion will follow in Chapter 12.

anthropological scholarship (Hastrup and Elsass, 1990; Shore and Wright, 1996). Applied work is often unpublished because there is a split between theory and practice which is said to be linked to masculine ideas of science which exclude advocacy, activism and commitment from "real science" and determine what counts as publishable material. However one argument for doing native applied anthropology is that the problems studied are part of the lives of the researchers which makes it reasonable to address them professionally regardless of their theoretical interest (Rappaport, 1993). To advocate an applied anthropological approach means examining one's values as a researcher, seeing if they are relevant and making them explicit. Secondly the researcher's values must be appropriate to the discipline; they should be of sufficiently high generality to avoid subordination to any particular social or political agenda or party (Rappaport, 1993). Thirdly the anthropological account needs to be a precise, accurate and well-grounded account that stands up to hostile and critical scrutiny (Rappaport, 1993). Praxis does not guarantee truth nor do good hypotheses guarantee effective practice (Kay, 1994). A praxis approach focuses analysis on how theory is transformed by actions that are inherently instrumental and strategic in nature (Warry, 1992).

Cernea (1995) claims that 'Science begins with application, so that in order to be of use, research must be inspired to establish what the relevant issues are and then apply the necessary remedies'.

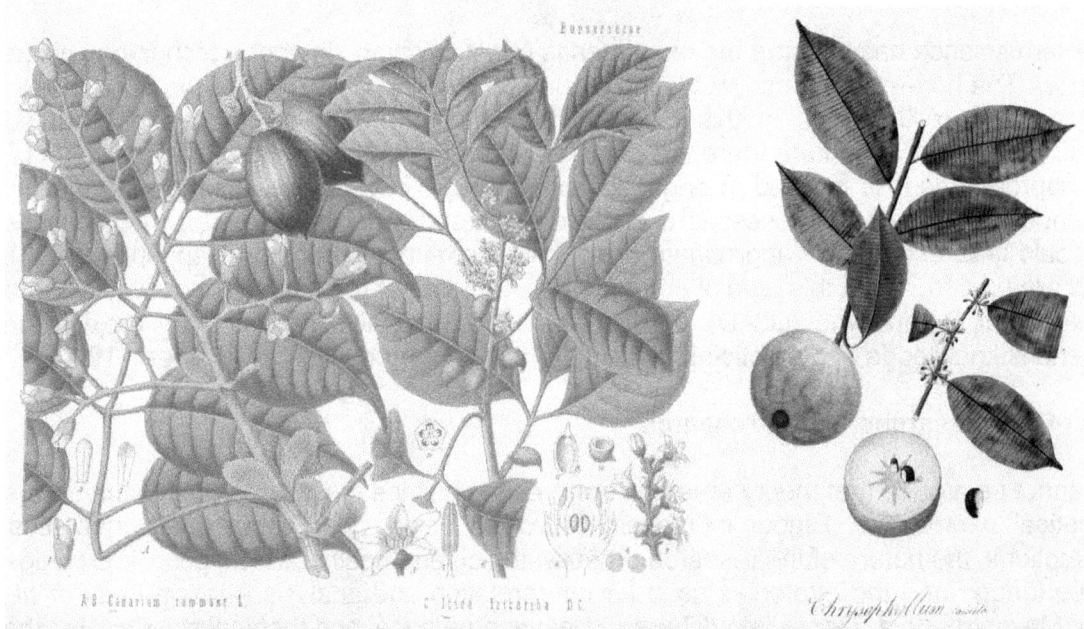

Figure 12. Protium icicariba
Figure 13. Chrysophllum cainito

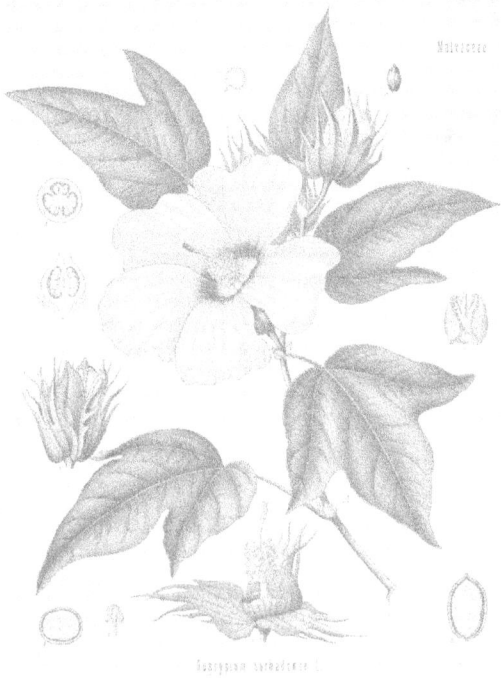

Figure 14. Gossypium barbadense
Figure 15.Sphinx Lineata/ Portulaca oleracea

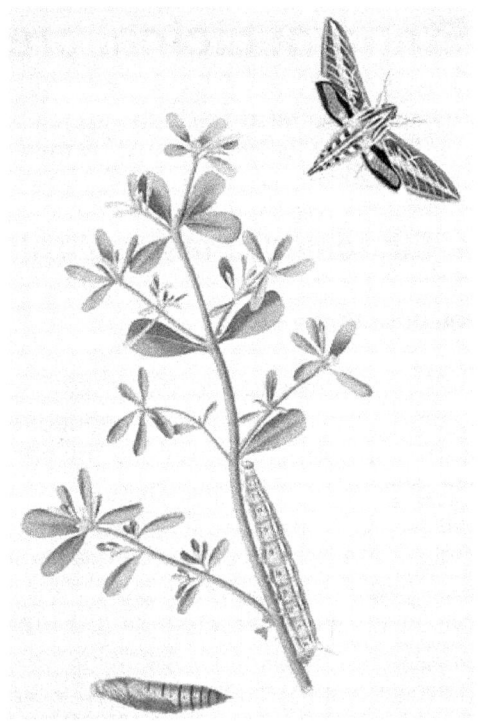

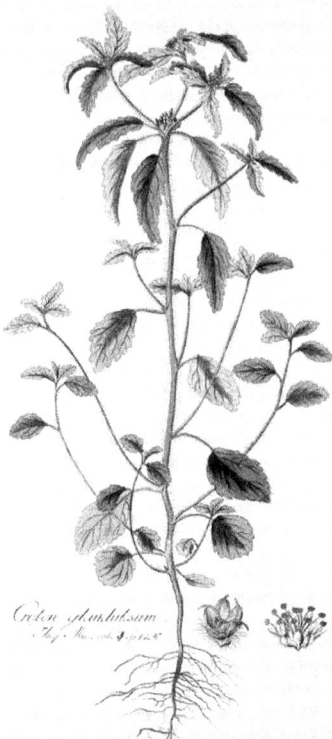

Figure 16. Hyptis verticillata
Figure 17. Theobroma cacao
Figure 18. Croton glandulosus

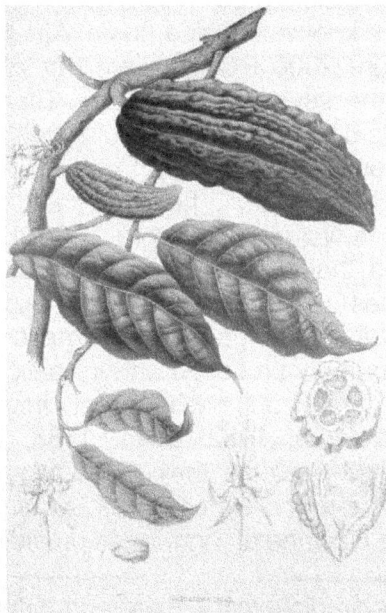

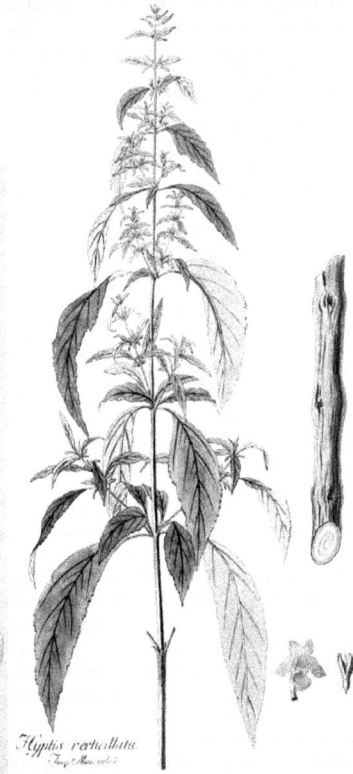

Ethnomedicinal creolization

The continuing reference to the sacred world means that the world has not become a disenchanted one that is no longer mediated by mysteries and miracles or sacraments and saints (Rapport and Overing, 2000).

4. Ethnomedicinal creolization

Introduction

Cultures are situated historically, and should be viewed in a theoretical framework that critically examines their embeddedness in social, economic and political structures (Baer, 1997). The Amerindians came by canoe to Trinidad and Tobago from the Orinoco delta; the Spanish were looking for gold; the Africans were abducted by slave traders; the French were displaced by the French Revolution and by the capture of other Caribbean islands by the British; the British came with the colonial establishment, and the other settlers saw Trinidad as a place to make a new start in the New World (Besson, 2000). Caribbean folk medicine is based on this marriage-á-cinq: European folk medicine; scientific medicine; African-based practices; Amerindian medicine and Indian-based medicine; a product of inter-group borrowing or medical syncretism (Laguerre, 1987). Folk medicine is called 'bush medicine' in the West Indies (Dennis, 1988). This term may have British origins. The term Creole usually refers to things of local/West Indian origin and is sometimes used to contrast East Indian from African/European elements (Aho and Minott, 1997).

A medical system is 'the pattern of social institutions and cultural traditions that evolve from deliberate behaviour to enhance health' (Laguerre, 1987). One aspect of folk medicinal beliefs that is ancient and globally known is the Doctrine of Signatures. Paracelsus (Theophrastus Bombast von Hohenheim, 1490 - 1541) developed this Doctrine from a much older set of beliefs. The belief was known in China, India, Africa and South America, and in some places it was present before 2000 BC (Nyazema et al., 1994). Nicholas Culpeper spread the belief in England in the seventeenth century (Blunt and Raphael, 1994). The Doctrine claims that features made by God identify the plant with a specific disease or part of the body or more simply 'like cures like' (Sofowora, 1982; Etkin, 1988). For example plants with heart-shaped leaves are good for treating heart disease; plants exuding a milky juice are believed to increase lactation in women (Sofowora, 1982; Etkin, 1988). In Belize and in Amazonian Ecuador it is believed that pain is cured by producing pain therefore stinging nettles are used to cure headaches[9] (Arnason et al., 1980; Davis and Yost, 1983). A belief that plants growing in dark places should be good for rheumatism led to the use of the willow Salix species, whose bark subsequently produced salicin -salicyclic acid- aspirin (Nyazema et al., 1994). Hausa, Zimbabwean and Israeli healers treat circulatory ailments and jaundice with red and yellow plants (Sofowora, 1982; Etkin, 1988; Nyazema et al., 1994). In Zimbabwe three of six plants used because they produce red coloured decoctions had antischistosoma activity comparable to the expensive praziquantel (Nyazema et al., 1994). There are many illustrations of the Doctrine of Signatures providing false leads.

Another global belief is the hot/cold dichotomy. People in different cultures throughout the world for example Amerindian, Chinese, East Indian, Portuguese and Spanish view illnesses, symptoms and remedies as 'hot' or 'cold' (Aho and Minott, 1977). The British

---

[9] A recent study at the Plymouth Postgraduate Medical School in Devon found that stinging nettles (Urtica dioica) produced anaesthesia when used by patients with osteoarthritis of the thumb (Randall et al., 2000).

expression "feed a cold, starve a fever' is a well-known example of a hot/cold classification (Butt Colson and de Armellada, 1983).

The process of syncretism in medicine consists of the adoptions and adaptations that are made selectively from incoming systems (Butt Colson and de Armellada, 1983). Essential, indigenous elements may be reinforced and modified by incoming ideas, but basic structures, objectives and characteristics of the indigenous remain identifiable and a continuity is achieved (Butt Colson and de Armellada, 1983). Syncretism in Caribbean medicine is defined by Brodwin (1998) as participation in four health cultures at once: globalised scientific biomedicine, its historical form derived from the former colonial power (British, Dutch, French, Spanish), the local island variant, and the syncretic set of popular folk medicine which has grown out of much older European, African and Amerindian traditions (Brodwin, 1998). Folk medicine as a system includes: home remedies; folk aetiologies of disease; preventative medicine; reproductive techniques; medicinal properties of plants; anatomical knowledge, and healers (Laguerre, 1987).
Folk remedies fall into several classes: certain well-known European medicinal herbs introduced by the early Spaniard colonists that are still commonly cultivated; indigenous wild and cultivated plants, the uses of which have been adopted from the Amerindians; and ornamental or other plants of relatively recent introduction for which curative uses have been invented without any historical basis (Morton, 1975). This invention would have been facilitated by the widespread introduction of plant species from all over the world for ornamental and medicinal reasons (Bayley, 1949).

The naturalistic system refers to the ethnomedicinal beliefs in which natural causes like cold, heat, wind, dampness and an upset in the balance of the basic body elements are the major causes of illness (Dressler, 1980; Butt Colson and de Armellada, 1983). A disturbed physical equilibrium gives rise to disease. Treatments and responses to illness are empirically based, determined by signs and symptoms and explainable within the natural order of things (Berlin and Berlin, 1994). Self treatment or treatment by a herbalist or someone knowledgeable is the norm (Berlin and Berlin, 1994).

Trinidad and Tobago folk medicine has a historical classification of diseases into hot and cold. Some researchers consider that the hot-cold concept of health and illness is absent in Spanish folk medicine and did not exist at the folk level in the past (Tan, 1989). These beliefs are now widespread in Latin America and the Caribbean, and according to Foster (1953) were derived from the élite and scholarly Hippocratic-galenic traditions that were brought to the Spanish colonies by Spanish physicians and clergy. Spanish medical practice at the time of Columbus was based on classical Greek and Roman medicine with diffusions from Arab medicine. Other Hippocratic principles are the oppositions of raw / cooked, hot /cold, wet / dry, sweet / sour. In addition, wellbeing is determined by a balance between different elements, bile, phlegm, and blood (Strobel, 1985).

There is research documenting an Amerindian system of hot and cold beliefs that differs from the Hippocratic tradition in that it encompassed the whole cosmos (Messer, 1987; Peña, 1999). There were only two elements and the concepts of warm and cold were not humours or physical elements (Peña, 1999). Everything that was masculine, celestial or came from above was considered warm; everything that was feminine came from below and was cold (Peña, 1999). Messer (1987) and Butt Colson and de Armellada (1983) accept the influence of Hispanic humoral medicine on post-16th century Mesoamerican indigenous thought, however Aztec, Mayan and Zapotec medicinal and cosmological systems have different hot-cold concepts. Butt Colson and de Armellada (1983) also argue that several major, widespread categories of illness and treatments also have a mainly indigenous, Amerindian derivation.

Butt Colson and de Armellada (1983) base their argument on ethnographic data derived from remote, mostly unacculturated Amerindian societies of the recent past and of today and historical evidence in 17th century literature on Carib peoples. Butt Colson and de Armellada (1983) focus on the following points: the existence amongst these Amerindians, as amongst many Latin American Creole and peasant groups, of certain specific and distinctive forms and interpretations of illness, their causation's and cures. These include the binary oppositions of hot and cold, the notion of imbalance accompanying the concept of the mediate and harmonious state; soul loss through shock and fright; the capture of the soul; whirlwind or cold air sickness and illness from contagious and powerful forces. However the Amerindian cosmovision had sufficient in common with the European theory to facilitate syncretism where coincidences occurred such as the hot/cold, bitter/sweet, high/low and strong/weak oppositions (Butt Colson and de Armellada, 1983).

Hot/cold theories are found in Asia (Ayurvedic medicine), Latin America and parts of Africa. The Trinidadian hot/cold system is not humoral in the sense that balance must be established between hot and cold, it is cathartic in that remedies are taken to remove heat from the system (Littlewood, 1988). Heat comes from the sun, work, sleeping, burns, cooking, and reproductive activities. Linked to the hot/cold dichotomy is a system of blood beliefs where an excess or lack of cold or heat in the body through exposure or diet causes illness. Blood then becomes 'bad' or dirty. Illnesses with skin changes such as chicken pox, measles, rashes, urticaria, impetigo, ringworm, eczema, are associated with 'too much heat in the body' (Bayley, 1949; Aho and Minott, 1977; Mitchell, 1983).

This may derive from the Aztec classification of 'heat' or 'hot' illnesses manifesting themselves as irritation, and the idea that an overheated state rendered one vulnerable to illness (Messer, 1987). Female *Warao* herbalists in Eastern Venezuela use the concept of bad blood (Wilbert, 1983). This concept is also used by Spanish New Mexicans (Conway and Slocumb, 1979). Another Aztec theory is that fever was caused by internal problems which could be eliminated with diuretics, purgatives or digestives (Ortiz de Montellano, 1975). These 'hot' conditions are treated externally with cool lotions like bay rum (the commercial preparation of *Pimenta racemosa*), limacol and milk of magnesia or bush teas. They are also treated internally with bushes classified as cool such as *Stachytarpheta jamaicensis*, *Ageratum conyzoides* or *Chamaesyce hirta* (Aho and Minott, 1977). Other illnesses linked to 'overheated' or 'hot/bad blood' or 'hot food' are fever, pressure and headaches (Bayley, 1949; Aho and Minott, 1977; Mitchell, 1983). Eating cold foods when the body is 'hot' can lead to illness. Also ironing as a 'hot' activity and then opening the fridge can lead to 'colds'. Teas are used for 'cooling' if there is too much 'heat' in the body. Cooling teas are used prophylatically when they are taken to keep the body healthy by cooling the 'system', or the bladder, meaning that they remove the 'heat' or impurities in the system (Littlewood, 1988). Cooling teas become treatment when they are taken for undiagnosed or unspecified illnesses or when feeling unwell. Purges reduce the heat further and 'clean the blood' or remove unwanted foetuses. Purges are also used to remove internal parasites and for reproductive problems. 'Cold' is associated with experiencing a sudden change in temperature, drafts or getting wet (Mitchell, 1983). Parts of the body associated with 'coldness' are the mole (fontanelle), chest, head, back, womb, eyes, ears and knee, phlegm, discharge and arthritic pain (Mitchell, 1983). Aching is associated with 'cold' in the Aztec system and several illnesses are attributed to the unhealthy penetration of excess cold and moisture (Messer, 1987). Liniments, poultices and laxatives are used for cold and for gas (wind) (Mitchell, 1983). Illnesses associated with coldness are influenza, asthma and the common cold (Aho and Minott, 1977). There are also 'hot' plants to stimulate the blood or to treat 'cold' illnesses, and 'hot' external applications like 'soft candle' 'grated nutmeg' and hot poultices (Laguerre, 1987; Littlewood, 1993). 'Hot' teas used for colds and fevers are *Leonotis nepetaefolia* and *Chromolaena odorata* (Aho and Minott, 1977).

Gas (wind) is associated with pain in the stomach but also in the joints and back and with pain that travels around the body (Mitchell, 1983; Littlewood, 1988). Medicines are administered in accordance with the identity between cause and effect. Expulsion of disease causing impurities is the primary mechanism by which bodily equilibrium is restored (Mitchell, 1983). Folk medicines achieve cures through 'bitterness', 'cutting', 'cooling', 'building', 'purging or washing out', and 'drawing out' (Mitchell, 1983).

Personalistic explanations of illness are explained by the active aggression of some agent which might be human, non-human, or supernatural like souls, deities, demons, ancestors and sorcerers (Dressler, 1980; Davis and Yost, 1983). The sick person is a victim of aggression or punishment directed against him for reasons that concern only him (Butt Colson and de Armellada, 1983). Dressler (1980) wrongly subsumes all personalistic beliefs under the African-based tradition of Obeah. Wrongly because *Warao* [Amerindian] personalistic explanations dominate over those of natural causation and some of these explanations persist in the Caribbean (Wilbert, 1983a&b). Obeah is a form of sorcery usually associated with evil; it is not legally practised. Obeah can be used to cause illness or misfortune or to worsen existing illnesses. Diagnosis of personalistic conditions is based on the retrospective presumption of an etiologic agent and a person with special knowledge or powers is necessary for treatment (Berlin and Berlin, 1994). Obeah is explained more fully in the section on African-based knowledge.

In Trinidad and Tobago Asian-based spiritual healing comes from Hindu priests who 'jharay' the individual or animal using special leaves. For Christians spiritually originated illness is treated by faith healers such as 'Shouters', Shangoists or Spiritual Baptists, or with Spanish-romanic prayers, *Scoparia dulcis* and candles (Aho and Minott, 1977). 'Shouters', Shangoists or Spiritual Baptists are syncretic combinations of African Yoruba practices and Roman Catholicism. Shango priests often incorporate bush remedies in their healing practices with prayers and rituals (Aho and Minott, 1977). The role of the Shango leader (often a woman) as a bush healer is as important as her role of religious leader (Mischel, 1959). Maljo is more closely linked to ethnoveterinary medicine than Obeah. Maljo or 'Mal yeux', also called 'bad eye' or 'blight' is another aspect of the personalistic system of ethnomedical beliefs. It occurs when a jealous or envious person looks at a person or animal and verbally admires it. Afterwards the living object begins to decline and could die. In Mesoamerican cultures infants are conceived to be cool, have sweet blood and to be vulnerable (attractive) to witchcraft and the evil eye which are both hot concepts in these cultures (Messer, 1987). In Trinidad and Tobago calves and kids have red pieces of cloth around their necks to prevent them from mal yeux, other animals have a blue spot painted on, sometimes with blue wound spray (Negasunt™ or other blue-coloured sprays used for myiasis prevention and treatment). To protect growing plants [from evil spirits], there are blue coloured bottles attached to poles in visible places, in the gardens or plots.

Gender roles may lie behind the Caribbean construction of the malady of Maljo or 'Mal yeux', also called 'bad eye' or 'blight'. This aspect of the personalistic system of ethnomedical beliefs occurs when a jealous or envious person looks at a person or animal and verbally admires it. Afterwards the living object begins to decline and could die. Unfortunately, the dominant gender code and the structural subordination of women make both real and symbolic threats to children's health all too common. Because Caribbean masculinity emphasises fathering children but not necessarily supporting them, there is keen competition among women for husbands and providers (Brodwin, 1998). Women regard each other with suspicion and jealousy, and such emotions fuel accusations of pathogenic attacks on their children (Brodwin, 1998).

Heinrich et al. (1992) record the properties of medicinal plants according to indigenous criteria: hot like onions, hot like chilli, sweet, bitter, astringent, burning, gelatinous, foaming, sour, aromatic (cooling). In her article, Strobel quotes a Guyanese respondent claiming that "quinine tablets are sour because sourness works on the gall bladder, which is the site of malaria." Strobel (1985) uses this example to demonstrate that western medicine is transformed and reinterpreted according to Creole criteria. Western medical interventions are simply considered more complex than the traditional Creole philosophy (Strobel, 1985; Littlewood, 1988). The Creole medical system is fairly flexible and fits the philosophy 'according to the circumstances' (Strobel, 1985; Littlewood, 1988). Strobel (1985) considers that traditional Creole medicine is a global approach and people utilise all available health care alternatives in a pragmatic way (Hill, 1985). Preventive medicine is practised by keeping the body in balance through proper use of diet, drinking 'bush' teas to help keep the blood 'clean' and keeping the hot/cold balance by avoiding certain behaviours or situations like taking a bath when the body is hot (Hill, 1985).

In Creole medicine there is a progression beginning with an individualised prevention of illness and ending with a specialised therapy. Home remedies are tried for minor illnesses, or if visiting the doctor is inconvenient due to distance or long waits at the medical facilities. When home remedies fail, specialists are called in after discussion with family, friends and neighbours (Hill, 1985). Conversely folk medicine is tried if biomedicine fails. If a natural cause is not immediately apparent, a supernatural explanation is used (Mischel, 1959; Strobel, 1985). The process of elimination is important in the diagnosis of the illness (Strobel, 1985). There are two more essential points of this medical system: (1) there is no barrier between mystical and scientific interpretations; (2) everyone has to determine what works for him/herself. These two Hippocratic traditions have been incorporated into Creole philosophy, which has a concept of the body as an integral part of the universe (Strobel, 1985).

Creolization

Creoleness, hybridity, mestizaje etc stands for the ethnic plurality of the Caribbean and other colonised places (Price and Price, 1997; Balutansky, 1997). Creolization in the Caribbean is the cultural construct that distils the dehumanising experiences of Caribbean history into a self-consciously de-centred Caribbean identity (Balutansky, 1997). Creolization as cultural syncretism gives rise to the subversive and transformative creativity of the Caribbean (Balutansky, 1997). Creolization in language emerged when ocean-borne trade of various European nations brought those citizens in touch with those in Africa the Caribbean and the Pacific (Richards, 1996). Community networks developed of people from different language groups and a pidgin language often developed into a fully formed Creole tongue that made communication possible between the groups of different origins (Richards, 1996). An analogous process in agrarian development and in folk knowledge development would be the exploitation of synergy between external and indigenous elements in the elaboration of local technologies and this synergy is a cross-cultural unceasing transformation (Richards, 1996). Technology development by immigrants would then involve matching available knowledge from different sources to available ethnomedicinal knowledge for emergent health needs. Good Creolization therefore means that the origin of an idea is not important, only that it works in the local context (Richards, 1996). Bles is one Caribbean Creole disease that is called a culture-bound syndrome in Biomedicine. It affects children and its main causes are traumas like falls, shocks and exertion (Vilayleck, 1996). Another Caribbean Creole disease found is marasmi, translated into biomedicine as infant malnutrition. One East Indian element that is resorted to by the Creole population in Trinidad and has become partly Creolised is jharay.

Origins of folk medicine

Have traditional medicinal practices deviated from those of the source continents Africa, India, South America and Europe? McClure (1982) traces the belief that purges can prevent disease caused by food to the ancient Egyptians. Some of the literature traces folk medicine only to its African roots. Mahabir (1991) complains of this in his justification for focusing solely on the Indian heritage. Even though similarity of use is not sufficient to establish the origin of particular cultural features, each case study compares ethnoveterinary practices to ethnmedicinal practices in India, Africa, South America, Europe and Africa. Tracing the origins of the folk medicine knowledge becomes important in the verification process, why things are done in certain ways, and if there are any theories behind the practice. For instance one of my sources indicated that the Hindu period of mourning is **9** days. There are also Hindu practices where ground Neem or leaves and flowers are offered for **9** days. A herbalist mentioned 'malomay for cooling, and for a clean out, take for **9** days then take a purge out'. In Catalonia and Almería, Spain, prayers are often associated with the administration of herbal remedies and the number **9**, and other odd numbers, is utilised to decide the number of plant parts to use or the period of consumption of the medicine (Martínez-Lirola et al., 1996; Bonet et al., 1999). When chronic illnesses are treated in Almería, Spain, treatment is usually interrupted every **9** days for a week's "rest" (Martínez-Lirola et al., 1996).

Sofowora (1982) details the collection of *Ageratum conyzoides*, which is collected at night to use in treating a child who cries too often for no known cause and witchcraft is suspected. In the dead of night the plant identified in the day is approached, **9** or 7 (for male or female respectively). *Aframomum melegueta* seeds are chewed and spat on the plant while the appropriate incantations are recited, the plant is then harvested (Sofowora, 1982). Nine is also a magic number in Belize (Arnason et al., 1980). Morton (1981) claims it is an important Maya number used for leaves of a plant, drops of a medicine or days to take a medicine. The Amerindian community practises the nine-night wake. In Dominica and other islands a person is buried within 24 hours in a token affair. However a large and festive wake is held 8 days later, these are important social and community events (Banks, 1956). However there may be other reasons for the number **9** being an important one in Trinidad and Tobago culture, for example the novenas or nine days/nights of prayer and nine first Fridays in the Roman Catholic religion.

Supernatural emic can sometimes indicate etic efficacy (McCorkle and Mathias-Mundy, 1992). The mosquito bush or duppy/jumbie basil (*Ocimum micranthum*) received one local name from its odour (the methyl cinnamate in the essential oil) the chemical is now reputed to be a mosquito repellent (Bayley, 1949). In previous decades nothing was known of yellow fever, and it was thought to be spread by the malignant vapours or duppies that came from the swamps (Bayley, 1949). It was noticed that when the *Ocimum micranthum* plant was broken and hung in the house, (probably to keep for medicinal purposes like colds and cooling), the duppies/jumbies kept away.

The written text in the following sections describes the diverse background of the knowledge, and who in which group possessed knowledge and why. The historical descriptions of the Trinidad and Tobago population suggest the diverse background of the knowledge base and the fact that the 'local' knowledge is in fact mobile and utilisable in other places. This is important given the struggle between science which claims universal applicability, and non science, which is sometimes assumed to be the opposite (Latour, 1986).

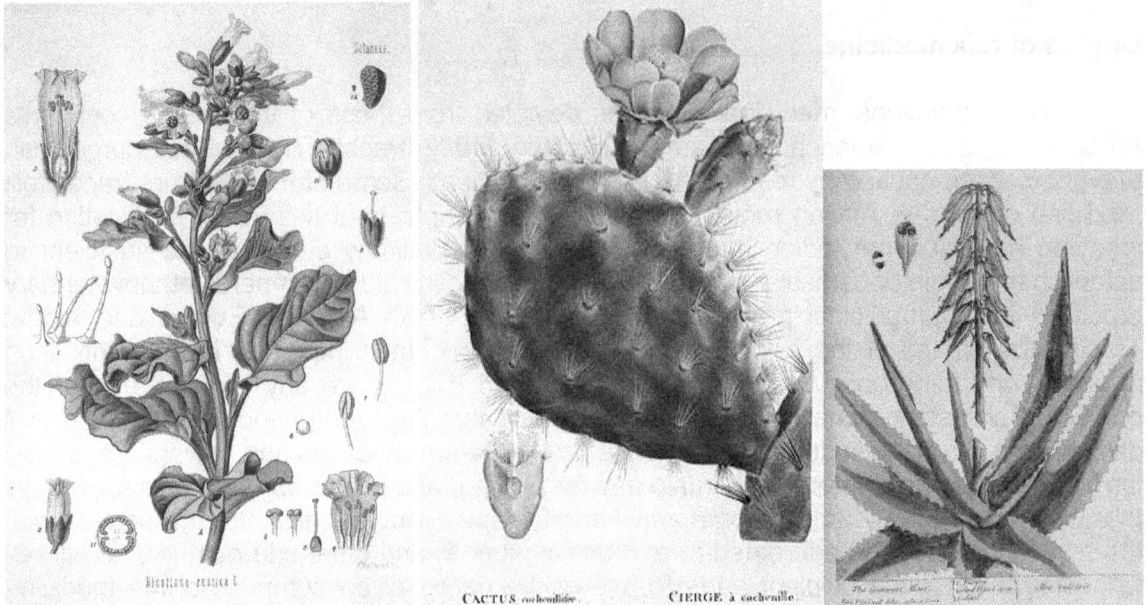

Figure 19. Nicotiana rustica
Figure 20. Nopalea cochenillifera
Figure 21. Aloe vera

Amerindian-based knowledge

Genetic research has suggested that present-day North and South Amerindians originated from the same single migration of an ancient Asian population in the Pleistocene (Pena, 1999). There is considerable controversy over the origins of Amerindian culture (Haslip-Viera *et al.*, 1997). According to Paquette and Engerman (1996):
1. The word Taino did not have emic value for any West Indian society (that is, as a term of self-ascribed social identity) and was not used by the Spanish. No distinction between Taino and Sub-Taino culture has been established. At the time of Columbus no West Indian society called themselves Carib.
2. There were many similarities and differences among the various inhabitants of the Greater Antilles and different languages may have been spoken during the time of Columbus; but the historically known languages from Trinidad to Cuba were Arawakan.
3. The ethnographic reality of the terms *Guanahuacabibes*, *Igneri* and *Lucayans* has not been established.

When Cristòbal Còlon 'discovered' Trinidad/Cairi in the 1498 there were several Amerindian tribes; the *Shebaio, Aruacas, Nepoio, Yao, Pariagoto, Chaimas, Tamanaques, Chaguanes, Salives, Quaquas* and *Caraibes*. These Meso Indians (population 10,000 - 40,000) lived in coastal and riverine villages and were fishermen, hunters and gatherers (Borde, 1876). Sir Walter Ralegh recorded similar and different names for these groups according to Lovén (1935). His names were *Jaois* living in Parico, *Arawacs* living in on the south coast at Punta Carao, *Saluaios* living in the southwest between Carao and Curiapan, *Nepoyos* (alternate names *Nepeio, Napoy, Nipujo, Nipiju, Mabouye* according to Boomert) located in the southeast and east in Carao and Punta Galera and *Carinepagotos* living in Spanish Citie/Port of Spain. This last group Whitehead calls those-who-live-at-carinepa and claims

40

that they like the *arwacas* were allied to the Spanish. Boomert (2000) claims the Nepoyo are now extinct. Lovén (1935) claimed that the *Jaois* and the *Arawacs* came to Trinidad from Guiana. Boomert (2000) adds another group the *Tivitiva* (*Tibitibe*, *Tibetebe* = bivalves, mud people) living on Trinidad's west coast as well as on the mainland. This group had subgroups called the *Ciawani* (*Seawano*, *Chaguanas*) and the *Waraweeti* (alternate names *Warao*, *Waraowitu*, *Warouw*, *Warrau*, *Guarano*, *Warrahoun*). Boomert also claims that the *Chaima* came to Trinidad in the late 17th century as represented by the place name Carapachaima.

Whitehead (1997) quotes the 1596 text by Lawrence Keymis (A *relation of the Second Voyage to Guiana*) in which the cacique *Wareo* tells Keymis that he was chased by the Spanish and the *Arwaccas* from his home in Moruga and that the *Yao* had left Trinidad for the Amazon before the 1600s because the Spanish were "borrowing[10]" their wives[11]. Jean Mocquet called the *Yao* '*Caripou*' (Whitehead 1997: 62). *Suppoyo*, *Nepoyo* and *Orinoquepon*i leaders and populations, like the *Yao*, were also absorbed or disappeared after resettling on the mainland. Interestingly Keymis calls the *Arwaccas* a "vagabound nation of Indians, which finding no certaine place of abode of their owne, do for the most part serve and follow the Spaniards". Whitehead (1997:45) claims that the alliance of the *aruacas* with the Spanish resulted in hostility towards them. He gives further details of how the groupings of *caribes*/*Karinya* and *aruacas* came into being as a reaction to Spanish and other European incursions in the region and also to European tendencies to simplify Amerindian complexity. For example *Warao* captured in the Delta in 1712 were settled by the Spanish in North Trinidad encomiendas (Boomert 2000: 89).

Lovén (1935) wrote that Sedeño landed in Trinidad in the *Chacomar* district in 1519. He went again with an army in 1532, and recorded that he fought against only two Amerindian provinces; *Camuaurao* (north Trinidad) under the war-chief *Baucumar* and *Chacomar* under *Marauna*[12]. Boomert (2000) claims that Sedeño arranged an alliance with *Maruana* (*Maluana*) of *Chacomar* (on the south coast close to Punta Curao[13]) and this created conflicts with the other tribes who were resisting Spanish settlement. Lovén quotes historical documents claiming that some of the Trinidadian tribes were at war with each other, some of the combatants had allies in the Antilles and the warfare facilitated the settlement of the Spanish (Lovén, 1935: 42). Whitehead (1997) writes that de Berrío attempted an alliance with the cacique *Morequito*, the successor to *Topiawari* and then later on with the *Nepoyo* cacique *Carapana*[14]. The cacique *Cantyman* helped the English capture San José. *Wannawanare* assisted Ralegh in the capture of San José in 1595 because he had been tortured by de Berrío and liberated by Ralegh (Boomert, 2000). Amerindians made many alliances with the Spanish, Dutch and English (including Ralegh) in the continuing struggle over the Caribbean (Whitehead, 1997). For example the *Nepoio* settled in Trinidad during de Berrío's time and the *Yaio* created the village of *Parico* (*Paracoa*) close to the Guapo River (Boomert, 2000). Amerindians also took advantage of weaknesses in the enemy. *Yao* king *Anacajoury* used his knowledge of the illnesses affecting the settlement party of Charles Leigh in 1604 to plan an attack on them.

---

[10] The beginning of Amerindian-Spanish creolization.

[11] Boomert (2000) claims that the Amerindians of Trinidad and Guiana had matrilineal inheritance increasing the seriousness of this "borrowing".

[12] Many caciques present in Trinidad were named after their district or village (Lovén, 1935: 38).

[13] The Amerindian village of Carao, Cayao, Carowa existed until the mid 17th century (Boomert, 2000). The current Curao point is close to Moruga.

[14] Carapana spent his boyhood in the Yaio village of Parico in southwest Trinidad and made alliances with de Berrío which brought him many followers anxious to obtain Spanish trade goods and presents. He susequently quarrelled with the Spanish when they made his followers employees and took many Nepoio women. The Spanish then facilitated his decline (Boomert, 2000). See Boomert (2000) for more on Carapana and other caciques.

Amerindians constructed small round earthen mounds known as montones on cleared plots to provide a bed for root crops such as cassava, *Xanthosoma sagittifolium, Xanthosoma jacquinii*, arrowroot (*Maranta arundinacea*), topi tambo (*Calathea allouia*) and *Zamia debilis*, beans, squash, cotton and maize (Newsom, 1993). Arrowroot rhizomes were mashed and used medicinally as poultices and to draw the poison out of arrow-derived wounds (Sanderson, 2005). Homegardens contained fruit trees such as mammee apple (*Mammea americana*), tobacco, avocado (*Persea americana*), *Pouteria campechiana*, manzanillas, *Bixa orellana*, calabash (*Crescentia cujete*)[15], genip (*Genipa americana*) and the snuff producing tree cohoba (*Piptadenia peregrina*) (Newsom, 1993). Other plants used by Amerindians include *Mastichodendron foetidissimum*, balata (*Manilkara bidentata*), *Oenothera* sp., and *Portulaca* sp. They used woods such as button mangrove (*Conocarpus erecta*), *Bourreria* sp., *Bumelia* sp., *Casearia* sp., white mangrove (*Laguncularia racemosa*), the parasitic Scotch attorney (*Clusia rosea*), *Ficus* sp., *Tabebeuia* sp., *Acacia* sp., lignum vitae (*Guaiacum* sp.), *Croton* sp., *Exostema* sp., *Erythroxylum* sp., *Annona* spp., *Coccoloba* sp., and *Capparis* sp. (Newsom, 1993). Mesoamerica is also home to sapote (*Casimiroa edulis* and *Diospyros digyna*), *Spondias mombin* and bottle gourds (*Lagenaria siceraria*). Columbus first recorded sweet potato and cassava on November 4, 1492. Las Casas paraphrases Columbus' diary thus: "full of *mames* that are like carrots; which have a flavour like chestnuts; these are what are called *ajes* and *batatas* which are very tasty" (Morison, 1963). Sweet potato is said to originate in tropical northwestern South America and had spread across the Caribbean before the 1490s (Sanderson, 2005).

Bixa orellana is very important to Amerindian culture. Lovén (1935) claims that the Amerindians in the southwest of Trinidad wore only *bija* (roucou and carapa oil) and that Baucumar went to war entirely painted with *bija*. Other Amerindian groups painted themselves black with genipa especially when they had unburied corpses (Lovén 1935: 49). Also important were engraved, polished or painted gourds used for eating and drinking vessels (Lovén 1935: 249). Amerindians also brought domesticates like guinea pigs (*Cavia porcellus*) and dogs to the Caribbean (Siegel, 1991). Columbus first mentioned the "dog that did not bark/*perros que no ladran*" on the island of Cuba on 28 October, 1492. To the Spaniards they resembled *gozcos* a breed on their peninsula. Amerindians also used these dogs for food (Morison, 1963).

Amerindians do not operate from the dualisms that separate humans from spirits, animals, plants or things; mind and body, thinking and feeling or nature and culture (Lawrence, 1998; McCorkle and Green, 1998). They practised a universal belief in spirits of nature but deities were not worshiped (Besson, 2000). Medicine men served as curers and advisors due to their ability to contact spirits. The Aztecs considered work to be 'heating' and drank refreshing or cooling beverages before work in order to keep themselves cool (Messer, 1987). Concepts such as moisture and winds tied to concepts of illness and the idea of 'readjustment' of body heat through administration of herbs, potions and massage are also linked to Amerindian beliefs (Messer, 1987).

Bitterness is often associated with heat and strength while coolness is associated with weakness in describing the hot/cold quality of herbs or, for the use of the curers, who drink bitter brews to increase their resistance to illness and evil (Messer, 1987).
Amerindian culture was almost completely Hispanicized by the Catholic missionaries of the Cisterciensan and Capuchin orders, who set up missions along the east and south coasts of Trinidad.

---

[15] Spanish-speaking Trinidadians calls calabash *talparo* or *totúmo* which are Amerindian derived names (Boomert, 2000: 96).

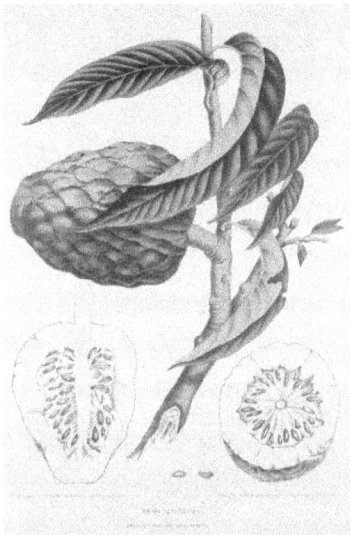

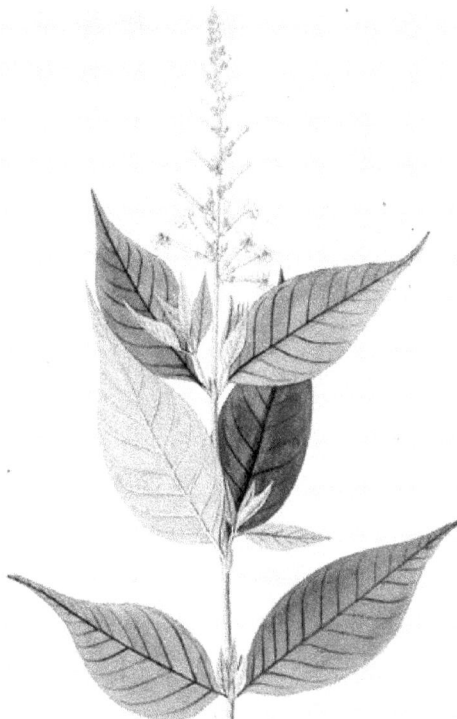

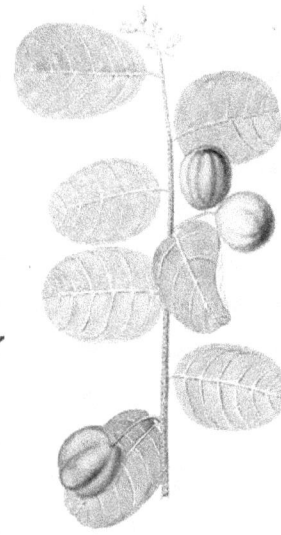

Figure 22. Annona reticulata
Figure 23. Barleria hirsuta
Figure 24. Chrysobalanus icaco

Some Amerindians re-crossed the Gulf of Paria to the mainland, but those who stayed accepted the culture and Catholic faith and gradually became assimilated (Banks, 1956). An example of their assimilation by the missionaries is the continuing celebration of the Santa Rosa festival in Arima. Siparia and Arima were established by the Spanish Capuchins who came from the Santa Maria province of Aragon in 1756 - 1758. In 1757, the Capuchins friars dedicated their Arima mission to the first New World saint, Santa Rosa. In 1787, the Arima mission was enlarged to accommodate the Amerindian people who had been displaced from Tacarigua, Caura and Arouca (Besson, 2000). By the 1770s, Amerindians were racially mixed with the Spaniards, mestizos and Africans. The Spanish-Amerindian mixtures came to be known as the cocoa panyols.

Brereton (1981) has written that the Amerindians influenced the lifestyle of rural Trinidadians before they disappeared, especially through the Spanish and the 'peóns' of Venezuelan origin. Also from the Amerindians comes the use of plants to excite dogs to hunt (Honychurch, 1986). Other aspects are rituals that include *Nicotiana tabacum*, and the significance attached to dreams (Butt Colson and de Armellada, 1983). The intoxication of fish before capture is considered to come from the Amerindians (Borde, 1876). However ichthyotoxic (fish killing) plants were used in Spain before 1255 and are still used there and in South East Asia (Álvarez Arias, 2000). The use of lignum vitae (*Guaiacum offinale*), for women's problems and sexually transmitted diseases may have Amerindian origins (Lawrence, 1998)[16]. Amerindian origins were seen in Tobago in the first phase of the research. An individual remedy to induce oestrus included cedar bark (*Cedrela odorata*). The Tacanas in the Bolivian Amazon use a decoction of cedar bark for post partum haemorrhage (Bourdy *et al.*, 2000). Amerindian culture also has personalistic explanations for sickness (Banks, 1956; Davis and Yost, 1983). There is an underlying aspect of their culture claiming

---

[16] In 1603, Bartholomew Gilbert set sail for Nevis from London in the 50-ton *Elizabeth*, to cut lignum vitae and buy tobacco from the Amerindians (Appleby, 1996).

43

that all human relationships are potentially dangerous (Banks, 1956). It is claimed that this theme underlies their couvade[17] and other rituals and purifications and the Amerindian theory of sickness.

Whitehead (1997: 59) records that Spanish oral tradition recorded by Ralegh from his interrogation of de Berrío posits a Guianan invasion of Peru and claims that the ceramic culture of the Amazon is America's oldest. However in contrast to the 'inscriptions' of the Europeans that shaped what they 'discovered' (Amazons, cannibals, etc) in the West Indies, the Amerindians had none. This is well illustrated by Waterton (1973: 111):

> I could find no monuments or marks of antiquity amongst these Indians; so that, after penetrating to the Rio Branco from the shores of the Western Ocean, had anybody questioned me on this subject I should have answered, I have seen nothing amongst these Indians which tells me that they have existed here for a century; though, for aught I know to the contrary, they may have been here before the Redemption, but their total want of civilisation has assimilated them to the forests in which they wander. Thus an aged tree falls and moulders into dust and you cannot tell what was its appearance, its beauties, or its diseases amongst the neighbouring trees; another has shot up in its place, and after Nature has had her course it will make way for a successor in its turn. So it is with the Indian of Guiana. He is now laid low in the dust; he has left no record behind him, either on parchment or on a stone or in earthenware to say what he has done. Perhaps the place where his buried ruins lie was unhealthy, and the survivors have left it long ago and gone far away into the wilds. All that you can say is, the trees where I stand appear lower and smaller than the rest, and from this I conjecture that some Indians may have had a settlement here formerly. Were I by chance to meet the son of the father who moulders here, he could tell me that his father was famous for slaying tigers and serpents and caymen, and noted in the chase of the tapir and wild boar, but that he remembers little or nothing of his grandfather.

European-based knowledge

In the late eighteenth century thousands of British, French, Spanish, Dutch and other European seamen were coming through the Caribbean annually, spending several weeks putting together a cargo for the return voyage. Rates of desertion and discharge were 30 – 40% from British ships arriving from Africa (Scott, 1996). In the late 1780s, approximately 21,000 "Jack Tars" came through the Caribbean annually (Scott, 1996). Sailors in the 17th century carried *Capsicum* on their voyages to protect against scurvy probably not knowing or caring that the herbalists Matthiolus (c. 1570) and Dodonaeus (1644) warned against its use (Pickersgill, 2005). The religious orders, especially the Dominicans, Franciscans and Augustinians, Capuchins, tried to establish themselves in Trinidad from 1591 (Besson, 2000). The last Aragon Capuchin came to Trinidad in 1758 (Besson, 2000). The friars organised missions at several areas which are still the major villages and towns in Trinidad (Besson, 2000). Spanish padres sent seeds of Amerindian plants to monastery gardens in Europe and may have been responsible for the rapid spread of *Capsicum* across the Iberian Peninsula (Pickersgill, 2005). The name *Aloe barbadensis* comes from the practice of Jesuit priests sending the plants from the mainland to the Spanish islands of Jamaica and Barbados (Pickersgill, 2005).

In the late 1700s, the settlers started to arrive in Puerto d'España. Trinidad was still a province of the Caracas captaincy-general in the late 1700s and a royal decree of 1783 openly invited discontented French settlers and held out special dispensations for those bringing slaves with them (Scott, 1996). The French plantation owners who came with

---

[17] Couvade (Fr. *couver*, "to hatch"), widespread custom among native peoples, whereby the father, during or immediately after the birth of a child, complains of having labor pains, and is accorded the treatment usually shown to pregnant women. The social function of couvade is held to be the assertion by the father of his role in reproduction or of his legal rights to the child. The underlying belief is that the souls of babies are weakly attached to their bodies and the couvade and practices of rest and dieting protect the soul for the first nine days after birth (Taylor, 1950; Butt Colson and de Armellada, 1983).

their slaves and families were driven from their estates in Grenada, Martinique and Guadeloupe by the tumultuous times and the conquering British.

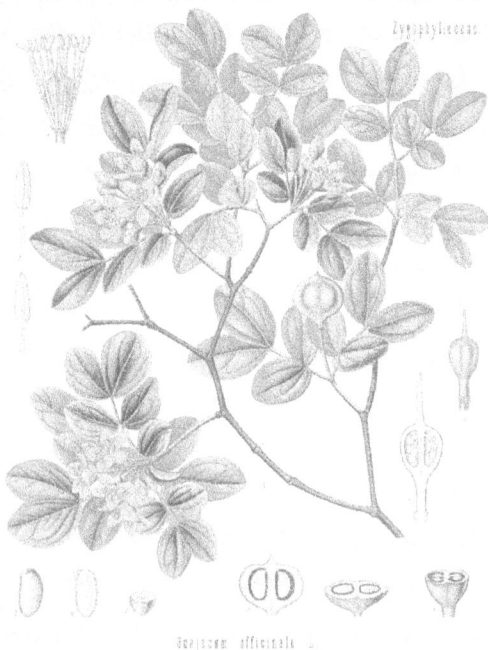

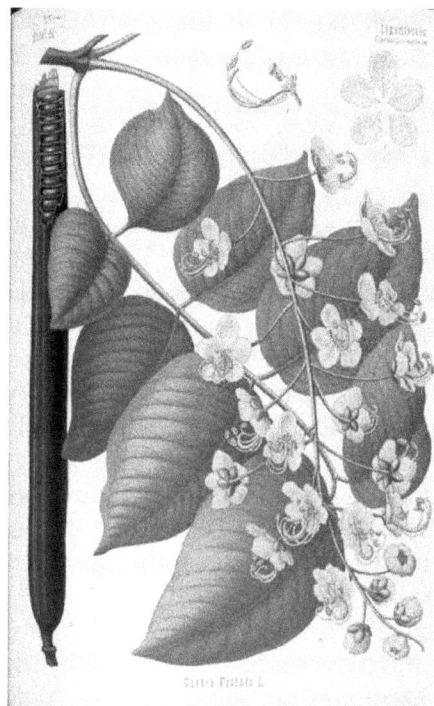

Figure 25. Guajacum officinale
Figure 26. Cassia fistula

Some were French royalists who fled from the French Revolution in France and its aftermath in the Caribbean; others were serving with the British forces in the Caribbean. Amongst these were the Count of Lopinot and his four sons, Chevalier de Verteuil, Chevalier de Bruny, Marquis de Montrichard and Vicomte de Bragelonne (Besson, 2000). These Chevaliers had a profound influence on social attitudes. The French did not discover or conquer Trinidad but because they constituted a large proportion of the population (twenty Frenchmen to every Spaniard) and were the elite, they influenced the culture of the society (Joseph, 1837). Newspapers in the British colonies were published in English and French (Scott, 1996). French words are still part of the local dialect of Trinidad, often as "Patois."

The term "French Creole" should but does not always include the free people of colour, the children of the French planters of the early times with their African slaves, and later, their mulatto, quadroon and octoroon mistresses (Besson, 2000). Some of these children were recognised by their fathers and legitimised and freed, receiving educations at French universities and inheriting land and property, their children becoming in turn the doctors, lawyers and school masters in the latter part of the 19th century. The entrenched social conservatism of the planters in Guadeloupe and Martinique increased the dissatisfaction of the free coloureds in those islands. After serving their eight years in the militias they left for Trinidad to gain access to land for small coffee plantations. Artists and artisans, "éclaires et mécontents" also left (Pérotin-Dumon, 1996). These minority groups, their aspirations and their effect on folk medicine are examined in Chapter 12.

In 1832, the population of Trinidad consisted of 3,683 whites, 16,302 mixed, about 700 Amerindians, 20,265 slaves and 4,615 'Aliens and Strangers' (Besson, 2000). Several English and Scottish merchants and their families settled and ran the import-export trade in the post-Cedula years (1783-97). The British aquired the islands of Dominica, St. Vincent, Grenada and Tobago from the French in 1763 as part of the treaty of Paris (Engerman, 1996). The English community comprised of expatriates who only came to Trinidad to govern and work, but not to settle, while many of the Catholic English and Irish intermarried with the French Creole population. Charles Warner served as Attorney General between the 1840s and the 1860s. He was responsible for the "Anglicisation" of this period (English textbooks, English laws, English schooling, Anglican Church) and became the "bête noire" of the French Creoles and the Catholics (Besson, 2000).

The first group of Portuguese came to Trinidad as early as 1630 as explorers bound for Brazil. Portuguese Sephardic Jews came in the late 18th century. Madeirans escaped from economic straits and religious persecution in 1846 and 1847. The Portuguese opened dry goods stores, rum shops and adjoining small groceries on the estates (Besson, 2000). With continuous immigration to reunite families the entire Portuguese community comprised 2000 members by the turn of the 20th century. Eventually the Portuguese were absorbed by intermarriage into the larger Roman Catholic community, consisting of Afro-French, Afro-Spanish, Irish and English settlers (Besson, 2000).

Madeira was colonised by the Portuguese in the 15th century and slaves and indentured labourers were brought to the islands. According to Rivera and Obón (1995), there were no natives in the islands to teach the newcomers about the local herbs.
However folk medicine was vital because of the lack of doctors and was almost exclusively in the hands of older women. Looking for ethnomedicinal origins in Madeira is complex because of the movement of plants and people. Madeiran ethnopharmacology is based on 39 native Macronesian species, 151 Mid-European and Mediterranean species used similarly to those in Portugal, and 69 exotic species from the African Portuguese colonies, Brazil and the West Indies (Rivera and Obón, 1995).

Some research on the European influence on folk medicine has been conducted (Bennett and Prance, 2000).There are 216 introduced species that are used by populations in northern South America (Brazil, Colombia, Ecuador and Peru). Twenty-one percent of these plants are of European origin, fourteen percent are from Eurasia and seventeen percent are of Mediterranean origin. Asprey and Thornton (1953-1955) claim that the name *semen contra* now used in the West Indies as the Creole name for the introduced European plant *Chenopodium ambrosioides* was originally one of the names of the drug Santonica derived from the introduced European plant *Artemesia cina* B. *Artemesia* was also used as an anthelmintic but perhaps less effectively. Spanish traditions were handed down from the original colonial heritage but are reinforced by visits and migrants escaping the turbulent politics of Venezuela. Bruni *et al. (*1997) claim that the use of the stigma and styles of *Zea mays* as a diuretic is found only in those parts of Italy where the Spanish influence was strong. This ethnomedicinal use is also found in Trinidad and in Latin America and is still found in Spain (Wong, 1976; Girón *et al.*, 1991; Bonet *et al.*, 1992; Raja *et al.*, 1997; Blanco *et al.*, 1999). Multiple plant mixtures are used in Caribbean folk medicine especially in 'lochs' for respiratory problems. A similar practice is seen in Murcia and Cartagena, Spain where the guiding principle is: '*the more plants used, the more the medicinal properties are increased*' (Alcazar *et al.*, 1990).

Hispanic prayers are used in Latin America for healing and against mal yeux. These spanish-romanic prayers, like the 'oracion' prayer are used during 'santowah' (santigual) which is the Spanish equivalent of jharay. The ceremony includes sweet broom (*Scoparia dulcis*) which is used to sprinkle holy water. Some of the prayers kept secret in Trinidad can be found for sale in Cuban shops in Miami (S. Moodie-Kublalsingh, Institute of Languages, University of The West Indies, pers. comm. August, 2000). Moodie (1982) claims that these prayers (magic rather than religion) came to the New World with the conquistadors. In

Almería, Spain, folk magical plant therapy for warts, evil eye, hepatic ailments or swellings consist of a ritual in which an incantation ("prayer") is recited and a plant (*Malva* species, *Marrubium* species, etc.) is used (Martínez-Lirola *et al.*, 1996). In Tuscany the concept of the evil eye exists and *Foeniculum vulgare* is put into a red cloth and hung on the animal (Pieroni, 2000). Red cloths are also used in Trinidad and Tobago.

Some 'French Creoles' were amateur naturalists and one, T.W. Carr, compared the native *Parthenium hysterophorus* to the European *Artemisia* in appearance and smell, calling it 'country wormwood' or 'absinthe bâtarde des antilles' in his flora. In Trinidad rashes are bathed with St. John's bush (*Justicia secunda*, Acanthaceae). It is claimed that this plant imparts a red colour to the bath water. In Europe the red pigment from crushed flowers of St. John's wort (*Hypericum perforatum*) represents the blood of St. John at his beheading, because the herb is in full flower on June 24th, St. John's Day.

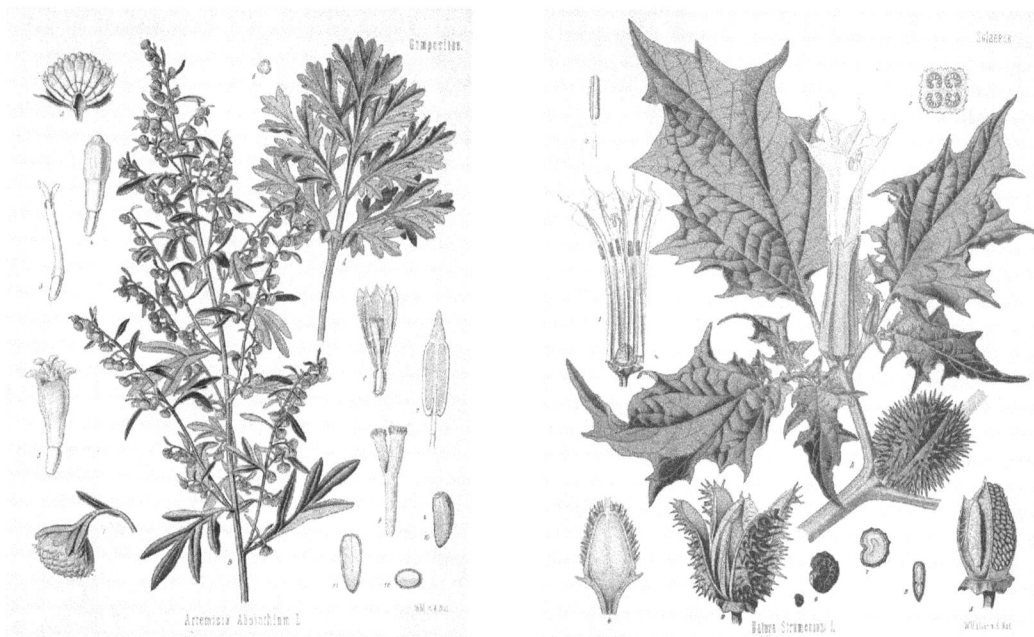

Figure 27. *Artemisia absinthium*
Figure 28. *Datura stramonium*

Chinese-based knowledge

Chinese Tartars (192 men and one woman) were brought to Trinidad on the 12 October 1806, on a ship called the 'Fortitude'. These men were brought to cultivate tea but most were dissatisfied with local conditions and returned on the 'Fortitude' (Joseph, 1837; Besson, 2000). The 23 who stayed made a living as entrepreneurs and creolized. Emancipation of slaves in 1838 created a labour shortage.
To fill this shortage 2,500 mainly male Chinese were brought legitimately to Trinidad as indentured workers, or were 'shanghaied' (abducted by European traders). Punti traders described Hakka prisoners as pigs on the bills of lading and shipped them to the Caribbean and South America. All of these immigrants arrived between 1853 and 1866. Almost 9,000 more Chinese immigrants came voluntarily from British Guyana to Trinidad over the next century (Besson, 2000). The Chinese soon left indentureship to become entrepreneurs and family members from China joined them (Besson, 2000). Harris (1991) has recorded the use of medicinal plants by the Chinese community in Trinidad.

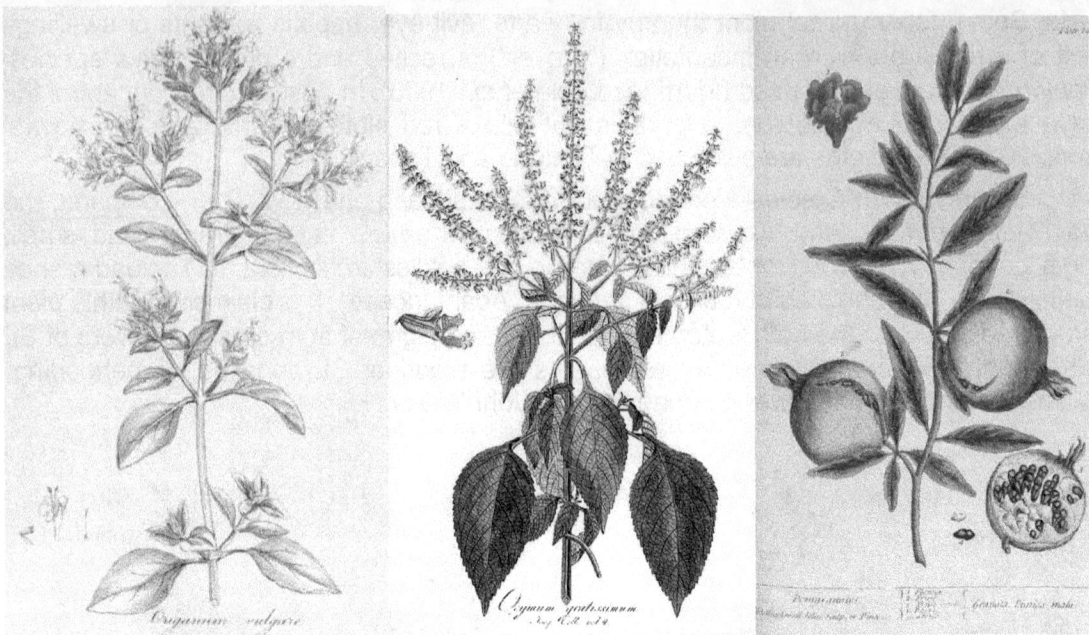

Figure 29. Origanum vulgare
Figure 30. Ocimum gratissimum
Figure 31. Punica granata

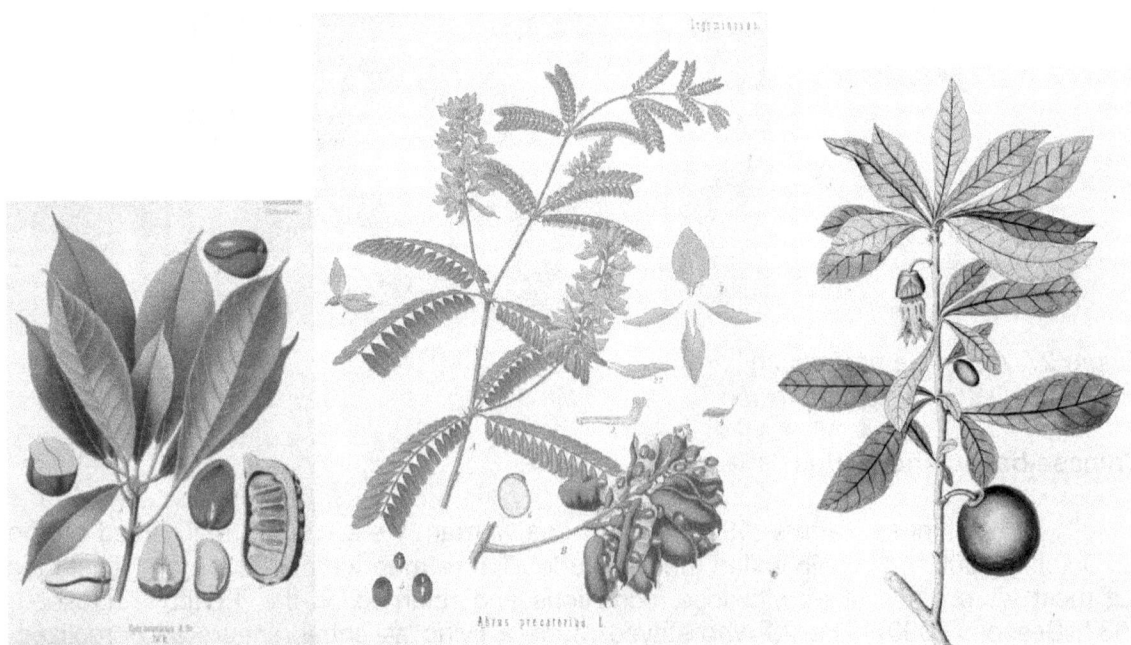

Figure 32. Cola acuminata
Figure 33. Abrus precatorius
Figure 34. Crescentia cujete

African-based knowledge

de las Casas sailed with Columbus' third voyage of 1498. In 1510, he was ordained as a priest and gave up his own Amerindian slaves. In 1515, de las Casas urged Cardinal Ximenes to send a commission of inquiry to the West Indies to investigate the demise of the Amerindians. African slaves were proposed as an alternative that was readily acceded to. The majority of the slaves came from the Bight of Biafra and Central Africa. Smaller numbers came from the Gold coast and the Windward coast (Lans, 1996). Personalistic explanations of sickness of African origin are subsumed under the term Obeah. An Obeahman is sought for illness caused or influenced by another human. Obeah includes healing as well as a whole range of 'magic' that is used for success in love, career and harming enemies. Obeah is associated with male practitioners, can be counteracted by another practitioner, by the use of talismans or by Catholic prayers (Littlewood, 1988). According to Honychurch (1986) *Theretia neriifolia*, *Abrus precatorius*, *Hippomane mancinella*, *Nerium oleander* have associations with Obeah and can only be cut at certain times of the moon. Some brews are left overnight in the dew to acquire maximum efficacy (Bayley, 1949).

Table 1 shows the diverse background of those of African origin who came to Trinidad in 1813, and also those from the other Caribbean islands owned by different European powers. In the early years of slavery many of the slaves were born in Martinique and Guadeloupe and possessed an African-French-Caribbean culture that included Patois as the main language. The movement of French slaves in the 1780s and 1790s to Trinidad gave it the reputation as a sanctuary similar to Puerto Rico leading to complains by absentee lobbyists in London (Scott, 1996). The royal cédula dated 14 April 1789 instructed Spanish colonies to welcome runaway French and British slaves who could show a "legitimate" claim to freedom and protect them from their former owners, José María Chacón, governor of Trinidad, publicized the decree in August of that year (Scott, 1996). Runaway slaves were multilingual with French and English added to their original languages. New slaves arriving from Africa had some impact on this culture. One example of the Creolization process is given: surelle means sour in Old French while sorrel is a sweetened drink made at Christmas time from *Hibiscus sabdariffa*. *Hibiscus sabdariffa* is used for hot and cold drinks in Sudan and Egypt (Ali *et al.*, 1991). Specialists in folk medicine may have been among those abducted from Africa. All of these factors would increase the probability of borrowing medical knowledge from other groups, the medical syncretism described by Laguerre (1987).

Table 1. Birthplaces of African-born and Creole slaves, Trinidad, 1813

Africans	Number	%
Senegambia	1500	10.7
Sierra Leone	599	4.3
Windward Coast	882	6.3
Gold Coast	1093	7.8
Bight of Benin	1075	7.7
Bight of Biafra	5509	39.4
Central Africa	2555	18.3
Mozambique	11	0.1
Unidentified	756	5.4
Subtotal	13980	100.0
Creoles Trinidad	7064	60.7
British colonies	2563	22.0
French colonies	1575	13.5
Spanish colonies	118	1.0
Unidentified	373	2.7
Subtotal	11629	100.0
Total	25673	

Source: Higman, 1979.

Indian-based knowledge

When the Portuguese indentured labour like the Chinese before them left the plantations to become entrepreneurs, the planters in Trinidad asked the British government and the local authorities to bring people from India to work on the plantations. On May 1845 the first ship, the Fatel Rozack brought 225 Indians to Trinidad. After that there was a steady influx of 141,615 people and their knowledge from 1845-1917 (Weller, 1968). The great majority came from the United Provinces of Agra and Oudh and Bihar (Weller, 1968). Hindi or a variant (especially Bhojpuri) was their main language and Hinduism their main religion. A significant minority were Moslem. The majority were simple country folk from traditional communities of village India. Table 2 shows their provinces of origin.

The Indians entered a system of indentureship. After five years of plantation work they had a choice of a free return passage to India or a small parcel of land in Trinidad to live on. In 1853 the Trinidad Government began to change the free return passage guarantee and more immigrants and their children stayed (Weller, 1968; Mohammed, 1995). Successive waves of immigrants strengthened the Indo-knowledge base and also brought plants and animals. Settlers added Indian culture to the Trinidad mosaic. 'Vaidyas' (physicians) may have come to Trinidad and Tobago in the closing years of indenture in the early 1900s. Trinidad Planters complained that labourers were recruited who were unfit for agricultural work such as jewellers, silversmiths, barbers and similar castes; such people only went '*to swell the ranks of ineffectives on arrival*' (Weller, 1968). These immigrants may have had a greater Ayurvedic knowledge. According to Samaroo (1975) and LaGuerre (1984) some Brahmins disguised their caste to escape from the strife in the UP and Bihar States and from the 1857 Mutiny.

Table 2. Origin of Indian immigrants to Trinidad from 1908

PLACE	NUMBER OF IMMIGRANTS
BENGAL/ AMJERE/ BOMBAY/MADRAS/ OTHERS	5
BIHAR	120
UNITED PROVINCES OF AGRA AND OUDH	1248
CENTRAL PROVINCES & PUNJAB	13
CENTRAL INDIA & NATIVE STATES	78
OUDH	983
TOTAL	2,447

Source: Weller, 1968.

These Brahmins resumed their traditional roles in Trinidad and Tobago as professionals either during or after indentureship ended, recreating an Indian knowledge network under Trinidad and Tobago conditions. Occasional recent Indian migrants would have reinforced the existing Trinidad knowledge. The type of healers found in Trinidad now are the "Ojhas" and "masseurs" (Mustapha, 1977). The "Ojhas' (Hindu pundit or Muslim imam), have magico-religious forms of healing and the 'masseurs' provide more a physical type of healing called 'cracking' 'rubbing' and 'vein pulling'. In 'vein pulling' pain is believed to originate from one 'vein' lapping over another, or by a twisted 'vein'. The masseur grasps the patient's vein with his fingers, pulls upwards and puts it back in place. This causes considerable pain and the entire leg becomes numb for a few minutes (Mustapha, 1977). The masseur's ability to massage away pains affecting the muscular and skeletal system is learnt by experience, and from their fathers. The skilled ones are visited before the medical practitioner. The majority of these healers see people at their homes (Mustapha, 1977). There are few differences between folk medicine among Hindus and Muslims in the local knowledge network. The Muslim minority may have absorbed the Hindu practices (Mustapha, 1977). The experience and the ability of the healer to cure a particular ailment and his availability at the time needed are what matters, religion is less important.

There are personalistic explanations for some illnesses in Indian populations. Recovery from this type of sickness would mean a prayer-based healing called 'jharay' which involves praying on the sick person [or animal] or on the food eaten by him/her (Mustapha, 1977). Illnesses are regarded as evil spirits taking possession of the body and bringing about an abnormal state. Priest healing or 'jharay' involves praying on the sick person [or animal] or on the food eaten by him/her. Depending on the religion of the priest/healer the prayer is taken from the 'Gita', 'Vedas' or the 'Quran' (Mustapha, 1977). There is a general form of 'jharay' used to cure any kind of illness, and there are specific kinds for curing special diseases, like jaundice, headache and toothache (Mustapha, 1977). The general form of 'jharay' is used in curing diseases of the mind brought about by evil spirits. It is also used to dispel fear, 'najar' (mal jeux), fever, sores, insect stings, and safe delivery of babies (Mustapha, 1977). Aho and Minott (1977) described one Hindu-based jharay ceremony. The healer used a pinch of salt, five bird peppers (*Capsicum annum*), five grains of garlic (*Allium sativum*), five mustard seeds, and five cocoyea broomsticks (*Cocos nucifera*).

These ingredients are passed over the baby from head to toe five times. Each time she repeats in Hindi, "who maljo is this, go back to them; leave my baby alone." At the end of this prayer she throws all the ingredients into a nearby fire made for this purpose. No one can look at the fire otherwise the maljo will attach itself to the looker. The ritualised fire symbolises the burning up of the maljo inflicting the baby. Well-known Ayurvedic plants/foods/spices are black pepper (*Piper nigrum*), long pepper (*Piper longum*) and ginger (*Zingiber officinalis*) (Eigner and Scholz, 1999). Plant uses still considered East Indian-based are those associated with Hindu and Moslem rituals like Phagwa. Datur (*Datura stramomium*) flower is boiled for Phagwa. Datur is also associated with intoxication more dangerous than that of alcohol. Turmeric (*Curcuma domestica*) is used to prepare Hindu brides as in India (Scartezzini and Speroni, 2000). Tulsi (*Ocimum sanctum*) is used in Hindu rituals.

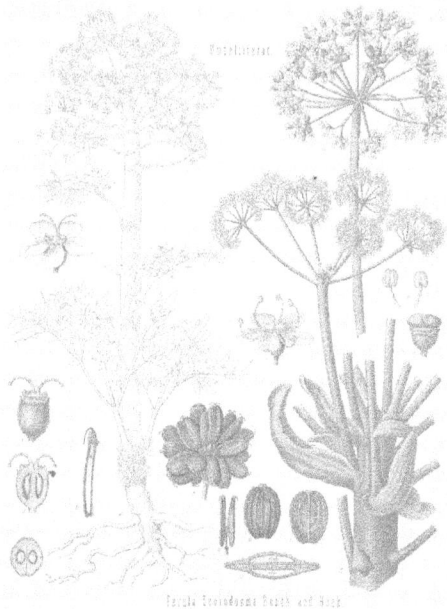

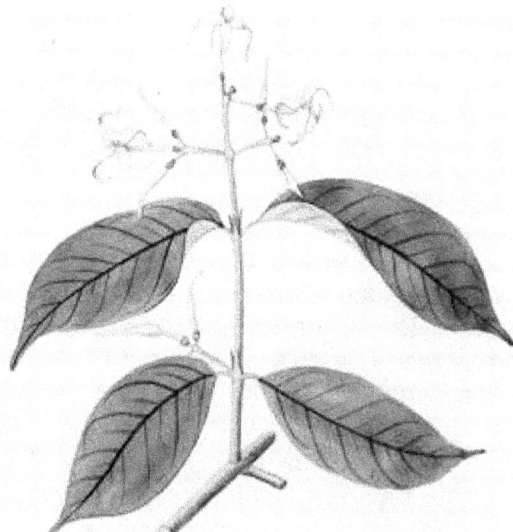

Figure 35 .*Ferula assafoetida*
Figure 36. *Coffea occidentalis*

Inscriptions

'By working on papers alone, on fragile inscriptions which are immensely less than the things from which they are extracted, it is still possible to dominate all things, and all people. What is insignificant for all other cultures becomes the most significant, the only significant aspect of reality' (Latour, 1986). Latour's phrase becomes important when considering two research questions: are the folk/ethnoveterinary medicinal practices derived from a body of knowledge that is ancient, coherent and global in nature? Do the different traditional medical systems that exist in Caribbean folk medicine share a common explanatory model? Commonalities in ethnomedicine are partly derived from the movement of peoples and plants from place to place. For example *Aloe vera* and *Punica granatum* are reputed to have been introduced to ancient Egypt from Eastern Africa and South - West Asia respectively (Reeves, 1992). Another aspect of the explanation lies in the 'inscriptions' that have been copied and recopied since Egyptians wrote on papyri.

Early recognised compilers of existing and current herbal knowledge were the Greeks Hippocrates, Aristotle, Theophrastus (b. 370 BC), Dioscorides and Galen. Roman writers were Pliny and Celsus (Kay, 1996). Dioscorides (Pedianos Dioskurides) included the writings of the herbalist Krateuas, physician to Mithridates VI King of Pontus from 120 to 63 BC in his <u>De Materia Medica</u> (<u>Codex Vindobonensis</u>) (Blunt and Raphael, 1994). <u>De Materia Medica</u> was translated into several languages and Turkish, Arabic and Hebrew names were added to it throughout the centuries (Blunt and Raphael, 1994). Latin manuscripts of <u>De Materia Medica</u> were combined with a Latin herbal by Apuleius Platonicus and were incorporated into the Anglo-Saxon codex <u>Cotton Vitellius C.III</u>. These early Greek and Roman compilations became the backbone of European medical theory and were translated by the Arabs Avicenna (Ibn Sīnā, 980 - 1037), the Persian Rhazes (Rāzi, 865 - 925) and the Jewish Maimonides (Kay, 1996). Translations of Greek medical handbooks and manuscripts into Arabic took place in the eighth and ninth centuries. Arabic folk medicine developed from the conflict between the magic-based medicine of the Bedouins, the Arabic translations of the Hellenic medicine and Ayurvedic medicine (Slikkerveer, 1990). Spanish folk medicine was influenced by the Arabs from 711 to 1492 (Hernández-Bermejo and García Sánchez, 1998). Translations of the early Roman-Greek compilations were made into German by Hieronymus Bock whose herbal published in 1546 was called <u>Kreuter Buch</u>. A Dutch translation <u>Pemptades</u> by Rembert Dodoens (1517-1585) was translated by Charles de L'Écluse (Carolus Clusius, 1526-1609), and was published in English by Henry Lyte in 1578 as <u>A Nievve Herball</u>. This became John Gerard's (1545 - 1612) <u>Herball or General Hiftorie of Plantes</u> (Blunt and Raphael, 1994; Kay, 1996). Each new work was a compilation of existing texts with new additions.

Women's folk knowledge existed in undocumented parallel with these texts (Kay, 1996). Forty-four drugs, diluents, flavouring agents and emollients mentioned by Discorides are still listed in the official pharmacopoeias of Europe (Blunt and Raphael, 1994). The Pilgrims took Gerard's work to the United States of America where it influenced American folk medicine (Kay, 1996). Francisco Hernandez, physician to Phillip II of Spain spent the years 1571 - 1577 gathering information in Mexico and then wrote <u>Rerum Medicarum Novae Hispaniae Thesaurus</u>, many versions of which have been published including one by Francisco Ximenez. Both Hernandez and Ximenez fitted Aztec ethnomedicinal information into the European concepts of disease such as "warm", "cold", and "moist", but it is not clear that the Aztecs used these categories (Ortiz de Montellano, 1975). Juan de Esteyneffer's (Johann Steinhöfer) <u>Florilegio medicinal de todas las enfermedas</u> compiled European texts and added 35 Mexican plants. This Florilegio is still used by Mexican healers. Martin de la Cruz wrote an herbal in Nahauatl which was translated into Latin by Juan Badiano as

<u>Libellus de medicinalibus indorum herbis</u> or <u>Codex Barberini, Latin 241</u> and given to King Carlos V in 1552 (Heinrich et al., 2005). It was apparently written in haste and influenced by the European occupation of the previous 30 years. Fray Bernadino de Sahagún's used ethnographic methods to compile his codices that then became the <u>Historia General de las Cosas de Nueva Espana</u>, published in 1793 (Heinrich et al., 2005). Castore Durante published his <u>Herbario Nuovo</u> in 1585 describing medicinal plants from Europe and the East and West Indies. It was translated into German in 1609 and Italian editions were published for the next century. In Trinidad and Tobago a similar process took place.

Ewen (1896) translated parts of Dr. de Grosourdy's <u>El Medico Botanico Criollo</u> and published his translation in the <u>Journal of the Trinidad Field Naturalists' Club 1894 - 1896</u> as the '*Economic uses of the Compositae*'. Ewen was one of the writers who saw similarities between European plants like 'wormwood' (*Artemisia absinthium*) and the native 'wild wormwood' (*Parthenium hysterophorus*).

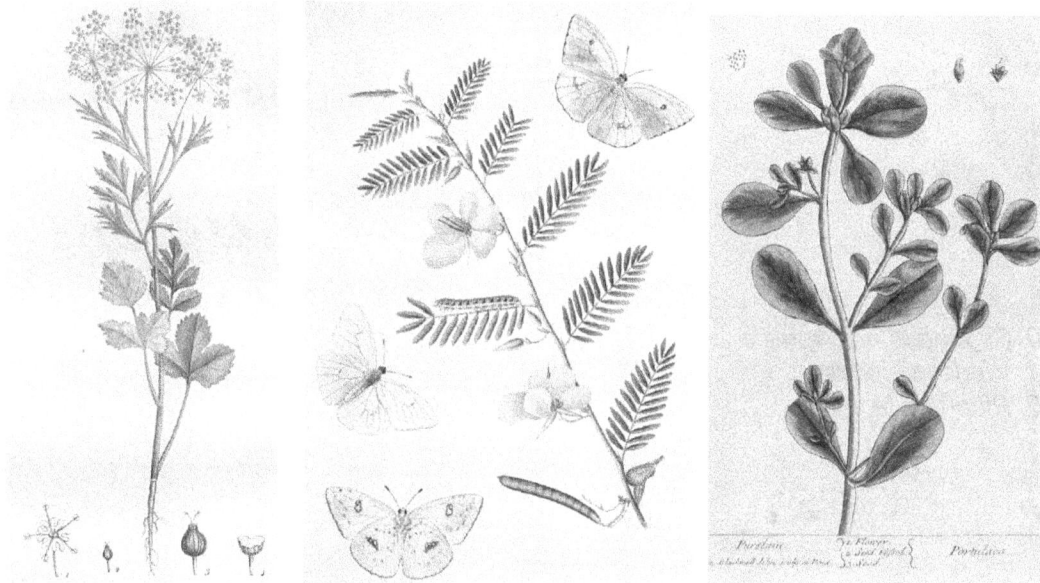

Figure 37. Pimpinella anisum
Figure 38.Cassia Chamæcrista/Papilio eubule
Figure 39. Portulaca oleracea

The syncretism process in Jamaica is described fully by Sheridan (1991). The medical profession in Jamaica ranged from Creole doctresses to Fellows of Royal Colleges of Physicians and Surgeons (like William Wright) and included charlatans and quacks; but the health of slaves was principally dealt with by overseers and knowledgeable slaves (Sheridan, 1991). Thomas Thistlewood who was born in Lincolnshire left journals and papers of his days as an overseer/plantation owner from 1750 to 1786. Thistlewood copied descriptions of medicinal plants from <u>The Useful Family Herbal</u> by John Hill, M.D., 2nd ed., London, 1755; he also had a copy of <u>Several Chirurgical Treatises</u> by Richard Wisewan, London, 1676. In addition to these texts Thistlewood acquired medical knowledge from befriended medical staff in Jamaica and had a garden of local medicinal plants (Sheridan, 1991). Thistlewood combined all of his knowledge and experience into a journal entry called <u>Receipts for a Physick</u>, 1770. Dr. William Wright, Thistlewood's contemporary combined Creole and European medicine with the collection of native Jamaican medicinal plants. Wright included 149 plants in his <u>Herbaria</u> written from 1773 -1813. Ralegh conducted research on the botanic pharmacopoeia while in the Tower[18] and his cordial was recorded by Nicaise Le Lebvre in the 1965 <u>Discours sur le Grand Cordial de Sr Walter Rawleigh par N. le Febvre</u> (Whitehead, 1997). The cordial provided a temporary reprieve from death for King James's son Henry. This brief history gives a partial explanation of some of the parallels in folk knowledge found in different cultures.

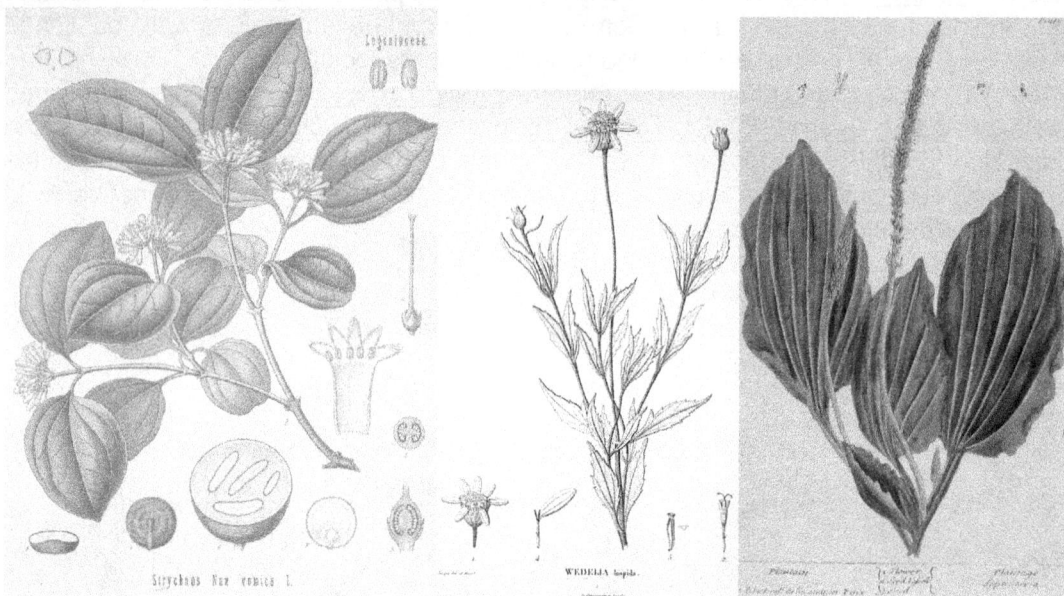

Figure 40. Strychnos nux-vomica
Figure 41. Wedelia hispida
Figure 42. Plantago latifolia

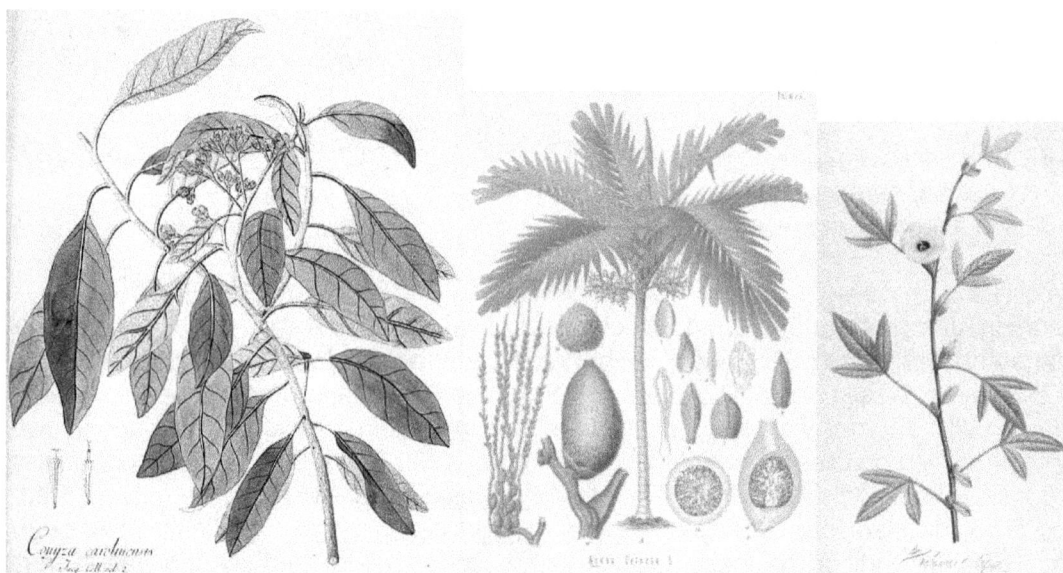

Figure 43. Pluchea carolinensis
Figure 44. Areca catechu
Figure 45. Hibiscus sabdariffa

---

[18] *Topiawari*'s only son *Cayoworaco* (*Iwiakanarie Gualtero*), *Leonard Ragapo* and *Harry* went back to the Mother Country with Ralegh in 1595 and then returned to Guiana to positions of influence (Whitehead, 1997).

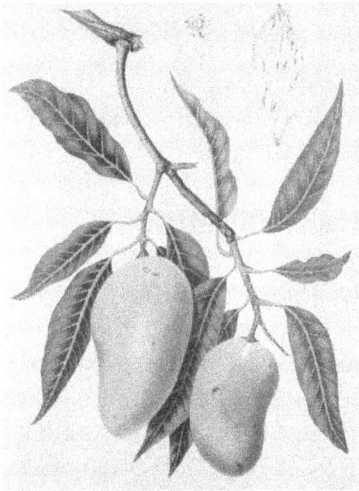

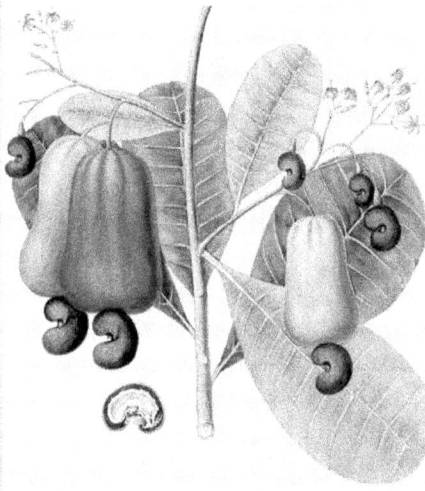

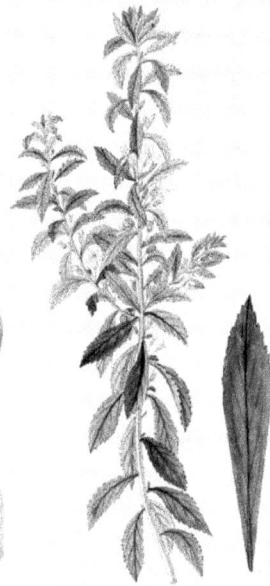

Figure 46. Mangifera indica
Figure 47. Anacardium occidentale
Figure 48. Capraria biflora

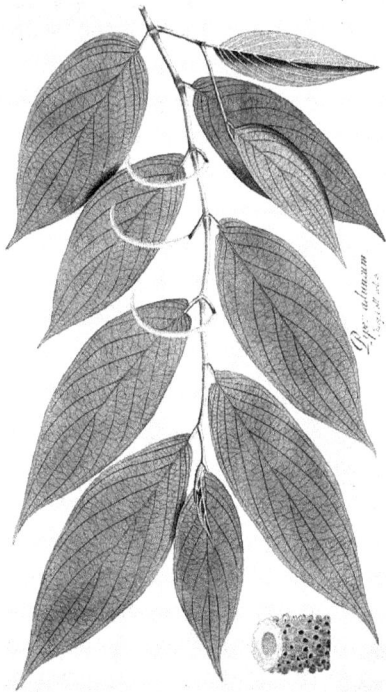

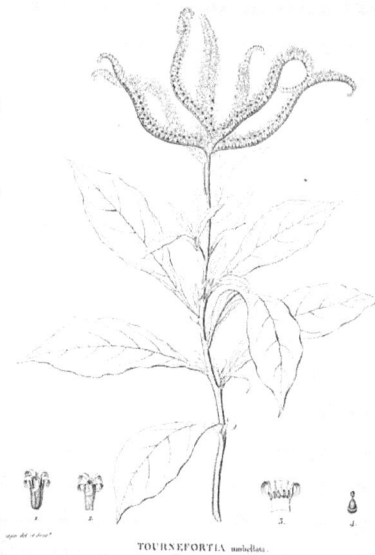

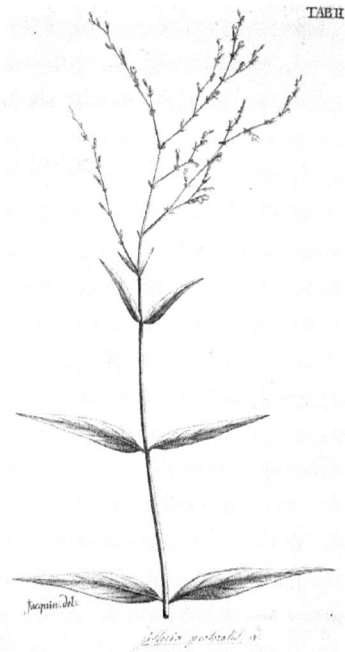

Figure 49. Piper aduncum
Figure 50. Tournefortia umbellata
Figure 51.Justicia pectoralis

Methods: data collection and non-experimental validation

Many things afterward become mere superstition, which were originally knowledge. You cannot warm-up the old superstitions. You must make a fresh start with genuine knowledge. This knowledge, however, must be gained in a spiritual way - not through the mere physical world-of-the-senses (Rudolf Steiner, 1924. Koberwitz Lecture 6)

5. Methods, data collection and non-experimental validation

Method refers to techniques for gathering research material (Maynard, 1994). Praxis research requires non-alienating methodologies that are dialogic and participatory in nature (Warry, 1992). There is considerable intracultural variability, rather than cultural homogeneity in Trinidad and Tobago. Hence there was no attempt to have the data be 'representative' of the nation as a whole, but of its constituent parts. The flexible Creole medical system and its highly individualised nature imply that identical recipes of multiple plant remedies are unlikely to be obtained. In order for pharmacological evaluation to have a sound basis, the ethnomedical information has to be complete (Souza Brito, 1996). Important considerations are who diagnosed the disease (practitioner, patient, researcher) and what were the criteria used for diagnosing the disease reported (Croom, 1983). Cognitive phenomena will include, how farmers and hunters classify livestock diseases and how they conceptualise the interrelationships, functions, and malfunctions of different organs and physiological systems (Mathias and McCorkle, 1997). This information is important since these cognitive processes guide selection of therapeutic (curative), prophylactic (preventive), or other (sale, slaughter) practices in response to disease (Mathias and McCorkle, 1997).

Second phase data collection

The methods include those associated with data collection, and those linked to non-experimental validation. Time and financial constraints limited the number of sites where data could be collected, and the number of respondents within each study site. The research did not need prior approval or official contacts or a department.

The researcher's status was an insider-observer in some respects. The outsider perspective was based on University studies abroad. As an insider the mother of a friend lent her files of newspaper clippings on medicinal plants and her pressed samples of medicinal plants. Insiders are more cognisant and accepting of complexity and internal variation, better able to understand nuances of language use and less likely to be duped or mistrusted (Wolf, 1996). The researcher was an insider /outsider to the veterinarians as a friend/acquaintance who had a cat boarding at the school for two years. Three veterinarians were occasional participants in the research, one collected information from 34 clients. Some of the staff of the Veterinary school became co-authors in publications based on the first phase of the research. Little hand-made gift bags were given to most respondents in the second research phase.

In order to gain access to the study population the researcher worked through previously known individuals and from previously existing social networks in building a snowball sample (Nalven, 1987). Known people helped in the creation of some networks, by suggesting people who could be interviewed. When respondents in the horse racing industry were contacted it was discovered that they already knew about the research from the initial contact. The process was facilitated by community-based contacts and occupationally based contacts obtained from newspapers. Snowball sampling led to community members who were well recognised as knowing more than the average person knows. Snowball sampling was used to generate a purposive sample of respondents who used ethnomedicines (8). Snowball sampling is part of link-tracing methodologies which take advantage of the social networks of identified respondents to provide a researcher with an ever-expanding set of potential contacts. Snowball sampling offers advantages if the aim of a study is primarily explorative, qualitative and descriptive and there is no intention to generalize the results to the wider population. Snowball sampling is used most frequently to conduct qualitative research, primarily through interviews. Secondly, snowball sampling is used as a more formal methodology for making inferences about a population of individuals who have been difficult to enumerate through the use of such methods as household surveys (8, 9, 10).

A purposive sample of ethnoveterinary key respondents was obtained. A purposive sample minimises negative outcomes. This networking approach was necessary because there was no sampling frame of persons involved in traditional healing. Participant observation and in-depth interviewing of key respondents are traditional anthropological approaches.

Interviews

Semi-structured interviews were conducted with 25 new key respondents, six herbalists, personnel associated with sporting animals, veterinarians, and six field staff of the Ministry of Agriculture from September 1996 to 2000. Three particularly knowledgeable respondents were interviewed five times over the four years. The majority of the interviews (95%) took place in Trinidad. In one swamp-based ethnic-Indian community, a female community member was paid to interview fellow community members. Two of five interviewed female herbalists sold herbs in the market and also to individuals. One male herbalist sold bottled herbal products to individuals.

3. Practitioners

The study included interviews with a few of the specialist healers who sell plants in the markets and on some of the main streets in the towns (Mischel, 1959). The largest category of respondents interviewed fell into the category of specialists in home remedies. These are practitioners who do not consider themselves to be healers, but who give remedies to friends and neighbours if they request one (Heinrich *et al.*, 1992). These practitioners know remedies for common or minor illnesses, whereas specialist groups such as midwives and some of the 'older heads' would have specialist knowledge. Some of the practitioners provided information including:

1. their training and background in the medicinal uses of plants, the type of practices they have, and their reputation in the community
2. people treated (e.g. self, family, surrounding community)
3. type of practice: general or specialist
4. diagnostic procedure (dreams, touch)
5. adjunct therapy (e.g. prayer, curing formulas, massage) (Croom, 1983).

10. Botanical identification

This was conducted in collaboration with the Herbarium of the University of the West Indies . The majority of the plants described in this research were authenticated or identified at the University of the West Indies Herbarium. Specimens were not deposited since some of the plants are common. Non-common plants were also not deposited by the Herbarium, due to that institution's policy. Collection of secondary data from the University of the West Indies (UWI) library, and other sources took place from 1996 onwards.

Non-experimental validation

Experts in the field consider that validation is still a weak point in ethnoveterinary medicine. Validation took place throughout the research process. This validation aspect of the research represents the fourth phase or reflecting phase in the research cycle. In knowledge-based action there are four major phrases: planning, acting, observing and reflecting (Masters, 1995).

Traditional validation is very costly. One factor leading to high costs is that multiple plant mixtures are sometimes used. Etkin (1993) advises that multiple plant mixtures need be taken into account in validation work since there are complex chemical interactions among constituents of a single plant and with mixtures of plants. Other considerations are whether some plants mixed together increase the availability of bioactive compounds, or if preparations diminish toxicity, while retaining therapeutic actions. Plant screening against microorganisms does not always evaluate a plant on its actual use (Heinrich *et al.*, 1992). This research has evaluated the ethnoveterinary plants using a non-experimental method (Browner *et al.*, 1988; Heinrich *et al.*, 1992). This method consisted of:

1. obtaining an accurate botanical identification
2. determining the extent to which the folk medicinal data can be understood in terms of bioscientific concepts and methods
3. searching the chemical / pharmaceutical literature for the plant's known chemical constituents
4. searching the pharmacological literature to determine the known physiological effects of either the crude plant, related species, or isolated chemical compounds that the plant is known to contain; and
5. assessing whether the plant use is based on empirically verifiable principles, for instance, if the plant is reputed to cause itching or bleeding, the etic assessment will determine if it contains chemical constituents that are capable of causing itching and bleeding. Or, whether symbolic aspects of healing (or hypnosis, social support, placebo) are of greater relevance (Heinrich *et al.*, 1992; Browner *et al.*, 1988).

The use of these multiple research methods has ensured that the prevalence of local diseases is linked to the identification of plants, and to any future research that seeks to develop plant based drugs. As such there will be no discrepancy between research objectives, future drug development and local needs. The multiple methods also ensured that medicinal plants are separated from religious and culturally – linked plants and that future clinical trials will be undertaken only on the medicinal plants. If ethnobotanical data, phytochemical and pharmacological information supports the folk use of a plant species, it can be grouped into the validation level with the highest degree of confidence. Plants at this level are very likely to be efficacious remedies (Heinrich *et al.*, 1992). Heinrich *et al.* (1992) established four levels of validity:

0.   If no information supports the use it indicates that the plant may be inactive.
1.   A plant (or closely related species of the same genus) which is used in geographically or temporally distinct areas in the treatment of similar illnesses attains the lowest level of validity, if no further phytochemical or pharmacological information validates the popular use. The use in other areas increases the likelihood that the plant is active against the illness.
2.   If in addition to the ethnobotanical data, phytochemical or pharmacological information also validates the use in Trinidad and Tobago, the plant is assigned a higher level of validity. Plants in this category may exert a physiological action on the patient and are more likely to be effective remedies than those at the lowest level of validity.
3.   If ethnobotanical, phytochemical and pharmacological data supports the folk use of the plant, it is grouped in the highest level of validity and are most likely to be effective remedies (Heinrich *et al.*, 1992).

This multi-method approach was necessary because the ordinary pastimes and practices of working people are often un-documented in history books and must be rescued and reconstituted from different sorts of data (Gould, 2000).

58

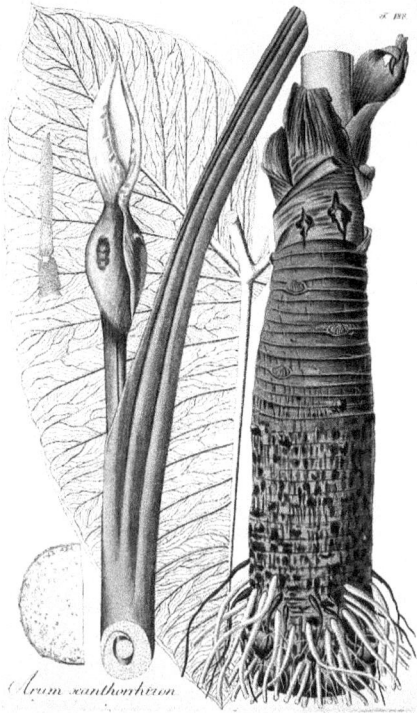

Figure 52. *Xanthosoma sagittifolium*
Figure 53.*Maranta arundinacea*

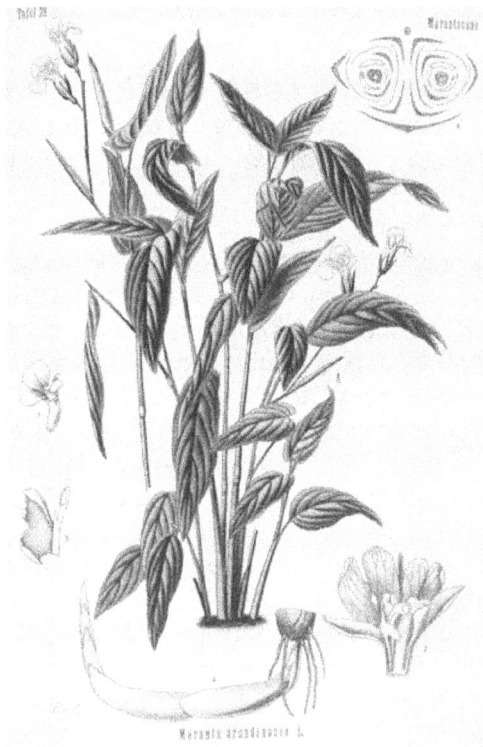

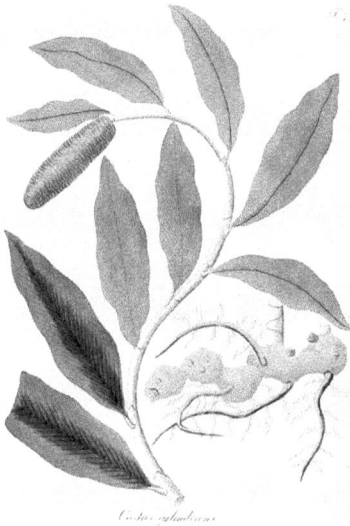

Figure 54. *Costus spicatus*
Figure 55. *Peperomia obtusifolia*
Figure 56. *Paspalum virgatum*

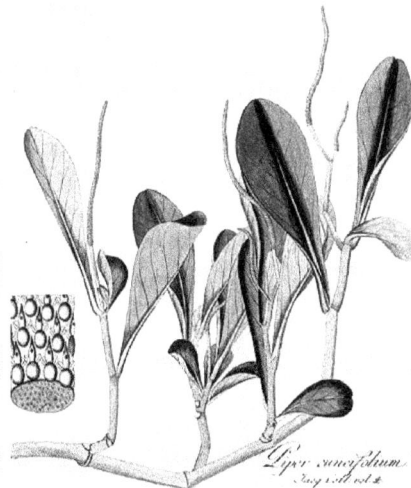

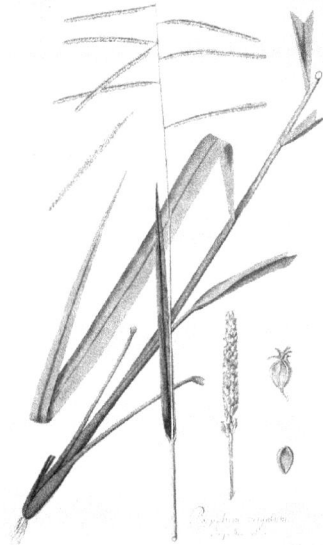

6. Introduction to the Case Studies

6. Introduction to the case studies

The results are divided into the following case studies:

1) Backyard animals   2) Horses   3) Ethnomedicine

Folk Medicinal Terms

The majority of folk medicine involves using the entire plant, or the flowers, leaves and roots of a variety of plants. Sometimes these are combined with drug store components (Inniss, 1910). Some non-plant cures are also called folk medicine. Folk medicine also has what Laguerre (1987) calls symbolic association, i.e. plants with yellow flowers, or yellow stems (*Cuscuta americana*) that are used as cures for jaundice. Folk medicine is based on tisanes, teas, tinctures and poultices. A tisane is a drink made by the addition of boiling water to fresh or dried unfermented plant material. A tisane can also be a mixture of folk medicine and drugstore ingredients. It consists of large amounts of plant parts and is given with sugar or epsom salts, in a specific dose for a specific time (Wong, 1976). A tincture is made by macerating or placing plant parts in alcohol either rum, vermouth or brandy. A decoction is prepared by placing the plant material in cold water and then bringing it to a boil, simmering for a certain period and then allowing the solution to stand for a further period (Sofowora, 1982). Pouring a given quantity of boiling water over a given weight of herbal material and infusing creates a tisane or infusion. This is called 'drawing' in local parlance. The tisane is left to steep covered for 10 – 15 minutes before straining (Wong, 1976). A tea is either a decoction or infusion of plant parts, and is made fresh each time. The separation between decoction and infusion is not clear-cut as was also found by Bonet *et al. (*1992, 1999). Teas are taken for 'cooling'. A loch is a decoction of flowers and a large amount of sugar, a syrup (Wong, 1976). Poultices are the most common means of external treatment. The leaves used are usually heated over a flame, or on a baking utensil, the painful area is rubbed with oil or paraffin (soft candle) and then the heated leaf is applied. Medicinal plants (folk medicine) are grown in house yards, are easily found in adjacent unutilised house plots, or are begged from neighbours. The most common folk medicine can be bought from women selling in the larger markets or on the streets in the cities. Due to increased urbanisation and spraying of weedkillers, some plants are not as common as they used to be.

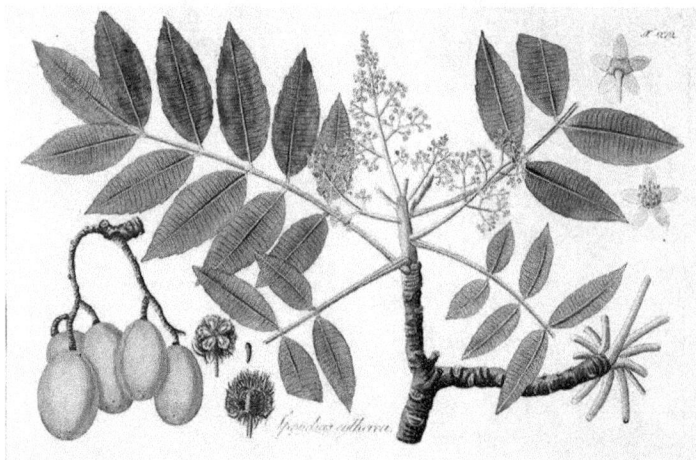

Figure 57.Spondius dulcis
Figure 58. Plantago angustifolia

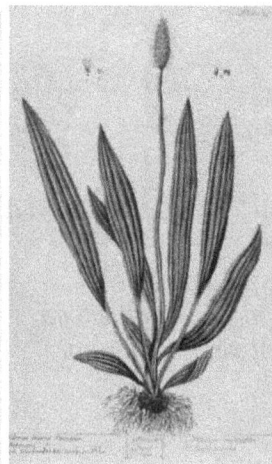

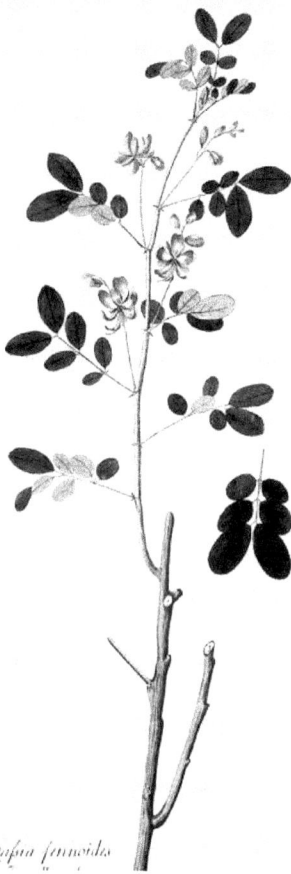

Cassia sennoides

Figure 59. Cassia sennoides
Figure 60. Mammea americana
Figure 61. Carica papaya

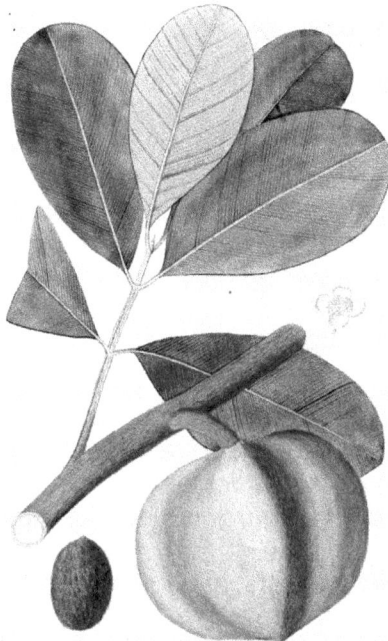

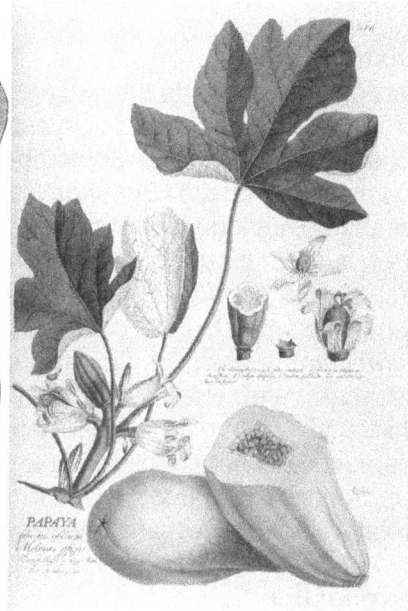

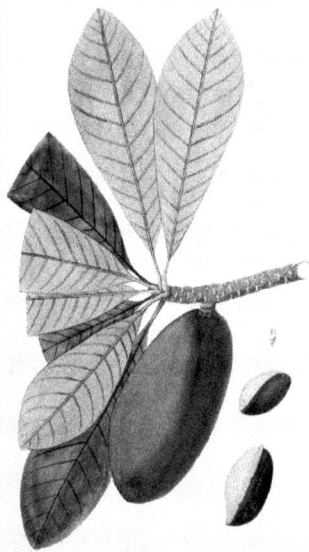

Figure 62. Manilkara zapota
Figure 63. Cissampelos pareira
Figure 64. Renealmia alpinia

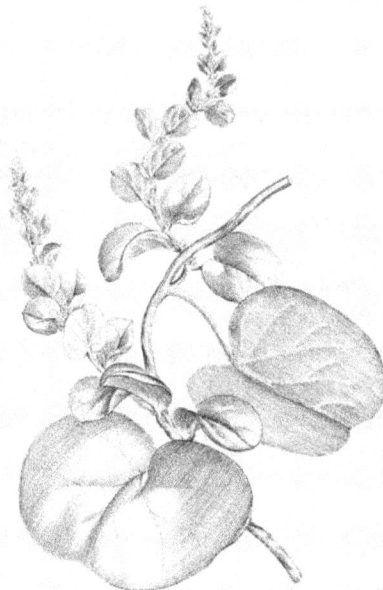

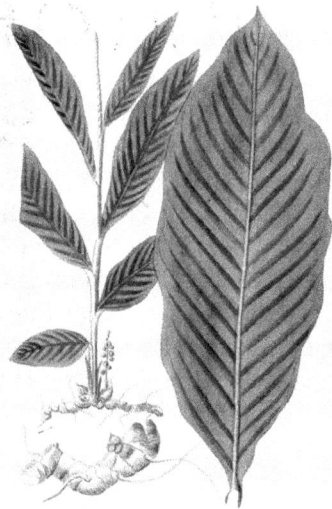

Case study 1: Backyard animals

Precisely among the 'weeds', so called, we often find the strongest curative herbs [they] are greatly influenced by the workings of the Moon (Steiner, 1924)

7. Case study 1: Backyard animals

Abstract
This chapter presents the findings of an exporatory study on ethnoveterinary medicines used for backyard pigs and backyard chickens in Trinidad and Tobago. Research data was collected from 1995 to September 2000. Six plants are used for backyard pigs. Crushed leaves of immortelle (*Erythrina pallida*, *E. micropteryx*) are used to remove dead piglets from the uterus. Leaf decoctions of bois canôt (*Cecropia peltata*) and bamboo (*Bambusa vulgaris*) are used for labour pains or leaves are fed as a post partum cleanser. Boiled green papaya fruit (*Carica papaya*) is fed to pigs to induce milk let down. The leaves and flowers of male papaya plants (*Carica papaya*) are fed to deworm pigs. Juice from sour orange (*Citrus aurantium*) is given to pigs to produce lean meat and coffee grounds are used for scours. Eyebright and planten leaves (*Plantago major*) are used for eye injuries of backyard chickens. Worm grass (*Chenopodium ambrosioides*) and cotton bush (*Gossypium* species) are used as anthelmintics. Aloe gel (*Aloe vera*) is used for internal injuries and the yellow sap from the cut *Aloe vera* leaf or the juice of *Citrus limonia* is used to purge the birds. A literature review revealed few toxicity concerns and the potential usefulness of the plants

Introduction

In 1997, the number of pig farms was estimated at 262, a reduction from 527 in the 1980s (CSO, 1997). 15,695 pigs worth TT$ 11,017,070 were sold from July to September 2002 (CSO, 2002). In 1995, the Agricultural Development Bank (ADB) and a national commercial bank sold 2500 non-performing agricultural loans (worth more than TT$300 million) to a newly created State enterprise. These loans were sold for 35 cents on every dollar of debt; and the 2,308 pig and poultry farmers concerned were not told beforehand (Trinidad Express Newspaper February 28, 1998). Concurrently the major meat processors were not providing any concessions. Small-scale Tobago pig farmers had already been put out of business in the 1990s. In the 1970s and 1980s, pig farmers in Tobago sold their animals to a state-owned marketing agency. This agency suffered financial constraints during the IMF-structural adjustment of the late 1980s and could not pay farmers for the meat supplied. Equipment failures at the agency led to the meat being discarded forcing farmers to engage in other economic activities. Outbreaks of *Brucella abortus* infection and rabies in Trinidad in 1997, in combination with the political climate in agriculture created a negative climate to conduct on-farm research. A decision was therefore made to focus on backyard pigs and to use snowball sampling to find the owners of these pigs.

Results

Eight plants and or products were used for medicinal purposes by backyard chicken owners. One of these plants (gru gru boeuf) was tentatively identified from the literature but eyebright has not yet been identified. Six plants were used for backyard pigs. The plants used for backyard pigs and backyard chickens in Trinidad and Tobago are presented alphabetically by botanical name in Table 3. The plant uses are grouped into categories below.

Table 3. Medicinal plants used for backyard pigs and backyard chickens in Trinidad and Tobago

Common name	Scientific name	Family	Plant part used	Use	No. of users
Aloes	*Aloe vera*	Liliaceae	Gel	Internal injuries in backyard chickens. 'Thinning the blood'	4 1
Aloes	*Aloe vera*	Liliaceae	Sap from cut leaf	Purgative agent for backyard chickens	4
Bamboo	*Bambusa vulgaris*	Poaceae	Leaf	Decoction to ease labour pains or fed for post partum cleansing	3
Papaya	*Carica papaya*	Caricaceae	Green fruit	Decoction to induce milk let down in pigs	2
Papaya	*Carica papaya*	Caricaceae	Leaves, flowers	Fed to deworm pigs	2
Bois canôt	*Cecropia peltata*	Cecropiaceae	Leaf	Decoction to ease labour pains in pigs or fed as a post partum cleanser	3
Worm grass	*Chenopodium ambrosioides*	Chenopodiaceae	Plant tops	Anthelmintic for backyard chickens	7
Sour orange	*Citrus aurantium*	Rutaceae	Juice, pulp	Juice included in pig diet before slaughter to reduce fat. Toughen and clean cocks skin	4
Lemon	*Citrus limonia*	Rutaceae	Juice, pulp	Used for upper respiratory problems and as a purgative in backyard chickens	6
Coffee	*C. arabica, C. robusta*	Rutaceae	Grounds	Given to scouring pigs in drinking water	3
Immortelle	*Erythrina pallida, E. micropteryx*	Fabaceae	Leaf	Crushed leaves added to drinking water to remove dead piglets from uterus	2
Cotton bush	*Gossypium sp.*	Malvaceae	Leaves	Anthelmintic for backyard chickens	3
Eyebright	Not yet identified	-	Leaves	Ocular injuries in backyard chickens	1
Planten	*Plantago major*	Plantaginaceae	Leaf juice	Ocular injuries in backyard chickens	2
Gru gru boeuf*	*Acrocomia aculeata** *A. ierensis**	Arecaceae	Kernel oil	Cheating by making skin greasy	No longer used

* Tentative identification

Respiratory problems
All the respondents used a combination of honey and sour orange or lemon (*Citrus* species) to treat upper respiratory problems in backyard chickens.

Deworming
Worm grass (*Chenopodium ambrosioides*) is used by all the respondents in the wet season, but in the dry season anthelmintics (developed for humans and dogs) were used for convenience. Most respondents gave the birds an undiluted infusion of *Chenopodium*

ambrosioides to drink and claimed to have no fixed dose. One respondent combined the Worm grass with Epsom salts and soft candle (whale oil). The ingredients were mixed and made into a little ball and pushed down the throat of the bird. The worm grass infusion or anthelmintic was given when the respondents saw worms in the faeces or brown-coloured stool. Three respondents gave a decoction of *Gossypium* species to backyard chickens as the drinking water. Caution about dosage (six plant-tops with young leaves for ten birds) was expressed. One person said that overdosing with *Gossypium* species is dangerous. The yellow sap under the green epidermis of the *Aloe vera* leaf is used to purge birds after deworming by four respondents. Two respondents remove the green skin from the *Aloe vera* leaf, two just cut off the end to collect the sap. All respondents purged birds with salt (sodium chloride), lemon juice or raw egg whites. Additionally one owner with a large flock of 300 birds gives aloes (*Aloe vera*) in the drinking water to the birds if they are likely to incur injuries from other birds. This is done five days before a likely injury to "thin down the blood." Two respondents fed the leaves and flowers of male papaya plants (*Carica papaya*) to deworm pigs.

Reproduction

Three respondents used leaf decoctions of bois canôt (*Cecropia peltata*) and bamboo (*Bambusa vulgaris*) for labour pains in pigs or leaves were fed as a post partum cleanser. The boiled green papaya fruit (*Carica papaya*) is fed to pigs to induce milk let down by two respondents. Two respondents used crushed leaves of immortelle (*Erythrina pallida, E. micropteryx*) in the drinking water to remove dead piglets from the uterus.

Husbandry

Four respondents gave sour orange juice (*Citrus aurantium*) to pigs to reduce the fat content of the meat. Three respondents give coffee grounds (*Coffee arabica, Coffee robusta*) to scouring pigs.

Discussion

All of the plants used for backyard pigs and backyard chickens are commonly known except for eyebright, which has not yet been identified. Eyebright and planten were reported as ocular medicines in a previous publication[19], but the eyebright plant was not seen and therefore not botanically identified. Worm grass and cotton bush are also used as anthelmintics for dogs (Lans *et al.*, 2000). Papaya seeds rather than leaves and flowers are also used as anthelmintics for dogs (Lans *et al.*, 2000). Some veterinarians interviewed in 1995 claimed that clients who used *Gossypium* species for their dogs sometimes lost puppies but that these puppies may have already been weak (Lans *et al.*, 2000). *Chenopodium* was so well known that respondents did not consider it 'new' information of interest to a researcher and had to be specifically asked if they used the plant.

In comparison with the information collected for dogs, commercial poultry and ruminants, very little information was collected on ethnoveterinary medicines used for pigs (Lans and Brown, 1998; Lans et al., 2000). Respondents raising backyard pigs claimed that these pigs did not become ill and that there were few diseases that affected pigs. One veterinarian said "it did not matter if the pigs became ill because they [the respondents] ate them anyway."

Dosages

Folk medicine in the Caribbean has had an extra-legal status (prescribing is not legal but also not prosecuted) that may account for the reluctance to provide details and specifics on dosages. It may be that drugs are given 'to effect', to achieve clinical improvement rather than complete elimination of the causative agent (Ibrahim, 1996).

An infusion of the fresh juice of *Aloe barbadensis* is used for urinary and bladder conditions and for cleaning the blood in Mexico (Nicholson and Arzeni, 1993). *Aloe vera* is used for supportive therapy and prophylaxis in commercial poultry production in Trinidad and Tobago and is used for internal injuries and as a purgative for ruminants (Brown and Lans, 1998; Lans and Brown, 1998).

Fresh *Aloe vera* leaves are used to obtain two components: (1) a bitter yellow juice (exudate) with high content of 1,8 dihydroxyanthraquinone derivatives (aloe emodin, chrysophanol) and their glycosides (aloins), which are used for their cathartic effects and, (2) a mucilaginous gel from the parenchymatous tissue, which has been used for topical treatment of skin burns and wounds (Vázquez *et al.*, 1996). *Aloe vera* has a significant influence on the proteoglycans and glycosaminoglycans in healing wounds and this healing may be related to mannose-6-phosphate and acemannan (Chithra *et al.,* 1998). Cinnamoyl-C-glucosylchromone in *Aloe barbadensis* contributes to its topical antiinflammatory activity (Hutter *et al.,* 1996).

Cecropia peltata) and *Bambusa vulgaris* are used as ethnoveterinary remedies for retained placenta in other species and the similar ethnoveterinary use for pigs may reflect this (Lans and Brown 1998). Consequently a short discussion of dietary factors related to retained placenta follows and the crude protein content of the leaves is provided for *Cecropia peltata*, *Bambusa* species and *Erythrina* species.

Dietary deficiencies result in increased oxidative stress and production of lipid peroxides (Michal *et al.,* 1994; Brzezinska-Siebodzinska *et al.,* 1994; Laven and Peters, 1996). Dietary polyunsaturated fatty acids and their role in the synthesis of prostaglandin and provision of energy before parturition may be related to retained placenta (Chassagne and Barnouin, 1992). Various studies indicate that retained placenta could be due to a prostaglandin ($PgF_{2\alpha}$) or an energy deficiency at parturition (Chassagne and Barnouin, 1992), or reduced blood glucose levels (Choudhury *et al.,* 1993) or the alteration of the arachidonic acid pathway (Kankofer *et al.,* 1996a&b; Kankofer and Maj, 1997).

Bamboo leaves are fed for retained placenta in ruminants in Trinbago (Lans and Brown, 1998). *Bambusa* species leaf decoctions are used as emmenagogues, to induce the lochia flow after childbirth and as abortifacients in India (Kapoor, 1990). *Bambusa* species were one component of two multi-plant herbal preparations evaluated for their effects on fertility in rats and buffaloes (Bhaskaran and Kshama, 1999; Deshpande *et al.,* 1999). *Bambusa* species fresh leaf juice had a weak ecbolic action on isolated human and rat uteri. Uterine stimulation was due to its action on cholinergic receptors (Kapoor, 1990). *Bambusa* species contains choline, betaine, proteolytic enzymes, diastatic and emulsyfying enzymes, and a cyanogentic glucoside (Kapoor, 1990). The crude protein content in bamboo species leaves ranged from 9 - 19% and the crude fibre content from 18 - 34% (Singh, 1999).

The leaves of *Bambusa arundinacea* are used as emmenogogues, for inflammations, for wound and for diarrhea in cattle (Muniappan and Sundararaj, 2003). The methanol extract of leaves showed the presence of flavonoids, glycosides, traces of alkaloids and phytosterols. The extract showed the absence of proteins, amino acids, tannins, fixed oils, volatile oils and steroids. A dose of 200 mg/kg (i.p.) of the methanol extract produced a significant antiinflammatory effect. The doses of 50, 100 and 200 mg/kg of the methanol extract showed ulcer score '0', which was highly significant when compared to the control animals

(Muniappan and Sundararaj, 2003). Histopathological studies were performed to confirm the ulcer score. There was no inflammation and ulceration. The gastric mucosa was normal which was comparable to the standard (Ranitidine). Further, the methanol extract of *Bambusa arundinacea* showed antihypersensitivity activity, immunosuppressive activity, wound healing property and antibacterial activity experimentally. The LD_{50} of the methanol extract was 1812.5 mg/kg (i.p.) and 2552.2 mg/kg (p.o.) (Muniappan and Sundararaj, 2003).

Carica papaya latex extract increased rat uterine contractile activity in proestrus and estrus stages of the oestrous cycle compared to metestrus and diestrus stages (Cherian, 2000). The crude papaya latex contained an uterotonic principle, which was suggested to be a combination of enzymes, alkaloids and other substances, which can evoke sustained contraction of the uterus by acting mainly on the α-adrenergic receptor population of the uterus at different stages (Cherian, 2000). The compounds responsible for the uterotonic activity may also be responsible for the induction of milk letdown by also stimulating contraction of the smooth muscle around the mammary alveoli. The fruit juice of ripe and unripened fruit of *Carica papaya* may contain antihypertensive agent(s) and showed significant antibacterial activity (Emeruwa, 1982; Eno *et al.*, 2000). The antibacterial and other properties of the plant may control the genital tract infections that may lead to retained placenta (Laven and Peters, 1996).

Carica papaya leaves contain papain, chymopapain and lysozyme proteolytic enzymes that may have anthelmintic effects (Oliver-Bever, 1986; Satrija *et al.*, 1995). Latex collected from young papaya fruits and sap demonstrated anthelmintic activity against *Ascaridia galli* and *Heterakis gallinae* infections in chickens; against *Heligmosomoides polygyrus* infections in mice; in sheep artificially infected with *Haemonchus contortus* (0.75 g /kg bodyweight); and against natural infection of *Ascaris suum* in pigs (Satrija *et al.*, 1994; Satrija *et al.*, 1995; Murdiati *et al.*, 1997; Singh and Nagaich, 1999). The anthelmintic principle of *Carica papaya* is said to be benzylisothiocyanate (Kumar *et al.*, 1991).

In Latin America *Cecropia peltata*) is used for diarrhoea, 'bad belly', as an emmenagogue and to 'wash out the babies' (Barrett, 1994; Duke, 2000). Artificially dried leaves of *Cecropia peltata* contain more than 14% (DM) protein (Madamba *et al.*, 1972). Free fatty acids including stearic, arachidic, behenic, lignoceric and cerotic acids were isolated from *Cecropia* species (Lachman-White *et al.*, 1992). *Cecropia pachystachya* Mart. is popularly called "ambay" and extensively used in herbal medicine of South America for cough and asthma. *Cecropia pachystachya* has cardiotonic and sedative properties (Consolini et al., 2006).

The fresh aerial parts of *Chenopodium ambrosioides* contain an essential oil that has ascaridol as its main component (Oliver-Bever, 1986). Ascaridol is a known anthelmintic however aqueous extracts of *Chenopodium ambrosioides* did not have any effect against an experimental infection of *Ascaridia galli* in chickens (Berchieri *et al.*, 1984).

Citrus species are used as supportive therapy for many disease conditions and for heat stress in commercial poultry in Trinidad and Tobago (Brown and Lans, 1998). Aqueous decoctions of *Citrus* species have shown antimycotic, antihemorrhagic and antibacterial activity (Robineau, 1991). The vitamin A and C content of *Citrus* species may also be useful. Vitamins A and C are antioxidants. Vitamin A is important for the health of epithelial, respiratory and ocular tissues. Vitamin C also helps poultry combat stressful conditions (Latshaw, 1991). Lemon was first taken to Europe in the 12th century and then to the West Indies in the 15th century by Columbus (Heinrich et al., 2005).

Four percent *Citrus* pectin added to the diet of forty pigs (divided into two groups of treatment and control) during the finishing period (71 to 103 kg live weight) produced a highly significant (p less than 0.01) increase of 125 g (15%) in their daily weight gain without affecting feed conversion (Lagreca and Marotta, 1985). The average thickness of back fat in pigs subjected to the pectin treatment was 2 mm (8%) less than in those of the control group. The juice of *Citrus aurantium* as administered by Trinidad's pig keepers contains fruit pulp that would be a source of pectin.

Coffee arabica is used in Nicaragua for stomach pain (Barrett, 1994). Spent coffee grounds contain tannins, crude protein, crude fibre, nitrogen-free extracts and fat (Campbell *et al.*, 1976; Wong and Wang, 1991; Rao Udayasekhara, 1996). Tannins and fibre would contribute to the anti-diarrhoeal effect (Duke, 2000). The need for treatment against scours is supported by the literature. Adesiyun and Cazabon (1996) found evidence of *Coxiella burnetii* and *Toxoplasma gondii* infection in 11.3% and 5.5% respectively of tested pig sera. *Listeria monoctytogenes* serotype 4, *Campylobacter* species and 19 *Salmonella* serotypes were isolated from pork carcasses at abattoirs in Trinidad (Cazabon *et al.,* 1978; Adesiyun and Krishnan, 1995). The prevalence of *Cryptosporidium* oocysts was 19.6% in piglets and 91.1% of faecal samples of piglets (2 to 8 weeks old) were positive for rotavirus antigen (Kaminjolo *et al.*, 1993; Kaminjolo and Adesiyun, 1994).

A bark decoction of *Erythrina* species is used in India and by the Tacanas in Bolivia, the Cabecar and Guaymi in Central America and in Peru for wounds, haemorrhage, dysmenorrhea, uterine haemorrhage and as a purgative (Hazlett, 1986; Kapoor, 1990; Jovel *et al.*, 1996; Bourdy *et al.,*, 2000). Similar uses are reported for Argentina, Ghana and Guinea (Oliver-Bever, 1986; Filipov, 1994). Leaves, stems and roots contain hydrocyanic acid. The bark contains isoflavones, resins, fatty acids, choline and the abortifacient compounds betaine and genistein (Duke, 2000; Dong-lei *et al.*, 2000). Leaves contain several alkaloids, a lectin and agglutinins (Cambie, 1997). *Erythrina* species plant parts showed sedative, analgesic and anti-inflammatory activity (Ratnasooriya and Dharmasiri, 1999; Saidu *et al.*, 2000). *Erythrina* species leaves are relatively high in protein content (at 19% DM) (Kunz Thomas and Diaz Carlos, 1995). *Erythrina velutina* and *Erythrina mulungu* are popularly used in Brazil for their effects on the central nervous system. Hydroalcoholic extracts of the stem bark of *Erythrina velutina* and *Erythrina mulungu* were shown to have depressant effects on the central nervous system, which partially corroborates the use of these species as tranquilizers in Brazilian popular medicine (Vasconcelos et al., 2004).

Gossypium species plant leaves and stems contain several insecticidal and pesticidal compounds such as α-phellandrene, α-pinene, camphene, chlorine, cyanidin, delphinidin, myrcene, catechin, rutin, quercetin, *p*-coumaric acid, palmitic acid and tannin (Duke, 2000). Although these compounds have insecticidal activity, Duke (2000) does not list them as vermifuges. The seeds and essential oil also contain compounds with insecticidal activity such as gossypol, ergosterol, farnesene, cadinene, betaine, linoleic acid and myristic acid (Duke, 2000). Morison (1963) claims that Columbus found *Gossypium microcarpum* and *G. punctatum* in 1492 but that *G. barbadense* was not present then.

Plantago major fresh leaf juice or bath is used for opthalmic reasons in Venezuela, France, Madeira and Mauritius (Morton, 1975; Novaretti and Lemordant, 1990; Rivera and Obón, 1995; Gurib-Fakim *et al.*, 1996; Jelager *et al.*, 1998). *Plantago major* plant extracts have several activities such as anti-inflammatory, analgesic, antioxidant, weak antibiotic, immunomodulating and expectorant (Matev *et al.*, 1982; Karpilovskaia *et al.*, 1989; Samuelsen, 2000). *Plantago major* was found to be active against *Salmonella typhi*, *Shigella dysenteriae*, *Shigella flexneri* and *Staphylococcus aureus* (Cáceres *et al.*, 1990; Navarro *et al.*, 1996). The fresh leaves of old plants of *Plantago major* that had gone to seed and were collected in early spring in Southern Ohio / Northern Kentucky contained 6 mg beta-carotene/100g and 19 mg /100g ascorbic acid (Samuelsen, 2000). Samuelsen (2000) reviewed the compounds in *Plantago major* that aid in wound healing. Plantamajoside and acteoside have antibacterial activities. Compounds with antioxidant and free radical scavenging activities are flavonoids and caffeic acid derivatives (plantamajoside and aceteoside). Pectic polysaccharides are immunostimulants. The long-chained saturated primary alcohols, present in the leaf wax, aid the healing of superficial wounds. Compounds with anti-inflammatory activity in *Plantago major* are baicalein, hispidulin, aucubin, oleanolic acid and ursolic acid (Ringbom *et al.*, 1998; Samuelsen, 2000).

This review of the ethnomedicinal literature indicates that ethnobotanical, phytochemical and/or pharmacological information provides some support of the ethnoveterinary use of the majority of the plants discussed in this chapter and they could be assigned to level 2 validity.

Conclusion

The following plants and uses are new to the published ethnoveterinary literature for Trinidad and Tobago: the use of immortelle (*Erythrina pallida, E. micropteryx*) and bois canôt (*Cecropia peltata*) for reproductive problems in pigs; boiled green papaya (*Carica papaya*) fruit fed to pigs to induce milk let down; sour orange juice (*Citrus aurantium*) used to reduce the fat content of pork; coffee grounds (*Coffee arabica, Coffee robusta*) for scouring; eyebright (not yet identified) and planten (*Plantago major*) leaves used for eye injuries in poultry.

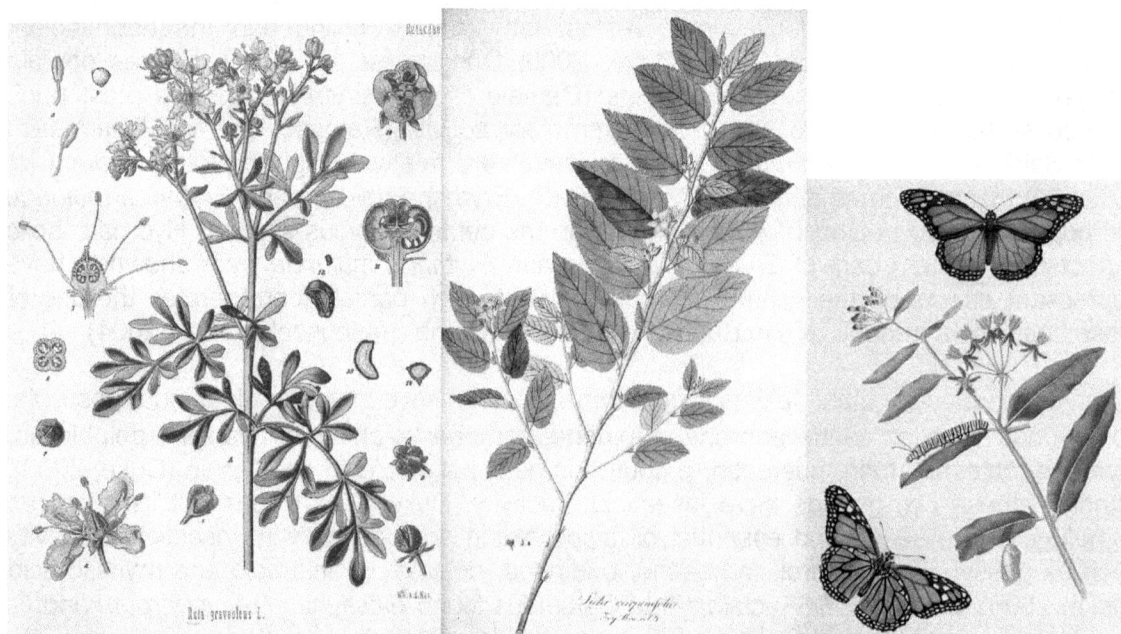

Figure 65. *Ruta graveolens*
Figure 66. *Sida carpinifolia*
Figure 67. *Asclepias curassavica /Papilio archippus*

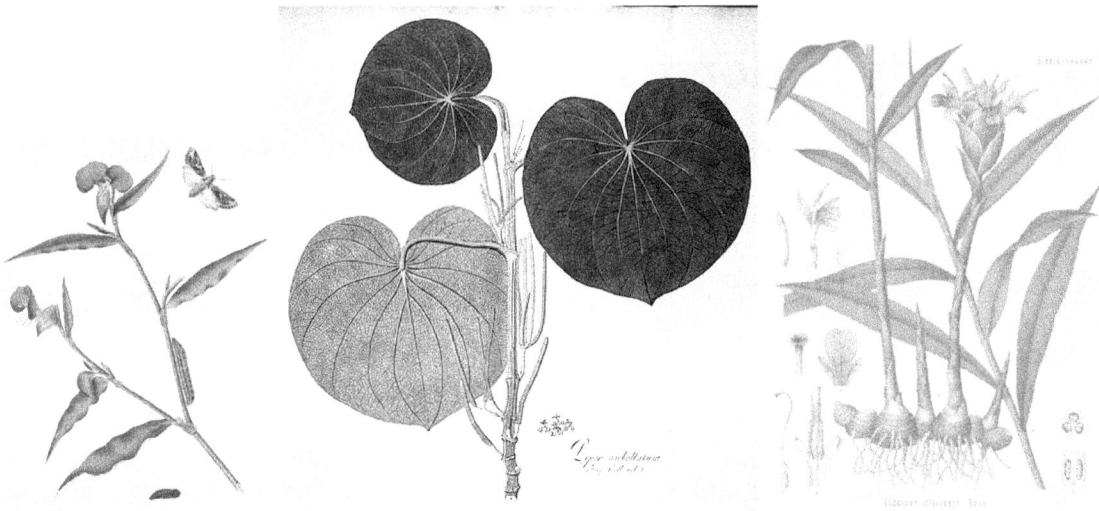

Figure 68. Commelina communis
Figure 69. Lepianthes peltata
Figure 70. Zingiber officinale

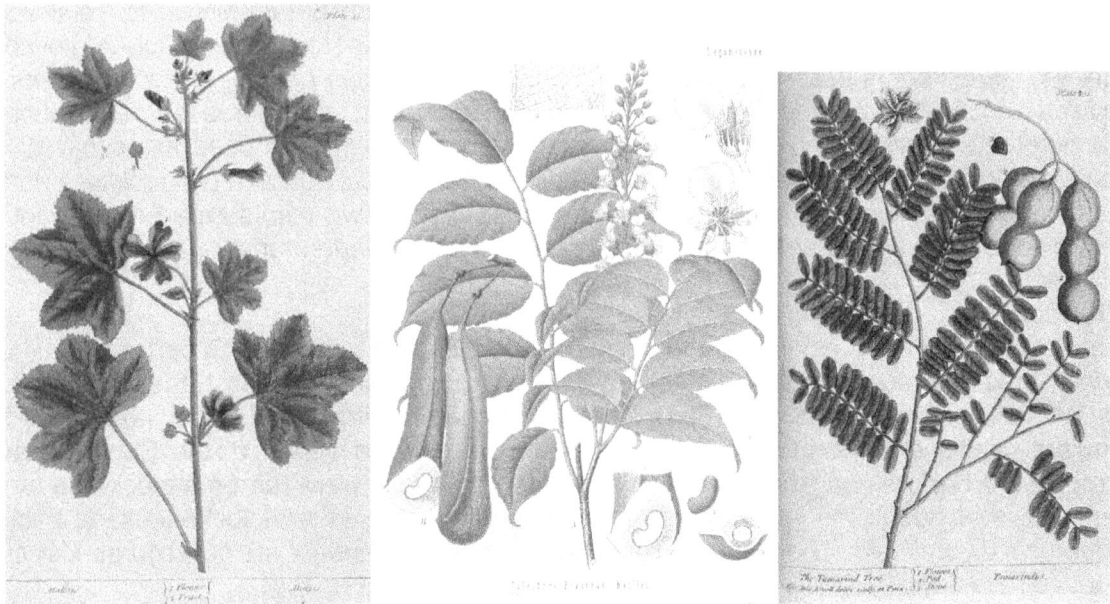

Figure 71. Malva vulgaris
Figure 72. Myrospermum pereirae
Figure 73. Tamarindus indica

Case study 2: Horses

The intellectual contribution of indigenous peoples is quietly regarded as suffering from the three "Q"s: quaint (with no currency or modern utility); quackery (it never worked or is probably carcinogenic); or quits (well on its way to extinction) (RAFI, 1995)

8. Case Study 2: Horses[20]

Abstract
Plants used as ethnoveterinary remedies for horses in Trinidad are also used in Caribbean folk medicine. Interviews with racehorse owners, trainers, breeders, jockeys and grooms determined that seventeen medicinal plants are used in equine ethnoveterinary medicine in Trinidad. *Psidium guajava* and *Musa* species are used for diarrhoea. *Aloe vera*, *Nopalea cochenillifera*, and *Ricinus communis* are used for tendon problems. *Panicum maximum* and *Cordia curassavica* are utilised for grooming. *Ricinus communis* and *Kalanchoe pinnata* are employed as poultices for hoof abscesses and sore joints. *Curcuma longa* is used for swellings.
Chenopodium ambrosioides is used as an anthelmintic. *Mucuna pruriens* is utilised as an irritant to enhance performance. *Curcuma longa* and *Aloe vera* are employed for retained placenta. *Momordica charantia* is used as a tonic, for skin rashes and for improved digestion. *Aloe vera* is used for digestive problems and *Cecropia peltata*, to treat bleeders. *Nopalea cochenillifera* and *Pimenta racemosa* are used to increase perspiration (diaphoretics/sudorifics) and hence cool horses. *Cecropia peltata* is used for respiratory problems. *Nasturtium officinale* is used to increase blood counts. *Pueraria phaseoloides* and *Stachytarpheta jamaicensis* are used as high protein feeds. Two plants called speedweed (*Oxalis corniculata* and *Desmodium* sp.) are used to enhance performance.

Introduction
Horse racing has been established in Trinidad since 1828 (Cozier and Robertson, 1994). Locally bred Thoroughbreds (Creoles) have been racing since at least the early 19th Century (Cozier and Robertson, 1994). The only utilised racetrack in Trinidad was moved from the capital city (Port of Spain), east to the refurbished venue at the Santa Rosa Complex (73 hectares) in Arima in 1993. Previously, all races were run on a clockwise turf track. However due to the influence of American-style racing, an anti-clockwise sand track surface circuit was laid. The Santa Rosa Complex hosts an annual racing Fixtures List of about 40 race days.

Results
The ethnoveterinary plants used for horses in Trinidad are summarised in Table 4. Nineteen plants are used. Dosages were often vague and terms like "some" or "enough" were used.

---

[20] Dr Karla Georges of the University of the West Indies, School of Veterinary Medicine contributed to this case study.

Table 4. Ethnoveterinary medicines used for horses in Trinidad

Scientific name	Family	Common Name	Plant part used	Use
Psidium guajava	Myrtaceae	Guava	Leaf, bud	Diarrhoea
Musa species	Musaceae	Banana	Fruit	Diarrhoea
Aloe vera	Liliaceae	Aloes	Leaf gel	Tendon problems
Nopalea cochenillifera	Cactaceae	Rachette	Joint	Tendon problems
Ricinus communis	Euphorbiaceae	Castor oil leaf	Leaf	Tendon problems
*Panicum maximum**	Poaceae	Wiz/ Guinea grass	Leaf	Grooming
Cordia curassavica	Boraginaceae	Black sage	Leafy branch	Grooming
Ricinus communis	Euphorbiaceae	Castor oil leaf	Leaf	Hoof problems, poultice
Kalanchoe pinnata	Crassulaceae	Wonder of the world	Leaf	Hoof problems, poultice
Curcuma longa	Zingiberaceae	Saffron	Rhizome	Swellings
C. ambrosioides	Chenopodiaceae	Worm grass	Leaf	Anthelmintic
Mucuna pruriens	Fabaceae	Cow itch	Leafy branch	Enhance performance
Nopalea cochenillifera	Cactaceae	Rachette	Joint	Inflammation
Curcuma longa	Zingiberaceae	Turmeric	Rhizome	Retained placenta
Aloe vera	Liliaceae	Aloes	Leaf gel	Retained placenta
Momordica charantia	Cucurbitaceae	Caraaili	Vine	Tonic, blood purifier
Aloe vera	Liliaceae	Aloes	Leaf gel	Digestive problems
Aloe vera	Liliaceae	Aloes	Leaf gel	Remove blood clots
Nopalea cochenillifera	Cactaceae	Rachette	Joint	Increase perspiration (Diaphoretic)
Pimenta racemosa	Myrtaceae	Bay leaves	Leaf	Diaphoretic
Cecropia peltata	Cecropiaceae	Bois canot	Leaf	Kidney problems
Nasturtium officinale	Brassicaceae	Water cress	Leaf	Increase blood count
Pueraria phaseoloides	Fabaceae	Kudzu	Leaf	High protein feed
Stachytarpheta jamaicensis	Verbenaceae	Vervine	Leaf	High protein feed
Aloe vera	Liliaceae	Aloes	Leaf gel	Blood in lungs

* Respondent identification was not confirmed.

Plants used for diarrhoea

Guava leaves, young fruits and/or buds (*Psidium guajava*) were boiled and mixed with mash or bran or a combination of both and given to the horse to eat by three respondents after orthodox treatments had been tried. One respondent used young green fruit of the banana (*Musa* sp.) including skins. This treatment was used once by each respondent for one horse. The banana fruit was boiled, crushed and mixed with the mash and this was given to the

71

horse to eat. Another respondent used eight kilos of carrots. One respondent reported a one-time use of stale cow dung, which was pushed down the horse's throat in order to obtain beneficial bacteria. Another respondent confirmed that horse or cow dung was used for diarrhea.

Plants used for tendonitis

Medicinal plants for tendonitis are preferred by those who believe that horses don't have much circulation from the knee down; therefore ice is of no value for swelling. One respondent claimed that treatment was based on the stage of injury. He believed that the herbal remedies were more effective in the first stages of injury and stressed that rest was the most important factor for the recovery process.

Tendon and ligament problems were described as the second biggest problem after respiratory problems. Horses with sprained tendons or ligaments have joints of rachette (*Nopalea cochenillifera*) applied directly to the injured area. The mucilage obtained from inside the rachette joints may be mixed with flour and or Epsom salts. Two respondents practice tendon splitting, or splitting of the affected suspensory ligament and the flexor tendon into the normal tissue above and below the lesion. Respondents do this to increase circulation to the affected area and thus enhance the healing process. Castor oil leaf (*Ricinus communis*) is quickly passed over a flame, and wrapped around the clay already placed on the injured tendon, which is then left to heal. Joints of rachette (*Nopalea cochenillifera*) can be split open and also be mixed with aloes (*Aloe vera*) or clay, and packed on to the tendon. This poultice is supposed to help with the healing process and to keep "heat" from the damaged tissue or injured joint out of the tendon. Alternatively, leaves of wonder of world (*Kalanchoe pinnata*) are used to remove the "heat" from the injured leg. Wonder of world is claimed to have antiinflammatory properties. The rest of the treatment consists of rest and some trainers use an ice pack. Enough ice is used to cover the leg.

Three interviewees blister flexor tendons or suspensory ligaments to help the healing process. The method consists of rubbing the tendon with iodine or mercuric iodine on a toothbrush. The tendon is rubbed for three days, left for three days, and then another cycle is started. After the raw scab comes off, aloes (*Aloe vera*) is applied to help the tissues and skin heal. Blistering agents' remove the hairs from the injured part, there is localised swelling, the skin sloughs off and subcutaneous necrosis can also occur. Blistering necessitates rest since a long healing period is required. Horses are not blistered above the knee. The iodine is said to act as a counter irritant, which brings blood to damaged part, and the increased circulation enhances the healing process.

Bucked shins are also blistered. Bucked shins were described as an injury in the forelimb of young horses after exercise. There is periostitis of the plantar surface of the third metacarpal (or metatarsal) bone. Horses with tendon injuries are also taken to the sea for exercise to take the weight off the legs. Alternatively the injured leg is placed in brine from salted pigtails; both practices are said to harden the tendon. This remedy is thought to be over 30 years old. Aloes (*Aloe vera*) is also used for soreness in horses' joints, the gel is made into a paste, applied and then the joint is bandaged. Poultices are made with river clay or white clay. Some buy the clay already prepared while others do their own preparation. Other poultices are made with a combination of clay, washing soap (hard bar) and glycerine and Epsom salts. The clay keeps the horses legs cool. Poultices are sometimes made with a combination of aloes, rachette, glycerine and Epsom salts, and are said to have a "drawing" effect.

Young castor oil leaves (*Ricinus communis*) or two to three young almond leaves (*Terminalia catappa*, identified from the literature) are warmed and the veins are crushed. These leaves are put on minor injuries and bandaged. It is said that oil runs out of *Ricinus communis* leaves and cools the "heat" or swelling in the leg. Horses with bad tendon injuries are treated with rachette and aloes. This particular treatment is called "sweating it down." The plants are grated and packed on the leg. In terms of dosages all respondents used sufficient plant material to cover the area being treated. The leg is then wrapped with a football sock that has had the toe cut off. The sock is then tied at the bottom. The plants are thus packed inside the sock. The sock is then wrapped with a bandage to keep it in place. An alternative treatment is to put aloes on first, then wrap a heated bois canôt (*Cecropia peltata*) leaf on the leg, which is then bandaged with cotton. This practice is repeated for a few months. Horses also have a decoction of bay leaves (*Pimenta racemosa*), indigo blue and a scent like lavender (owner preference for scent) rubbed on sore muscles.

Plants used for grooming
Wiz is the horse racing term for a ball of dried plant material used for grooming. A wiz may be made up of wild carailli leaves (*Momordica charantia*), elephant or guinea grass (*Panicum maximum*) or wild senna leaves (*Senna alata*). A bundle of this dry grass is beaten on a wall and stripped thin. It is then rolled into a ball and placed in the sun to dry. A wiz is best if left to age. This matted bundle is then rubbed on the horses' skin and is said to make the skin shiny. A wiz is used only on a clean horse. A bundle of branch tips of black sage (*Cordia curassavica*) (also called shining bush in the horse racing industry) is used before horses race to make the horse's coat shiny, as a coat cleaner and to remove the superficial dust. The dust from the horse's skin turns the bunch of leaves brown. A wet horse may be rubbed with wild carailli (*Momordica charantia*) or wild senna (*Senna alata*) leaves to cool them. Coconut oil (*Cocos nucifera*) is also used to make the coat shine. One respondent used carailli (*Momordica charantia*) for rashes. The carailli vine was boiled and the water was then used to sponge the horse.

Plants used for hoof problems and other injuries
Wonder of the world (*Kalanchoe pinnata*), young banana leaves (*Musa* species), or castor oil leaves (*Ricinus communis*) are rolled with a bottle to burst the plant veins. The leaves are then passed quickly over a flame to warm them. Soft candle (whale fat) and Epsom salts are pasted on and the leaves are then placed on top. The whole thing is then wrapped with vet wrap or Elastoplast®. Alternatively turmeric (*Curcuma longa*) is pounded and used. The entire foot is then placed in a bag or bandaged for three or four days and "sweated" for as long as it takes to draw the inflammation out. This practice is said to draw infections out of injuries like bruises from stones below the hoof. For cuts, aloes (*Aloe vera*) is bandaged on for two to three days.

Plants used as anthelmintics
Worm grass (*Chenopodium ambrosioides*) is used as an anthelmintic, but less so than in the past. The very infrequently used Leucaena (*Leucaena leucocephala*) is said to make hairs from the horses' tail drop off.

Plants used for enhanced performance
Horse's hind quarters are occasionally rubbed with cow itch (*Mucuna pruriens*), this is said to help them come out of the boxes faster, since the plant acts as an irritant. Bay leaf (*Pimenta racemosa*), is used to bathe horses on race day, this is said to carry heat into body, which makes them run faster to get away from the sun's heat. Two plants called speedweed (*Oxalis corniculata* and *Desmodium* sp.) are used to enhance performance. The plants are fed to horses with the rest of their feed and not given specifically before a race.

Plants used for anhydrosis

If it is felt that the animal is not sweating, or is dry coated, *Aloe vera* or two bois canot leaves (*Cecropia peltata*) or grated ratchette (*Nopalea cochenillifera*) is mixed with water and administered as a drench. Pepper leaves (*Capsicum annum, Capsicum frutescens*) may also be used. It is thought that this "heats" the horse which makes it drink more water. These practices are said to "cool down" the horse's system and bring out the "heat", the animal sweats a few hours later. In previous times horses were taken to the river to stand up in the water for an hour after the race.

Plants used for retained placenta

Horses with retained placenta are seen to have a black discharge three days post partum. These horses are given a 3-inch piece of aloes (*Aloe vera*) each day for three days, and then purged with castor oil (*Ricinus communis*). One respondent used linseed oil mixed with aloe vera gel twice weekly. About half of a large leaf of aloe was used. Another respondent used pounded turmeric rhizome (*Curcuma longa*). Tumeric is said to flush out the uterus. Horses are also given molasses water to drink, this is said to "clean them out." Horses are also given a combination of glycerine, Epsom salts and rachette (*Nopalea cochenillifera*) to remove inflammation.

Plants used for digestion

Aloes (*Aloe vera*) is boiled for five minutes and mixed with linseed oil. This is syringed down the horse's throat; some spit it out. Aloes is used for most internal problems and it is said to ease digestive problems. Subsequent to the administration of the *Aloe vera* the horse is given a purge with castor oil (*Ricinus communis*). Aloe leaves are also peeled and blended with water this mixture is then combined with honey, and given orally with a syringe. A decoction of caraaili (*Momordica charantia*) vine is given orally as a digestive aid. Rachette (*Nopalea cochenillifera*) joints are pounded up, put in water, and given to horses to drink, they "sweat it out" and this helps them reduce their temperature. Horses are also bathed with bay leaves (*Pimenta racemosa*) to make them feel cool. A decoction of one or two cups of bay leaves is added to a half bucket of water, this liquid is then used to sponge the horse. Alternatively they are sponged with bay rum (bay oil extracted from leaves of *P. racemosa*, alcohol and water).

Plants used for bleeders

Water cress (*Nasturtium officinale*) is put in horses' food to "increase their blood count." Vervine (*Stachytarpheta jamaicensis*) and kudzu (*Pueraria phaseoloides*) are fed as high protein feeds. Horses that collect blood in their lungs during or after a race are called "bleeders" (exercise induced pulmonary haemorrhage). To treat bleeders, honey and aloes are given orally. Sometimes the white of an egg is included. Additionally, pureed lemon juice is syringed into the horse's nostrils, this is said to curb bleeding by acting as an astringent.

Plants used for urinary problems

A decoction of bois canôt (*Cecropia peltata*) leaves is given as the drinking water. One respondent remembered seeing a veterinarian use the long stem of a pawpaw leaf (*Carica papaya*) as a catheter to clear a urinary blockage. To stimulate diuresis a decoction of the dry leaves of bois canôt (*Cecropia peltata*) is prepared in a bucket; a cup of this liquid in then put in the horses' drinking water. This is thought to assist in "cleaning out the bladder" of the horse.

Plants used for respiratory conditions

For bad head colds, horses are sweated or syringed with a cough medicine made of honey, garlic, and onion and boiled bois canôt leaves (*Cecropia peltata*). To "sweat" the horse heated bricks from a dirt oven are put into a bucket with Vicks, peppermint oil or Foyles Balsam™. The horse's head is put in the bag, and forced to inhale the steam.

Discussion

The Santa Rosa track has a turf course that is not used as frequently as the sand course. In the wet season the sand course is described as "sloppy." These track conditions may have led to the description of tendon problems as the second biggest problem after lung problems. Clay was used by Native American groups for broken bones in horses and humans (Lawrence, 1998). Firing and blistering are no longer recommended in orthodox veterinary medicine. Raudenbush et al. (2001) reported that peppermint odour had a positive effect on running speed. The use of cow itch on race day is considered an offence by the Trinidad and Tobago racing authority.

Review of the ethnomedicinal literature

The following is an ethnopharmacological review and evaluation (Heinrich et al. (1992).

Aloe vera emulsion (sap and gel mixed with mineral oil) has been used to treat patients with peptic ulcer (Yusuf et al., 2004). *Aloe vera* contains one of a few molecules that are known to possess both gastrointestinal mast cell stabilizing and gastrointestinal cytoprotective activity; hence its protective role in defence against gastrointestinal infections and injury (Penissi et al., 2003). Acemannan from *Aloe vera* has been used in inflammatory bowel disease therapy (Robinson, 1998).

Cecropia sciadophylla infusion is used in the Peruvian Amazon for kidney stones (Jovel et al., 1996). *C. obtusifolia* leaves are sold in Mexican herb markets for their antidiabetic properties. Extracts of the leaves showed hypoglycaemic activity (Perez et al., 1984). Free fatty acids including stearic, arachidic, behenic, lignoceric and cerotic acids were isolated from *Cecropia* species (Lachman-White et al., 1992).

Chenopodium ambrosioides (L.) infusions have been used for centuries in the Americas against intestinal worms. The aqueous infusion used as a vermifuge is safer than the use of the herb's essential oil (MacDonald et al., 2004)

Cordia species contain phenolic compounds (Ficarra et al., 1995) and terpenoid quinones (Lachman-White et al., 1992). Branches are reported to be resinous and leaves are aromatic and have stiff hairs on their upper sides (Morton, 1981).

Curcumin was given orally at a dose of 375 mg/3 times per day for a period of 6-22 months to eight patients suffering from idiopathic inflammatory orbital pseudotumours. Follow up lasted for 2 years at 3 monthly intervals. Four of five patients recovered completely. In one patient the swelling regressed but some limitation of movement persisted. There were no side effects or recurrence (Lal et al. 2000).

Desmodium adscendens is used to treat bronchial asthma in Ghana (Barreto, 2002). Studies have shown that butanolic extract inhibits contraction of the ileum and trachea in guinea pigs. Three active components (triterpenoid glycosides) were identified (McManus, 1993). An extract of *Desmodium grahami* produced a concentration-dependent inhibition of spontaneous ileum contractions (Rojas et al., 1999). In addition, the extract showed antimicrobial activity against pathogenic enterobacteria supporting its ethnomedical use for the treatment of gastrointestinal disorders. Three antimicrobial isoflavones were isolated from *Desmodium canum* (Monache et al., 1996).

Kalanchoe pinnata (syn. *Bryophyllum pinnatum*) has been used since 1921 in Germany as a sedative. Studies on *Kalanchoe pinnata* have shown the following *in vitro* effects in rodent tissue: positive inotropism, sedation, H1 antagonism (ileum, bronchial muscle, peripheral vasculature), and antimicrobial activity (Gwehenberger et al., 2004).

Leaf extracts (water, ethanol and methanol) of *Momordica charantia* have shown broad-spectrum antimicrobial activity, experimentally and clinically (Grover and Yadav, 2004). Extracts have immunomodulatory, analgesic and anti-inflammatory activities.

Mucuna pruriens is used as a stimulant tonic and diuretic in India (Ghosal et al., 1971; Deokule, 1991). Spicular hairs of the pod of *Mucuna pruriens* penetrate the skin causing intense irritation (Oliver Bever, 1986). Hairs contain 5-hydroxytryptamine (serotonin) and the itching produced by the hairs is due to the liberation of histamine in the epidermal layer of the skin (Oliver Bever, 1986).

Musa paradisiaca stem is used in India for diarrhoea (Ahmad and Beg, 2001). *Musa sapientum* var. Cavendishii contains soluble and insoluble dietary fibre that contributes to its hypo-cholesterolaemic effect (Horigome et al., 1992). A lectin was isolated from *Musa paradisiaca* (Koshte et al., 1990). Best et al. (1984) found that dried unripe plantain banana was anti-ulcerogenic due to its ability to stimulate growth of the gastric mucosa and was effective both as a prophylactic treatment and in healing ulcers already induced by aspirin. The active factor(s) were water soluble. Pannangpetch et al. (2001) found that extracts of both raw Hom bananas (*Musa sapientum* Linn.) and Palo bananas (Musa *paradisiaca*) protected the rat stomach from indomethacin-induced injuries, but Num Waa bananas (*Musa sapientum* Linn.) had no protective effect. The Hom banana extract (*Musa sapientum* Linn.) had a significant healing effect on acetic acid-induced ulcers.

Goda et al. (1999) found histamine release inhibitors (flavonols and megastigmanes) in watercress (*Nasturtium officinale*). Phenethyl isothiocyanate (PEITC) which is released upon chewing of watercress (*Nasturtium officinale*) is a chemoprotective agent (Hecht et al., 1995). Chen et al. (1996) found that consumption of watercress causes a decrease in the levels of oxidative metabolites of acetaminophen, probably due to inhibition of oxidative metabolism of this drug.

A double-blind, placebo-controlled, crossover trial of 64 healthy, young adult volunteers established that an extract of *Opuntia ficus indica* plant (a related species to *Nopalea cochenillifera*) lessens the inflammatory response to stressful stimuli by inhibiting the production of inflammatory mediators (Wiese et al., 2004).

The pounded bulbs of *Oxalis stricta* and *Oxalis violacea* were fed to horses by Pawnee Omaha and Ponca to make them fleet (Moerman, 1998). *Oxalis erythrorhiza* aerial parts decoction is used for hepatic and heart complains (Feresin et al., 2003). Ketoacids were reported from *Oxalis corniculata* and 2''-glucoisovitexin was isolated from *Oxalis acetosella* (Feresin et al., 2003). Five *Oxalis* species including *Oxalis corniculata* have been used to treat skin infections and unspecified microbial infections. Dichloromethane extracts of *Oxalis erythrorhiza* showed activity against methicillin-resistant and methicillin-sensitive strains of S. *aureus* as well as towards the dermatophytes *Microsporum canis*, *Trichophyton rubrum*, *Trichophyton mentagrophytes*, *Epidermophyton floccosum* and *Microsporum gypseum* (Feresin et al., 2003). The antimicrobial activity of alkyl phenols and the benzoquinone embelin, from hexane and dichloromethane extracts of *Oxalis erythrorhiza* was established. Embelin inhibits the dermatophytes *Epidermophyton floccosum*, *Microsporum canis*, *Trichophyton mentagrophytes* and *T. rubrum* and *Microsporum gypseum*.

Panicum maximum leaves contain ash, calcium, carbohydrates, carotene, chlorine, fat, fibre, HCN, iodine, iron, magnesium, oxalates, phosphorus, phytic acid, potassium, protein, sodium, sulphur, tocopherol (Duke, 2000).

The extract from leaves of *Pimenta racemosa* var. *ozua* showed antinociceptive activity, associated with an anti-inflammatory effect (Garcia et al., 2004). The anti-inflammatory activity of abietic acid, a diterpene from *Pimenta racemosa* var. *grissea*, was established *in-vivo* after oral or topical administration (Fernández et al., 2001).

Tona et al. (1999) and Olajide et al. (1999) found that plant extracts made of the leaves of *Psidium guajava* act as antidiarrhoeic agents by a triple pronounced antibacterial, antiamoebic and antispasmodic action (inhibition of intestinal motility). *Psidium guajava* leaves are mentioned in the Farmacopea Mexicana as astringents (Ankli et al., 1999). *Psidium guajava* plant parts contain cineol, tannins, triterpenes and flavonoids (Olajide et al., 1999).

The raw extract of castor oil contains 90% ricinoleic acid (Vieira et al., 2001). In an experimental model of blepharitis in the guinea-pig eyelid the pro-inflammatory and anti-inflammatory properties of ricinoleic acid became evident (Vieira et al., 2001). A 10-day, randomized, controlled experimental study compared the safety and efficacy of a prescription product, (both aerosol spray and ointment base, containing active ingredients: balsam of Peru, castor oil, and trypsin) used for the treatment of pressure ulcers and perineal dermatitis (Gray and Jones, 2004). Sixty healthy volunteers (> 65 years of age) submitted to intentional formation of two equivalent skin wounds (approx. 6 mm in diameter) using a laser; and served as their own control. Wounds were randomized to treatment with one of the balsam of Peru products or saline and evaluated every other day. Wounds treated with the ointment had significantly lower edema, scabbing, and erythema scores and higher epithelialization scores than the spray or saline managed wounds (Gray and Jones, 2004).

Stachytarpheta jamaicensis plant is rich in caffeic acid, stachytarphetin, chlorogenic acid, the hypotensive gamma-amino-butyric acid, flavones (luteolol and derivatives) and catechic tannins (Robineau, 1991; Heinrich et al., 1992).

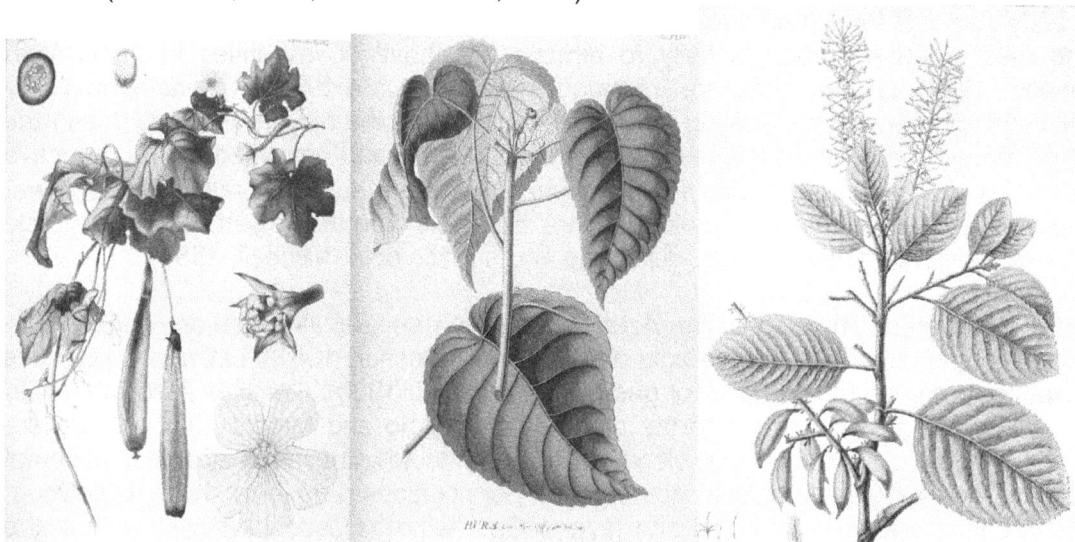

Figure 74. Luffa cylindrical
Figure 75. Hura sp.
Figure 76. Roupala monosperma

Case study 3: Ethnomedicine

Tout hazyé sé rimèd (every bush is a remedy) (INRA-CARDI, 1991)

9. Case study 3: Ethnomedicine

Background

There is little knowledge about the medicinal plant traditions of the people living in the Caribbean before the arrival of Columbus except for the practices documented by Father Bartolomé de las Casas. Caribbean folk medicine incorporates knowledge from Africa, Europe, India, and South America; a product of inter-group borrowing or medical syncretism. Several (approx. 30) of the total (>100) ethnomedicinal plant uses have already been recorded in an ethnomedicinal study in one rural community in the northern range of Trinidad (Wong, 1976). This chapter returns to the questions of whether ethnoveterinary medicine is a separate field from human folk medicine. Most ethnoveterinary medicines are derived from a similar ethnomedicinal use. However the ethnomedicinal plants listed below were not found to have a closely corresponding ethnoveterinary use during the research. The chapter also addresses the research question of tracing the ethnomedicinal practices to the original continents of Trinidad and Tobago's current population. In both the first and second phases of the research the plants kojoroot and gullyroot were said to be the same and also said to be different plants. In this book the same botanical name is used but the local name specified for the particular use is given.

The Trinidadian hot/cold system is not humoral in the sense that balance must be established between hot and cold, it is cathartic in that remedies are taken to remove heat from the system (Littlewood, 1988). Heat comes from the sun, work, sleeping, burns, cooking, and reproductive activities. Linked to the hot/cold dichotomy is a system of blood beliefs where an excess or lack of cold or heat in the body through exposure or diet causes illness. Blood then becomes 'bad' or dirty. Illnesses with skin changes such as chicken pox, measles, rashes, urticaria, impetigo, ringworm, eczema, are associated with 'too much heat in the body' (Bayley, 1949; Aho and Minott, 1977; Mitchell, 1983); and cooling teas are used. Cooling teas are used prophylatically to remove the 'heat' or impurities in the system (Littlewood, 1988). Cooling teas are treatment when they are taken for undiagnosed or unspecified illnesses or when feeling unwell. Purges reduce the heat further and 'clean the blood' or remove unwanted foetuses, or internal parasites and are used for reproductive problems. 'Cold' is associated with a sudden change in temperature, drafts or getting wet (Mitchell, 1983). Associated with 'coldness' are the mole (fontanelle), chest, head, back, womb, eyes, ears and knee, phlegm, discharge and arthritic pain (Mitchell, 1983).

Aching is associated with 'cold' in the Aztec system and several illnesses are attributed to the unhealthy penetration of excess cold and moisture (Messer, 1987). Liniments, poultices and laxatives are used for cold and for gas (wind) (Mitchell, 1983). Illnesses associated with coldness are influenza, asthma and the common cold (Aho and Minott, 1977). There are also 'hot' plants to stimulate the blood or to treat 'cold' illnesses, and 'hot' external applications like 'soft candle' 'grated nutmeg' and hot poultices (Laguerre, 1987; Littlewood, 1993). 'Hot' teas are used for colds and fevers. Gas (wind) is associated with pain in the stomach but also in the joints and back and with pain that travels around the body (Mitchell, 1983; Littlewood, 1988). Expulsion of disease causing impurities is the primary mechanism by which bodily equilibrium is restored (Mitchell, 1983). Folk medicines achieve cures through 'bitterness', 'cutting', 'cooling', 'building', 'purging or washing out', and 'drawing out'

(Mitchell, 1983). The section below focuses on the nineteen plants used for eye and dental problems and headaches; the thirteen plants used for diabetes, twenty for hypertension, four for jaundice and the forty-four plants used for urinary problems, "cooling" and high cholesterol levels.

Results

Three plants are used for eye problems (*Capraria biflora*, *Kalanchoe pinnata*, *Ocimum gratissimum*), five for headaches (*Acnistus arborescens*, *Lepianthes peltata*, *Musa* sp., *Ricinus communis*, *Senna occidentalis*), three for nervous conditions (*Annona muricata*, *Musa* sp., *Piper hispidum*), three to aid sleep (*Annona muricata*, *Citrus nobilis*, *Crescentia cujete*), five for problems in the mouth (*Aristolochia rugosa*, *Chrysobalanus icaco*, *Cocos nucifera*, *Spondias mombin* and *Tagetes patula*), one for ear problems (*Tagetes patula*), one as a brain tonic (*Rosmarinus officinalis*) and one as a narcotic (*Datura stramonium*). The plants represent 17 plant families. The ethnomedicinal plants used in Trinidad and Tobago for eye and dental problems and headaches are summarised in Table 5.

Table 5. Ethnomedicinal plants used for eye problems, headaches, dental problems, ect

Scientific name	Family	Common name	Plant part used	Use
A. arborescens	Solanaceae	Wild tobacco		Headache
Annona muricata	Annonaceae	Soursop	Leaves	Nerves, Sleep aid
Aristolochia rugosa	Aristolochiaceae	Mat root	Root	Toothache
Capraria biflora	Scrophulariaceae	Du thé pays	Leaves	Eye wash
C. icaco	Chrysobalanaceae	Ipecak		Tonsils
Citrus nobilis	Rutaceae	Portugal	Bud	Sleep aid for babies
Cocos nucifera	Arecaceae	Coconut	Root	Bleeding gums
Crescentia cujete	Bignoniaceae	Calabash	Leaves	Sleep aid
Datura stramonium	Solanaceae	Datur		Narcotic
Kalanchoe pinnata	Crassulaceae	Wonder/ world	Leaves	Eye problems
Lepianthes peltata	Piperaceae	Sun bush	Leaves	Headache
Musa species	Musaceae	Banana	Young leaf, green fruit	Tie on head for headache, Boil with skin for nerves, 'run down'
O. gratissimum	Lamiaceae	Fon bazin	Seeds	Clears eyes
Piper hispidum	Piperaceae	Candle bush	Leaves	Nerves
Ricinus communis	Euphorbiaceae	Castor oil leaf	Leaves	Tie on head for headache
R. officinalis	Lamiaceae	Rosemary		Brain tonic
Senna occidentalis	Caesalpiniaceae	Wild coffee	Leaves	Tie on for headaches
Spondias mombin	Anacardiaceae	Hogplum	Leaves	Mouthwash, tonsils, sore throat
Tagetes patula	Asteraceae	Marigold		Pain in ear, Toothache

Plants used for urinary problems

Forty-four plants are used for urinary problems, "cooling" and high cholesterol levels. They represent at least thirty plant families. The term "stoppage of water" means urinary retention. Three plants are used for bladder problems: *Costus scaber*, *Pilea microphylla* and *Cocos nucifera*. Two plants are used for high cholesterol levels: *Solanum melongena* and *Portulaca oleraceae*.

Several plants are used for "cooling": *Musa* species *Begonia humilis Bontia daphnoides*, *Cissus verticillata*, *Coleus aromaticus*, *Commelina elegans*, *Cuscuta americana*, *Cyperus rotundus*, *Desmodium canum*, *Entada polystachya*, *Justicia pectoralis*, *Momordica charantia*, *Peperomia pellucida*, *Ruellia tuberosa*, *Sansevieria guineensis*, *Stachytarpheta jamaicensis*, *Scoparia dulcis*, *Cassia alata*, *Capraria biflora*, *Kalachoe pinnata*, *Mimosa pudica* and *Solanum americanum*. *Bauhinia cumanensis*, *Bauhinia excisa* and *Capraria biflora* are used for gall stones, while *Hibiscus sabdariffa* is used to clean the liver and blood.

The following plants are used for kidney and bladder problems: *Kalachoe pinnata*, *Mimosa pudica*, *Chamaesyce hirta*, *Flemingia strobilifera*, *Peperomia rotundifolia*, *Petiveria alliacea*, *Nopalea cochenillifera*, *Apium graveolens*, *Cynodon dactylon*, *Zea mays*, *Theobroma cacao*, *Lepianthes peltata*, *Eleusine indica*, *Gomphrena globosa*, *Pityrogramma calomelanos* and *Vetiveria zizanioides*.

The results are summarized in Table 6.

Table 6. Ethnomedicinal plants used for "cooling", high cholesterol and urinary problems in Trinidad and Tobago

Scientific name	Family	Common name	Part used	Use
Apium graveolens	Apiaceae	Celery		Kidney tonic
Bauhinia cumanensis	Fabaceae	Monkey step	Bark	Gall stones
Begonia humilis	Begoniaceae	Lozeille		Cooling
Bontia daphnoides	Myoporaceae	Olive bush	Leaves	Cooling
Capraria biflora	Scrophulariaceae	Du thé pays	Leaves	Gall stones, cooling
Cassia alata	Fabaceae	Senna	Leaves	Cooling with cloves and ginger
Chamaesyce hirta	Euphorbiaceae	Mal nommée		Kidney problems
Cissus verticillata	Vitaceae	Blister bush	Vine	Cooling
Cocos nucifera	Arecaceae	Coconut	Root	Bladder stones
Coleus aromaticus	Lamiaceae	Spanish thyme	Leaves	Cooling
C. elegans	Commelinaceae	Water grass	Plant	Cooling
Costus scaber	Zingiberaceae	Wild cane		Cleans bladder
Cuscuta americana	Convolvulaceae	Love vine	Vine	Cooling
Cynodon dactylon	Poaceae	Dube		Stoppage of water

Table 6. Ethnomedicinal plants used for "cooling", high cholesterol and urinary problems in Trinidad and Tobago (cont.)

Scientific name	Family	Common name	Part used	Use
Cyperus rotundus	Cyperaceae	Nut grass		Cooling
Desmodium canum	Fabaceae	Sweet heart bush	Plant	Cooling
Eleusine indica	Poaceae	Dead man's grass	Root Leaves	Urinary
Entada polystachya	Fabaceae	Mayoc chapelle		Cooling
Flemingia strobilifera	Fabaceae	Kidney bush		Kidney problems
Gomphrena globosa	Amaranthaceae	Bachelor button	Leaves	Urinary problems
Hibiscus sabdariffa	Malvaceae	Sorrel	Flower & seed	Cleans liver and blood
Justicia pectoralis	Acanthaceae	Carpenter grass	Leaves	Cooling
Kalachoe pinnata	Crassulaceae	Wonder of the world	Leaves	Cooling, Bladder stones
Lepianthes peltata	Piperaceae	Lani bois	Leaves	Tea
Mimosa pudica	Fabaceae	Ti marie, mese marie		Cooling, Kidney problems
M. charantia	Cucurbitaceae	Caraaili	Vine	Cooling
Musa species	Musaceae	Banana	Dry leaf	Boil for cooling
N. cochenillifera	Cactaceae	Rachette	Joint	Kidney stones
Peperomia rotundifolia	Piperaceae	Giron fleur, mowon		Kidney problems
P. pellucida	Piperaceae	Shining bush		Cooling
Petiveria alliacea	Phytolaccaceae	Mapourite, kudjuruk		Kidney problems
Pilea microphylla	Urticaceae	Du thé bethelmay	Leaves	Bladder cleanser
Pityrogramma calomelanos	Pteridaceae	Fern		Urinary problems
Portulaca oleraceae	Portulacaceae	Pussley	Plant	Cholesterol, short breath
Ruellia tuberosa	Acanthaceae	Minny root	Root	Cooling
S. guineensis	Agavaceae	Langue bouef	Leaves	Cooling
Scoparia dulcis	Scrophulariaceae	Sweet broom	Plant	Cooling for babies
Solanum americanum	Solanaceae	Agouma, gouma	Plant	Cooling, provides iron
S. melongena	Solanaceae	Melongene	Fruit	Cholesterol
S. jamaicensis	Verbenaceae	Vervine	Leaves	Cooling
Theobroma cacao	Sterculiaceae	Cocoa	Core	Eat for urinary problems
Vetiveria zizanioides	Poaceae	Vetivert		Urinary problems
Zea mays	Poaceae	Corn silk	Stigma	Diuretic

Plants used for high blood pressure, diabetes and jaundice

Thirteen plants are used for diabetes, twenty for hypertension and four for jaundice.

Each of the thirty plants comes from a different plant family. Multiple-plant remedies are used for several conditions including one used for jaundice which combined white bachelor button (*Gomphrena globosa*), olive bush (*Bontia daphnoides)*, small white vere michelle (unidentified), and fine-stemmed rather than thick-stemmed love vine (*Cuscuta americana*).

Tournefortia hirsutissima is used for "cooling." The following plants are used to treat diabetes: *Antigonon leptopus, Bidens alba, Bidens pilosa, Bontia daphnoides, Carica papaya, Gomphrena globosa, Bixa orellana, Catharanthus roseus, Cocos nucifera, Laportea aestuans, Momordica charantia, Morus alba, Phyllanthus urinaria* and *Spiranthes acaulis*.

Apium graveolens is used as a heart tonic and the following plants are used for hypertension: *Aloe vera, Annona muricata, Artocarpus altilis, Bixa orellana, Bidens alba, Bidens pilosa, Bontia daphnoides, Carica papaya, Cecropia peltata, Citrus paradisa, Cola nitida, Crescentia cujete, Gomphrena globosa, Hibiscus sabdariffa, Kalanchoe pinnata, Nopalea cochenillifera, Morus alba, Ocimum campechianum, Passiflora quadrangularis, Persea americana* and *Tamarindus indicus*. Low blood pressure is treated with *Apium graveolens*.

Jaundice is treated with the following plants (many of which are also listed above): *Bixa orellana, Bontia daphnoides, Gomphrena globosa* and *Cuscuta americana*.

The ethnomedicinal plants used in Trinidad and Tobago for diabetes are summarised in Table 7.

Table 7. Ethnomedicinal plants used for high blood pressure and diabetes in Trinbago

Scientific name	Family	Common name	Plant part used	Use
Aloe vera	Liliaceae	Aloes	Leaf gel	High blood pressure
Annona muricata	Annonaceae	Soursop	Leaves	Hypertension
A. leptopus	Polygonaceae	Coralita	Vine	Diabetes
Apium graveolens	Apiaceae	Celery		Heart tonic, Low blood pressure
Artocarpus altilis	Moraceae	Breadfruit	Leaves	Hypertension
Bidens alba / Bidens pilosa	Asteraceae	Needle grass	Leafy branch	Hypertension, Diabetes
Bixa orellana	Bixaceae	Roucou	Leaves, root	Hypertension, Diabetes, Jaundice
Bontia daphnoides	Myoporaceae	Olive bush	Leaves	Diabetes, Jaundice, Hypertension
Carica papaya	Caricaceae	Papaya	Green fruit	Hypertension, Diabetes
C. roseus	Apocynaceae	Periwinkle		Diabetes
Cecropia peltata	Cecropiaceae	Bois canôt	Leaves	Hypertension
Citrus paradisi	Rutaceae	Grapefruit	Peel	Hypertension
Cocos nucifera	Arecaceae	Coconut	Shell, flower	Diabetes
Cola nitida	Sterculiaceae	Obie seed	Seed	Hypertension

Table 7. Ethnomedicinal plants used for high blood pressure and diabetes in Trinbago (cont.)

Scientific name	Family	Common name	Plant part used	Use
Crescentia cujete	Bignoniaceae	Calabash	Leaves	Hypertension
C. americana	Convolvulaceae	Love vine	Vine	Jaundice
G. globosa	Amaranthaceae	Bachelor button	Leaves	Jaundice, Diabetes, Hypertension
H. sabdariffa	Malvaceae	Sorrel	Leaf	Hypertension
Kalanchoe pinnata	Crassulaceae	W/ world	Leaf	Hypertension
Laportea aestuans	Urticaceae	Red stinging nettle	Leaves	Diabetes
M. charantia	Cucurbitaceae	Caraaili		Diabetes
Morus alba	Moraceae	Pawi bush		Diabetes, Hypertension
N. cochenillifera	Cactaceae	Rachette	Joint	Hypertension
O. campechianum	Lamiaceae	Ti bom	Leaves	Hypertension
P. quadrangularis	Passifloraceae	Barbadine	Leaves	Hypertension
Persea americana	Lauraceae	Avocado	Leaf	Hypertension
P. urinaria	Euphorbiaceae	Red seed under leaf		Diabetes
Spiranthes acaulis	Orchidaceae	Lapsogen		Early diabetes
T. indicus	Fabaceae	Tamarind	Seed	Hypertension
Tournefortia hirsutissima	Boraginaceae	Chigger[21] bush	Leaves	Cooling

Discussion

Non-experimental validation of plants used for eye problems, headaches, dental problems, etc.

Acnistus arborescens leaves have been used traditionally to treat cancerous growths (Kupchan *et al.*, 1965). Alcoholic extracts of dried leaves of *Acnistus arborescens* contained a novel steroidal tumour inhibitor (Kupchan *et al.*, 1965).

In 1492 Columbus was given a Christmas-time gift of "quinces" which may have been soursop (Morison, 1963). *Annona muricata* fruit and leaves are used in Caribbean traditional medicine for their tranquillizing and sedative properties (Hasrat *et al.*, 1997b). Bourne and Egbe (1979) found that an alcoholic extract from the ripe fruit of soursop (*Annona muricata*) decreased the motor activity and prolonged the barbiturate (thiopentone sodium) sleeping

---

[21] In Guiana there is a little insect in the grass and on the shrubs which the French call bete-rouge. It is of a beautiful scarlet colour, and so minute that you must bring your eye close to it before you can perceive it. It is most numerous in the rainy season. Its bite causes an intolerable itching. The best way to get rid of it is to rub the part affected with oil or rum. You must be careful not to scratch it. If you do so, and break the skin, you expose yourself to a sore (Waterton, 1973). Still more inconvenient, painful and annoying is another little pest called the chegoe. It attacks different parts of the body, but chiefly the feet, betwixt the toe-nails and the flesh. There it buries itself, and at first causes an itching not unpleasant. In a day or so, after examining the part, you perceive a place about the size of a pea, somewhat discoloured, rather of a blue appearance. Sometimes it happens that the itching is so trivial, you are not aware that the miner is at work. Time, they say, makes great discoveries. The discoloured part turns out to be the nest of the chegoe, containing hundreds of eggs, which, if allowed to hatch there, the young ones will soon begin to form other nests, and in time cause a spreading ulcer (Waterton, 1973).

time of rats. The study supported local claims of sedative properties (Bourne and Egbe, 1979). Studies showed that the fruit of *Annona muricata* possesses antidepressive effects (in contrast to sedative properties), possibly induced by alkaloids, benzyltetrahydroisoquinoline, annonaine, nornuciferine, asimilobine or reticuline (Hasrat *et al*, 1997b). In the French West Indies, PSP and atypical Parkinsonism predominated in patients who consumed herbal tea and fruits of the Annonaceae (custard apple or pawpaw family). Benzyltetrahydroisoquinolines (alkaloids), present in Annonaceae, are neurotoxic to the basal ganglia in animals (Caparros-Lefebvre and Elbaz, 1999). This analysis was based on small numbers of cases.

Aristolochia species are used in western Panama as analgesics (Joly *et al.*, 1987).

Capraria biflora is used as a bath tonic in Belize and Curaçao (Morton, 1968b; Arnason *et al.*, 1980).

The use of *Chrysobalanus icaco* as an astringent in Trinidad has been previously recorded (Wong, 1976). On his first voyage Columbus likened these fruit to coconuts (Morison, 1963). Ferdinand Columbus claimed that the inhabitants of Hispaniola called them caxina.

Citrus aurantifolia was found active against *Staphylococcus aureus* (Facey *et al.*, 1999).

Cocos nucifera nut shell is used as a rubefacient in India (Kapoor, 1990).

Crescentia cujete is used in Panama as a tranquiliser (Duke, 2000).

Datura stramonium is used as a narcotic in Pakistan and in the republic of Niger, alkaloids in the plant have an atropine-like effect (Djibo and Bouzou, 2000; Shinwari and Khan, 2000).

Kalanchoe pinnata is used for headaches by the Caribs in Guatemala (Girón *et al.*, 1991).

In the Caribbean and South America, warm *Lepianthes peltata* leaves are tied to the head and forehead to relieve headaches (Hodge and Taylor, 1957; Lachman-White *et al.*, 1992). *Lepianthes peltata* leaves are also applied to other areas for the relief of arthritic pains, hernia pains, liver pains and other inflammatory disorders (Lachman-White *et al.*, 1992; Mongelli *et al.*, 1999). *Lepianthes peltata* and *Lepianthes umbella* showed no mutagenicity (Felzenszwalb *et al.*, 1987). A catechol derivative (4-nerolidylcatechol) was isolated from the methanolic leaf extract (Mongelli *et al.*, 1999).

Musa paradisiaca is used for epilepsy in India and for fevers in Barbados (Handler and Jacoby, 1993; Ahmad and Beg, 2001). Heated leaves of *Musa* species are used for eye infections in Brazil and Indonesia (Milliken and Albert, 1996).

Ocimum micranthum was used as a wash for bloodshot eyes when the condition was caused by a blow (Asprey and Thornton, 1953-1955). *Ocimum* species seeds are put into the eye in Belize and Mexico (Arnason *et al.*, 1980; Ankli *et al.*, 1999). *Ocimum* species grown in Rwanda were found to be antimicrobially active against *Escherichia coli*, *Bacillus subtilis*, *Staphylococcus aureus* and *Trichophyton mentagrophytes* var. *interdigitale* (Janssen *et al.*, 1989). The essential oil (EO) and leaf extracts of *Ocimum gratissimum* inhibited *Staphylococcus aureus*, *Shigella* species, *Aeromonas sobria*, *Salmonella* species, *Plesiomonas shigelloides*, *Escherichia coli*, *Klebsiella* species and *Proteus mirabilis*. The endpoint was not reached for *Pseudomonas aeruginosa* (>=24 mg/ml). Eugenol was responsible for the observed antibacterial activity (Ilori *et al.*, 1996; Nakamura *et al.*, 1999).

Combinations with antibiotics potentiated the antibacterial activity of *Ocimum gratissimum* (Jedlickova *et al.*, 1992).

In Costa Rica *Piper marginatum* leaves are boiled and the tea is drunk to treat headaches (Hazlett, 1986). The plant and leaf contain ascorbic acid, beta-carotene, minerals, cepharadione-B, riboflavin, safrole and thiamin (Duke, 2000). Aqueous and ethanol extracts of aerial parts of *Piper auritum* have produced spasmogenic uterine stimulant and vasodilator effects (Gupta *et al.*, 1993).

Ricinus communis is put on the head for headache in Belize (Arnason *et al.*, 1980). Stems contain flavonoids, phenolic acids, triterpenes and phytosterols (Cambie, 1997).

Rosmarinus officinalis is used as a tonic in Venezuela (Morton, 1975).

Ferdinand Columbus claimed that the inhabitants of Hispaniola called the hogplum *hobi*. *Spondias mombin* contains long-chain phenolic acids, a long-chain phenol, two antivirally active ellagitannins and five 6-alkenylsalicylic acids (Corthout *et al.*, 1990 a & b; Corthout *et al.*, 1994). *Spondias mombin* has antibacterial and molluscicidal properties (Ajao *et al.* 1985; Corthout *et al.* 1994). *Spondias mombin* leaves were evaluated by Ayoka et al. (2006). The leaves were extracted with aqueous, methanol and ethanol solvents on hexobarbital-induced sleeping time and novelty-induced rearing (NIR) behaviours in mice and rats was tested (Ayoka et al., 2006). Their results suggested that the leaf extracts of *Spondias mombin* possess sedative and antidopaminergic effects.

Tagetes patula contains polyacetylenes, ellagic acid and thiophene derivatives. The leaves contain flavonoids (quercetagetin, patuletin, patulitrin, mannitol) (Cambie, 1997).

More data is necessary to evaluate the safety of the plants used for eye problems, headaches, dental problems and other conditions related to the head. *Annona muricata*, *Aristolochia rugosa* and *Datura stamonium* have validity for the folk uses described but also potentially serious side effects. The following plants have been understudied and therefore few claims can be made about their validity: *Lepianthes peltata*, *Musa species*, *Ocimum gratissimum*, *Piper hispidum*, *Ricinus communis*, *Senna occidentalis* and *Tagetes patula*. More studies are needed to establish the validity of the following plants for their respective uses: *Acnistus arborescens*, *Capraria biflora*, *Chrysobalanus icaco*, *Citrus nobilis*, *Cocos nucifera*, *Crescentia cujete*, *Kalanchoe pinnata*, *Rosmarinus officinalis* and *Spondias mombin*.

Non-experimental validation of plants used for urinary problems

Apium graveolens contains flavonoids and a furanocoumarin (bergaptene) (Lewis, 1989). It possesses antinociceptive and antiinflammatory effects. The latter may be due to the presence of volatile oils, flavonoids and resins (Atta and Alkofahi, 1998). The use of the plant extract for inflammation, pain and spasmodic colic is explained by these results.

Stems of *Bauhinia* species are ground, boiled in water and drunk to treat diarrhoea, dysentery or kidney disorders in Costa Rica, Brazil, French Guyana and Mexico (Jiu, 1966; Hazlett, 1986; Milliken and Albert, 1996).

Begonia species are used for dysentery, renal disorders and women's problems in Colombia and western Panama; for stomach aches, vomiting and diarrhoea by the Chocó Indians and by the Cabecar and Guaymi in Central America (Davis and Yost, 1983; Hazlett, 1986; Joly *et al.*, 1990; Laferriere, 1994). Anthocyanins have been found in flowers of *Begonia* species (Chirol and Jay, 1995).

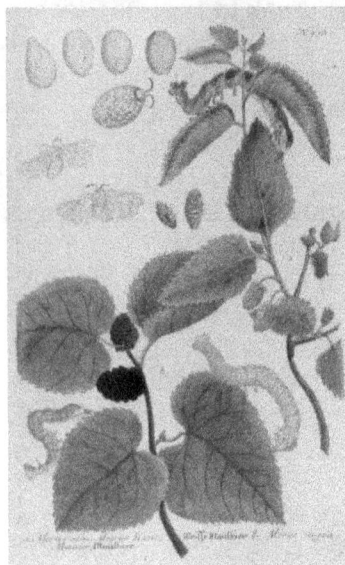

Figure 77. Morus alba
Figure 78. Acnistus arborescens
Figure 79. Annona squamosa

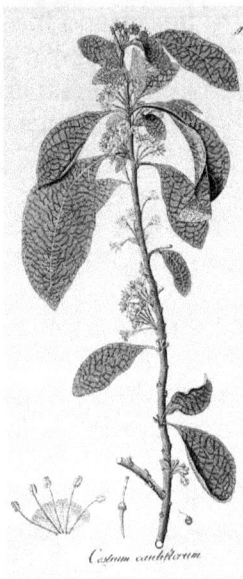

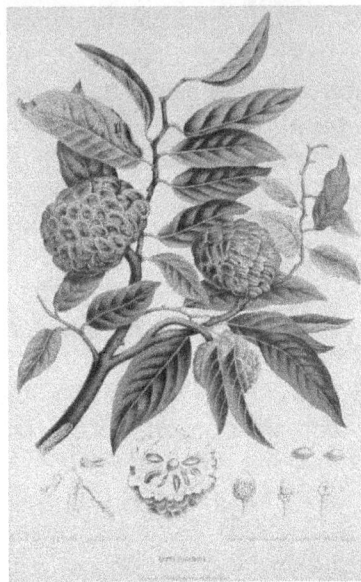

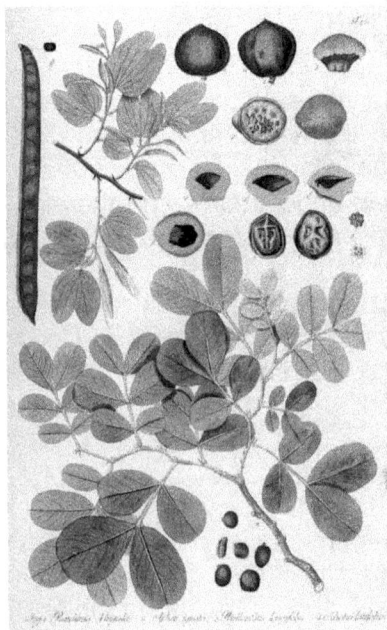

Figure 80. Bauhinia aculeata
Figure 81. Begonia humilis
Figure 82. Cyperus rotundus

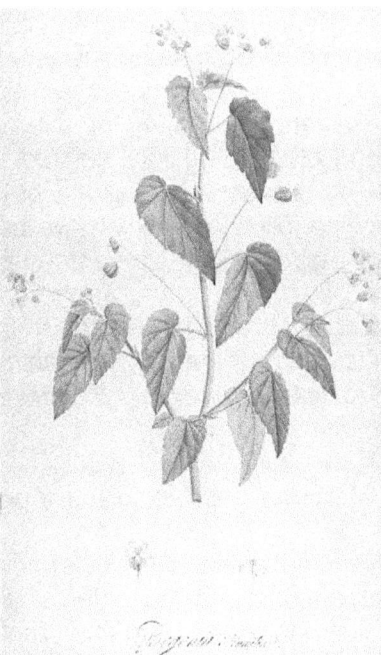

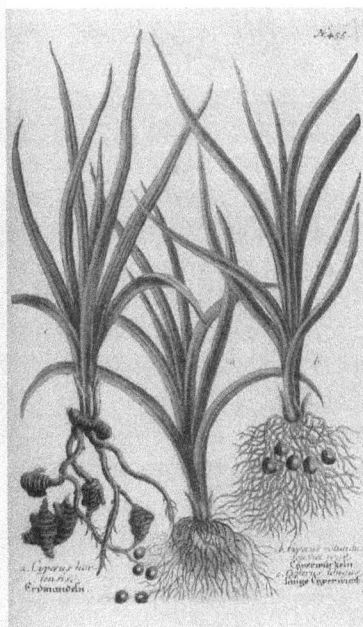

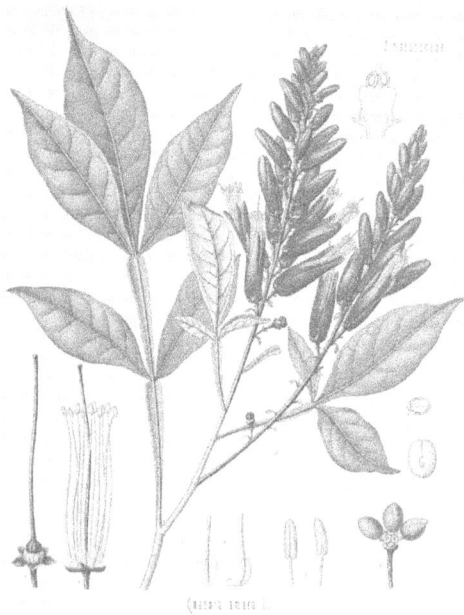

Figure 83. Quassia amara
Figure 84. Petiveria alliacea

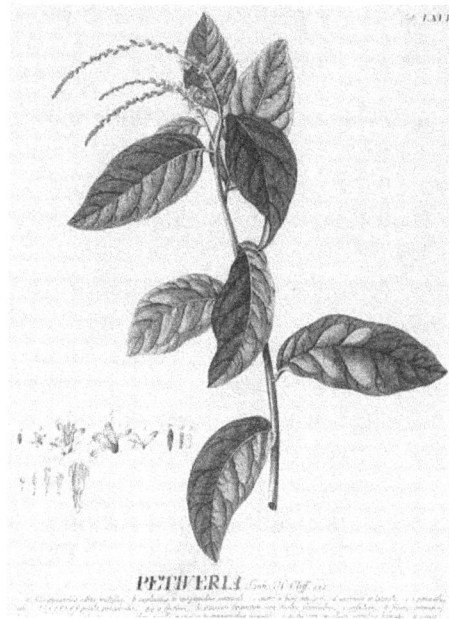

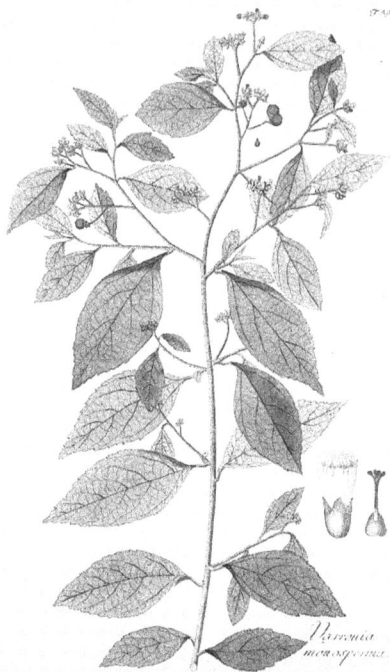

Figure 85. Cordia polycephala
Figure 86. Piper obtusifolium
Figure 87. Tournefortia glabra

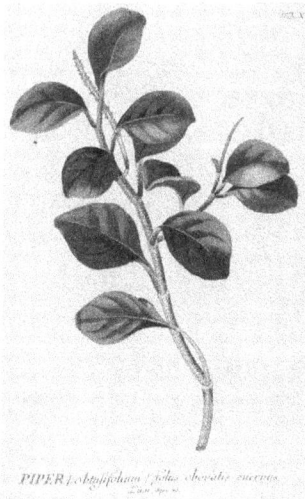

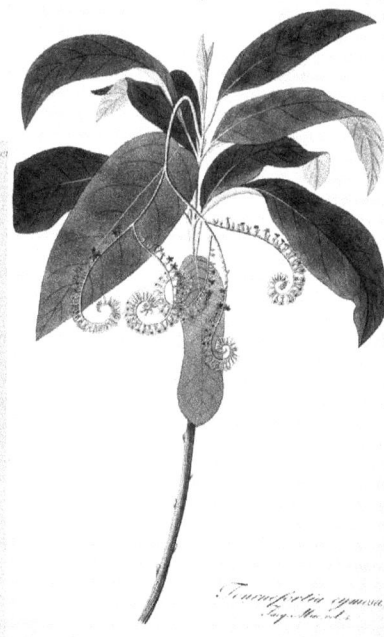

The ethnomedicinal use of *Bontia daphnoides* for hypertension and nephritis in Trinidad has been previously recorded (Wong, 1976). *Bontia daphnoides* contains (-)-epingaione, a sesquiterpene furan (Chinnock *et al.*, 1987).

Capraria biflora has been used ethnomedicinally as a diuretic, and for intestinal problems, hypertension and gonorrhoea (Comerford, 1996; Duke, 2000). The aerial parts of *Capraria biflora* contain sesquiterpenoids, caprariolides A-D (Collins *et al.*, 2000). *Capraria biflora* is

87

used in northern Venezuela, Cuba and Mexico for diarrhoea and to stop vomiting (Morton, 1968b, 1975).

Cassia alata tea is used for hypertension in Marie Galante (Honychurch, 1986).

Chamaesyce hirta is locally used in Africa, Australia, Mauritius, Rodrigues and Bolivia to treat numerous diseases, including hypertension, dysentery and oedema (Gurib-Fakim *et al.*, 1993; Bourdy *et al.*, 2000). The active component(s) in the water extract of *Chamaesyce hirta* leaf had a similar diuretic spectrum to that of acetazolamide a standard diuretic drug. These results validate the traditional use of *Chamaesyce hirta* by the Swahilis and Sukumas as a diuretic agent (Johnson *et al.*, 1999). Tona *et al.* (1999) found that the lyophilised aqueous extract of *Chamaesyce hirta* produced sedative properties at high doses (100 mg of dried plant/kg) and no toxic effects. These findings validate the traditional use of *Chamaesyce hirta* as a sedative with anxiolytic properties (Lanhers *et al.*, 1990; 1991).

Cissus sicyoides is used in Latin America for gonorrhoea, hypertension and inflammation (van den Berg, 1984; Garcia *et al.*, 1999b). *Cissus rubiginosa* is used as an antidiarrhoeal agent in Congolese folk medicine and has antibacterial activity (Longanga Otshudi *et al.*, 2000). *Cissus sicyoides* stems contain phenolic compounds. These latter compounds may be responsible for its activity against Gram-positive and Gram-negative microorganisms (Garcia *et al.*, 1999b).

Cocos nucifera root is used in India as a diuretic (Kapoor, 1990).

The use of *Coleus aromaticus* for stomach problems in Trinidad has been documented in Wong (1976).

The use of *Commelina elegans* in Trinidad for cystitis was documented by Wong (1976). *Commelina* species are used against diarrhoea, and as laxatives (Russo, 1992; Muñoz *et al.*, 2000b). *Commelina diffusa* contains anthocyanins (Cambie, 1997). *Commelina communis* contains n-hentriacontanol (Muñoz *et al.*, 2000b).

Cuscuta reflexa is used in Uttar Pradesh India for jaundice (Singh and Maheshwari, 1994). *Cuscuta americana* showed activity against *Staphylococcus aureus* (Verpoorte and Dihal, 1987). The hydroalcoholic extract of *Cuscuta americana* showed hepatotoxicity (Joyeux *et al.*, 1995).

Cynodon dactylon is used in West Bengal, Turkey, Pakistan, Mauritius and Rodrigues as a diuretic, for dropsy, gonorrhea and dysentery (Gurib-Fakim *et al.*, 1993; Mukhopadhyay *et al.*, 1995; Shinwari and Khan, 2000; Yeşilada *et al.*, 1999).

Cyperus rotundus is used as an analgesic in traditional Chinese medicine (Jeong *et al.*, 2000). In Mauritius and Rodrigues *Cyperus rotundus* decoction is used against dysentery and diarrhoea (Gurib-Fakim *et al.*, 1993). *Cyperus scariosus* root comprised one part of a polyherbal ayurvedic preparation that provided partial protection to rats with cisplatin-induced renal toxicity (Rao and Rao, 1998). The rhizome contains sesquiterpenes and monoterpene and aliphatic alcohols and shows antipyretic activity (Kapoor, 1990; Weenen *et al.*, 1990; Vedavathy and Rao, 1991; Thebtaranonth *et al.*, 1995; SunKee *et al.*, 2000).

Wong (1976) has documented the use of *Desmodium adscendens* and *Desmodium canum* in Trinidad as a depurative, and for oliguria, kidney disease and venereal disease. These uses are also current in Colombia, Mexico, Nicaragua and in Barbados where the ethnomedicinal use existed pre-1834 (Zamora-Martínez and Nieto de Pascual Pola, 1992; Handler and Jacoby, 1993; Barrett, 1994; Laferriere, 1994). *Desmodium adscendens* root decoction is used in Mauritius and Rodrigues as a bitter tonic and diuretic and is used for liver disorders in the Brazilian Amazon (Brandäo *et al.*, 1992; Gurib-Fakim *et al.*, 1993). *Desmodium styracifolium* was used as one component in a twelve-herb mixture used to successfully treat bovine urolithiasis (Sugimoto *et al.*, 1992). The ethanol extract of *Desmodium canum* roots contains antimicrobially active prenylated isoflavanones (desmodianones) (Monache *et al.*, 1996).

Eleusine indica was used as a 'blood cleanser' by the Caribs (Honychurch, 1986).

The use of *Entada polystachya* in Trinidad for venereal diseases and as a depurative has been recorded by Wong (1976). *Entada* species leaf decoctions are used in the Dutch East Indies, in Mauritius and Rodrigues and in Mali for bloody diarrhoea and abdominal cramps (Hirschhorn, 1983; Gurib-Fakim *et al.*, 1993; Occhiuto *et al.*, 1999). Extracts of *Entada abyssinica* (stem bark), showed activity against various *Candida* species (Fabry *et al.*, 1996). *Entada africana* exhibited antimicrobial activity against *Vibrio cholerae* (Akinsinde and Olukoya, 1995).

Flemingia strobilifera is used in India for dysentery and as a sedative (Nigam and Saxena, 1975; Duke, 2000). Roy and Tandon (1996) found antifluke activity in *Flemingia vestita*. Tandon *et al.* (1997) found *in vitro* vermifugal activity in *Flemingia vestita* probably caused by the isoflavone genistein.

Gomphrena globosa (white and rose coloured plants) are used for urinary problems in Trinidad and are used for dysentery in Venezuela (Morton, 1975).

Hibiscus sabdariffa has been used ethnomedicinally as a cholagogue, choleretic, diuretic, tea, tonic and laxative (Duke, 2000).

Justicia pectoralis contains coumarins (dihydrocoumarin and umbelliferone), betaine and 3-(2-hydroxyphenyl) propionic acid (de Vries *et al.*, 1988). Coumarin and umbelliferone are major constituents of the plant and have the ability to relax smooth muscle (MacRae and Towers, 1984).

Kalanchoe pinnata leaf infusion is used in Bolivia and Guatemala to treat inflammation and pain in the stomach (Girón *et al.*, 1991; Muñoz *et al.*, 2000a).

Mimosa pudica exhibited antimicrobial activity against *Vibrio cholerae* (Akinsinde and Olukoya, 1995). It was not found to be effective in either preventing stone deposition or dissolving preformed stones (experimental urolithiasis in rats) (Joyamma *et al.*, 1990). *Mimosa pudica* leaf infusion is used for diarrhoea (Hirschhorn, 1981; Barrett, 1994). *Mimosa pudica* leaves contain ascorbic acid, crocetin, mimosine, norepinephrine beta-carotene, minerals, crocetin-dimethyl-ether and thiamin (Duke, 2000).

'Bark' and 'trash' of *Musa sapientum* were used for 'stoppage of water' and 'sourness of stomach', 'bad belly' and diarrhoea in Jamaica and Nicaragua (Asprey and Thornton, 1953-1955; Barrett, 1994). The use for urinary problems finds parallels in Mayan traditional medical practice (Asprey and Thornton, 1953-1955).

Nopalea cochenillifera decoction is used for inflammation, as a laxative and for urinary problems in Mexico and the Caribbean (Sheridan, 1991; Honychurch, 1986; Duke, 2000).

Peperomia pellucida is used in Nicaragua for kidney problems and cooling (Barrett, 1994). The methanol extract of *Peperomia pellucida* aerial parts showed significant analgesic activity (Aziba *et al.*, 2001). *Peperomia pellucida* ethyl-acetate soluble extracts were active against Gram-positive and Gram-negative bacteria (Bojo *et al.*, 1997). *Peperomia pellucida* lowers uric acid in the blood and was endorsed by the Department of Health in the Philippines (de Guzman, 1998). *Peperomia pellucida* showed selective antifungal activity but failed to show any antiviral or cytotoxic activity (Ali *et al.*, 1996; Mohammed *et al.*, 1996).

Pilea microphylla is used as a diuretic in Brazil and is used for urinary problems in Guatemala (Comerford, 1996; Duke, 2000). *Pilea microphylla* was found active against *Staphylococcus aureus* (Facey *et al.*, 1999). *Pilea imparifolia* stem decoction is drunk for diarrhoea in western Panama (Joly *et al.*, 1987).

Pityrogramma calomelanos methanolic extract has cytotoxic properties (Sukumaran and Kuttan, 1991).

Portulaca oleracea and *Portulaca* species are used in Arabian countries, Almería, Spain, Peru, Madeira, Jordan, India, Pakistan, Nicaragua and Nepal as a diuretic, laxative, for blood purification, for reducing ulcers, for liver problems, tumours and inflammation (Barrett, 1994; Rivera and Obón, 1995; Martínez Lirola *et al.*, 1996; Chan *et al.*, 2000; Joshi and Joshi, 2000; Afifi and Abu-Irmaileh, 2000; Ahmad and Beg, 2001). Ethanolic extracts have analgesic and antiinflammatory activities comparable to the synthetic drug sodium diclofenac (Chan *et al.*, 2000). Previous studies have investigated muscle relaxant activity, effect on blood pressure, neuropharmacology and anticonvulsant activity (Chan *et al.*, 2000). The muscle relaxant properties of *Portulaca oleracea* are associated with high concentrations of potassium ions (Habtemariam *et al.*, 1993). The diterpenoid (pilosanone C) is found in *Portulaca pilosa* (Ohsaki *et al.*, 1995).

Ruellia species are used traditionally for sexually transmitted diseases. In Barbados *Ruellia tuberosa* is used for intestinal inflammation, blood disorders, cystitis and enteritis (Ahmad *et al.*, 1993; Handler and Jacoby, 1993). *Ruellia patula* yielded two lignan glycosides (Ahmad *et al.*, 1993).

Sansevieria guineensis originates in South Africa (Comerford, 1996; Franssen *et al.*, 1997). The methanol extract of the whole plant of *Sansevieria trifasciata* yielded 12 steroidal saponins and four pregnane glycosides (Mimaki *et al.*, 1996, 1997).

Scoparia dulcis was used in Barbados as a diuretic prior to 1834 (Handler and Jacoby, 1993). Freire *et al.* (1991) reported analgesic and antiinflammatory activity from water and ethanolic extracts of *Scoparia dulcis* related to the triterpene glutinol. The diterpene acid, scoparic acid A is a beta-glucuronidase inhibitor (Hayashi *et al.*, 1992). Antiviral diterpenoids and triterpenoids have been found in *Scoparia dulcis* (Mahato *et al.*, 1981; Morton, 1981; Asano *et al.*, 1990; Hayashi *et al.*, 1988, 1990; Heinrich *et al.*, 1992; Lachman-White *et al.*, 1992).

An infusion of the powdered or macerated *Solanum melongena* (eggplant) fruit is used to reduce serum cholesterol in Almería, Spain and Brazil (Martínez Lirola *et al.*, 1996; Guimaraes *et al.*, 2000). Flavonoids extracted from its fruits showed potent antioxidant activity and significant hypolipidemic action in normal and cholesterol fed rats. A significant increase in the concentrations of hepatic and faecal bile acids and faecal neutral sterols was also observed indicating a higher rate of degradation of cholesterol (Sudheesh *et al.*, 1997, 1999). *Solanum melongena* infusion reduced the blood levels of total and LDL cholesterol and of apolipoprotein B in humans. This effect was modest and transitory (Guimaraes *et al.*, 2000). *Solanum melongena* peels contain an anthocyanin (nasunin) which is a potent O2*-scavenger and iron chelator that can protect against lipid peroxidation (Noda *et al.*, 1998). A lipoxygenase was also found in eggplant fruits (Nakayama *et al.*, 1995). *Solanum surrattense* was included in a twelve-herb mixture used to effectively treat bovine urolithiasis (Sugimoto *et al.*, 1992). *Solanum americanum* leaf extracts were active against *Microsporum gypseum* and *Cryptococcus neoformans* and showed intraperitoneal subacute toxicity in mice (Cáceres *et al.*, 1998; Muñoz *et al.*, 2000a).

The analgesic effect of *Stachytarpheta jamaicensis* was evaluated in rats and showed a lesser effect than morphine (Robineau, 1991).

Theobroma cacao whole plant contains epicatechin, gentistic acid (2,5-dihydroxybenzoic acid) and leucocyanidins (Ortiz de Montellano, 1975). The leaves of *Theobroma cacao* contain chlorogenic acid, the flavonoid rutin, and glycosides of cyanidin). Seeds of *Theobroma cacao* contain caffeine (0.3%) and theobromine (1.5%) and p-hydroxybenzoic acid, syringic acid, vanillic acid and ferulic acid. Theobromine is a diuretic, stimulant and smooth muscle dilator (Ortiz de Montellano, 1975).

Vetiveria zizanioides is used by the Caribs in Guatemala for urinary infections (Girón *et al.*, 1991).

Zea mays corn silk or stigma/style has been included in the British Pharmaceutical Codex (1934) and the British Herbal Pharmacopoeia (1983, 1990). These monographs have listed the traditional uses of corn silk for cystitis, urethritis, nocturnal enuresis, prostatitis and for acute or chronic inflammation of the urinary system (Habtemariam, 1998). Studies have shown *in vivo* diuretic and hypotensive activity (Habtemariam, 1998). Corn silk contains amines, fixed oils, saponins, tannins, bitter glycosides, allantoin, cryptoxanthin, flavone and phytosterols including beta-sitosterol and stigmasterol. The last two compounds are known to have antiinflammatory activity *in vivo* and may have a beneficial effect in treating prostate problems (Habtemariam, 1998).

More data is necessary to evaluate the safety of the following plants used for urinary problems, "cooling" and high cholesterol levels: *Costus scaber*, *Cynodon dactylon*, *Entada polystachya*, *Flemingia strobilifera*, *Gomprena globosa*, *Justicia pectoralis*, *Lepianthes pelata*, *Momordica charantia*, *Nopalea cochenillifera*, *Petiveria alliacea*, *Pityrogramma calomelanos*, *Ruellia tuberosa*, *Sansevieriea guineensis*, *Stachytarpheta jamaicensis*, *Theobroma cacao* and *Vetiveria zizanioides*.
Few studies were found to support the use of the following plants for urinary problems: *Justicia pectoralis*, *Lepianthes pelata*, *Momordica charantia*, *Petiveria alliacea*, *Pityrogramma calomelanos*, *Ruellia tuberosa*, *Sansevieriea guineensis*, *Stachytarpheta jamaicensis*, *Theobroma cacao* and *Vetiveria zizanioides*.

The following plants have established analgesic or sedative effects: *Apium graveolens*, *Bauhinia cumanensis*, *Capraria biflora*, *Chamaesyce hirta* and *Portulaca oleraceae*. *Chamaesyce hirta*, *Cissus verticillata*, *Kalanchoe pinnata*, *Peperomia* spp., *Portulaca oleraceae*, *Scoparia dulcis*, and *Zea mays* have sufficient evidence to support their traditional use for urinary problems, cooling and high cholesterol. The use of eggplant extract as a hypocholesterolemic agent has some support but needs more study. *Cuscuta americana* also merits more study.

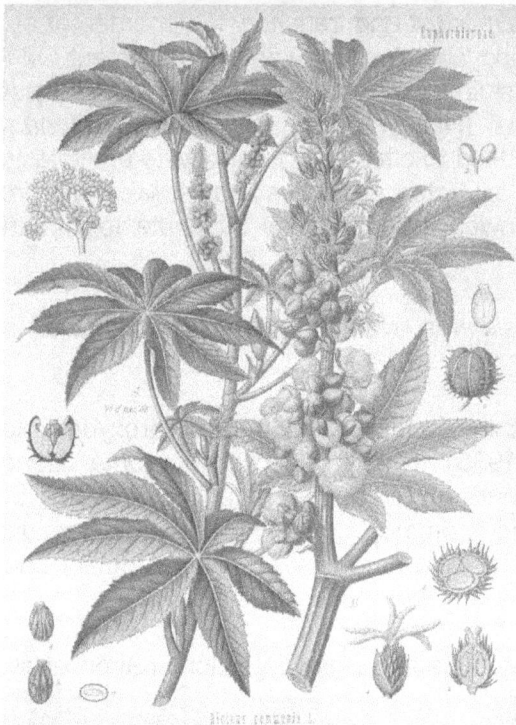

Figure 88. Ricinus communis
Figure 89.Aristolochia rugosa

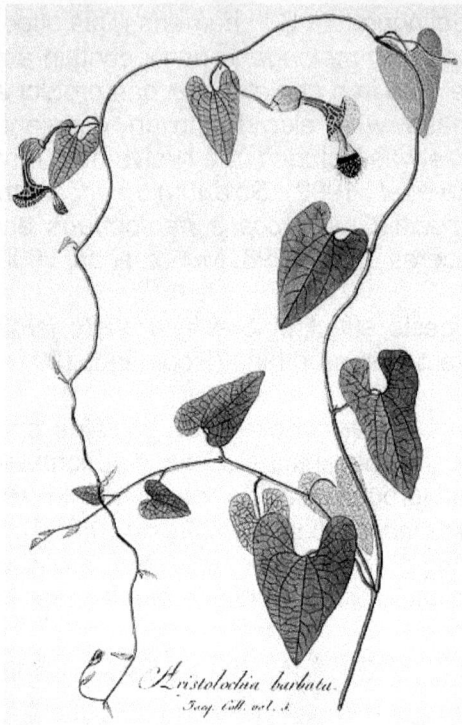

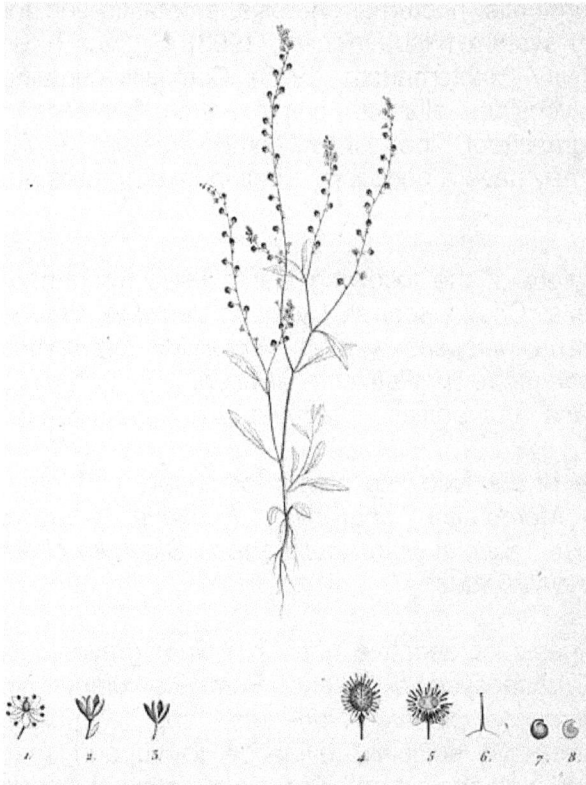

Figure 90. Microtea maypurensis
Figure 91. Dorstenia contrayerva

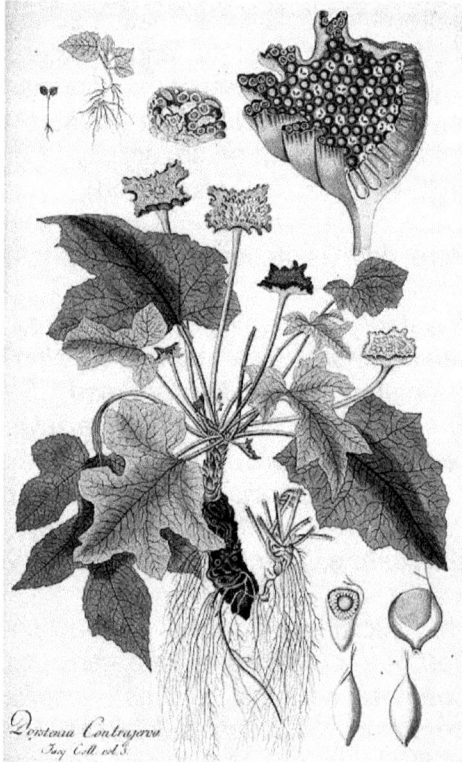

Non-experimental validation of plants used for high blood pressure, jaundice and diabetes

Alleyne and Cruickshank (1990) did not find any difference between non-users of informal medication and those who used it in addition to, or in replacement of, formal medication to control diabetes mellitus in Jamaica. However teas made from periwinkle (*Catharantus* species) and rice bitters (*Andrographics paniculata*) interfered with the control of diabetes. In a previous study, with more severe cases of diabetes, the authors found that formal medication gave better control of the diabetes than folk medicine teas (Alleyne *et al.*, 1979). Guilliford and Mahabir (1997) studied 622 people with diabetes mellitus in Trinidad and Tobago. Herbal remedies for diabetes were used by 152 (24%) of patients. Caraaili, aloes, olive bush and seed-under-leaf were the plants most frequently used. Patients who reported burning or numbness in the feet or feelings of tiredness, weakness, giddiness or dizziness used bush medicines more frequently than those who reported other symptoms (Guilliford and Mahabir, 1997). A small percentage of pregnant women treated at the Mount Hope Women's Hospital experienced hypertension (Ali, 1995).

Antigonon leptopus Hook & Arn is used in Mexico and Haiti (Zamora-Martínez and Nieto de Pascual Pola, 1992; Duke, 2000). The flowers contain several compounds and the plant contains flavonoids, alkaloids and saponins (Ahmad and Khan, 1991; Facey *et al.*, 1999; Duke, 2000).

Apium graveolens (celery) aqueous extract has an antihyperlipidemic property which was not due to 3-n-butylphthalide (BuPh) (BuPh was previously reported to produce the lipid-lowering action in celery) (Tsi *et al.*, 1995). Apigenin, isolated from *Apium graveolens*, relaxes rat thoracic aorta (Ko *et al.*, 1991). *Apium graveolens* has antiinflammatory activity (Al-Hindawi *et al.*, 1989).

Artocarpus altilis (Parkinson) Fosberg. (syn. *Artocarpus communis*) leaves were used in Jamaica for high blood pressure (Asprey and Thornton, 1953-1955). Leaves are used to treat liver diseases, hypertension, fevers and for their antiinflammatory and detoxifying properties (Lin *et al.*, 1992; Chen *et al.*, 1993). *Artocarpus altilis* contains camphorol, HCN, quercetin (Duke, 2000). Three prenylflavones and three flavonoids were isolated from the ethanol extract of dried stems (Chen *et al.*, 1993). Other constituents are listed by Dunstan *et al.* (1997). A geranylated chalcone was isolated from leaves of *Artocarpus incisus* and it showed potent 5-alpha-reductase inhibitory activity (Shimiz *et al.*, 2000). An extract of the leaves of *Artocarpus altilis* exerted a negative inotrophic effect on rat myocardium (Young *et al.*, 1993).

Bidens pilosa is used in western Cameroon and in Central America for the management of problems related to high blood pressure (Tan *et al.*, 2000). *Bidens pilosa* aqueous leaf extract possesses aortic smooth muscle relaxant activity (Dimo *et al.*, 1998). Several compounds are found in *Bidens* species including alkaloids, saponins, flavonoids (quercetin), polyacetylenes, triterpenes, sterols, flavones and sesquiterpenes (Hoffman and Hölzl, 1987; Hoffman and Hölzl, 1988; Sarg *et al.*, 1991; Alarcon de la Lastra *et al.*, 1994; Zulueta *et al.*, 1995; Alvarez *et al.*, 1996; Chin *et al.* 1996; Martin Calero *et al.*, 1996; Chippaux *et al.*, 1997; Brandão *et al.*, 1998; Alvarez *et al.*, 1999; Tan *et al.*, 2000). Sarg *et al.* (1991) and Ubillas *et al.* (2000) found that *Bidens pilosa* showed decrease of blood glucose possibly caused by polyacetylenic glucosides.

Bixa orellana is used in Trinidad and in Central America for diabetes, as a diuretic, for oliguria, as a purgative and for stomatitis (Duke, 2000). *Bixa orellana* root decoction is also used for diabetes by the Caribs of Guatemala (Girón *et al.*, 1991).

The ethnomedicinal use of *Bontia daphnoides* for hypertension and nephritis in Trinidad has been previously recorded (Wong, 1976). The use of *Bontia daphnoides* for jaundice may be related to its use for urinary problems as recorded by Wong (1976).

The fruit juice of unripened fruit of *Carica papaya* probably contains antihypertensive agent(s) which exhibit(s) alpha-adrenoceptor activity (Eno *et al.*, 2000).

Catharanthus roseus is used in Mauritius and Rodrigues for diabetes and fever (Gurib-Fakim *et al.*, 1993). Active principles are three alkaloids: leurosine, vindoline and vindolinine which are more potent than tolbutamide as hypoglycaemic agents (Oliver Bever, 1986).

Cecropia species are used for high blood pressure in Barbados and Panama and for diabetes in Mexico (Jiu, 1966; Honychurch, 1986; Caballero-George *et al.*, 2001).

Citrus sinensis root is used in Nicaragua for high blood pressure (Barrett, 1994). *Citrus aurantium* leaf decoction is taken for high blood pressure in Curaçao (Morton, 1968b). *Citrus* species are used in Spain as digestives (Vázquez *et al.*, 1997).

Cocos nucifera kernel is reported to contain a mannan (Kapoor, 1990). The juice from the flower stalk is used in India as a diuretic and laxative.

Cola nitida is chewed by Nigerians habitually. *Cola nitida* nuts contain a heart stimulant called kolanin, and also contain caffeine, theobromine and quinine which are associated with increased blood pressure (Osim and Udia, 1993).

The ethnomedicinal use of *Crescentia cujete* for high blood pressure in Trinidad has been previously recorded (Wong, 1976). *Crescentia cujete* is used for diabetes in Curaçao (Morton, 1968b). The pulp contains polyphenols, lipophile chromophores, quaternary alkaloids, hydrocyanic acid, crescentic, tartaric, citric, tannic and chlorogenic acids (Morton, 1968a; Robineau, 1991).

Cuscuta americana is used in India, Maderia, Mauritius and Rodrigues to 'purify the blood', against gout and for bilious conditions (Asprey and Thornton, 1953-1955; Gurib-Fakim *et al.*, 1993; Rivera and Obón, 1995). *Cuscuta reflexa* is used for jaundice in Pakistan (Shinwari and Khan, 2000). At high doses *Cuscuta* species can cause fatal gastro-intestinal toxicity (Muñoz *et al.*, 2000b).

Wong (1976) has recorded the use of *Gomphrena globosa* for oliguria, hypertension and diabetes in Trinidad. *Gomphrena martiana* and *Gomphrena boliviana* yielded five 5,6,7-trisubstituted flavones and a lipophilic flavonoid fraction (Pomilio *et al.*, 1992; Pomilio *et al.*, 1994). The ethnomedicinal use of *Gomphrena globosa* for jaundice may be related to its use for urinary problems as recorded by Wong (1976).

Hibiscus sabdariffa has been used ethnomedicinally as a cholagogue, choleretic, diuretic and for hypertension (Duke, 2000). *Hibiscus sabdariffa* contains flavanoids, polysaccharides and organic acids (Dafallah and al-Mustafa, 1996).

Laportea aestuans Chew and *Laportea crenulata* have been used ethnomedicinally for dysentery, oliguria, as a diuretic and for biliousness (Duke, 2000).

Momordia charantia is widely used in the Caribbean for hypertension and diabetes (Guilliford and Mahabir, 1997; Muñoz *et al.*, 2000a). In normal mice intraperitoneal administration of *Momordica charantia* aqueous extract improved glucose tolerance in normal mice after eight hours and reduced the level of hyperglycaemia in streptozotocin diabetic mice by 50% after five hours (Bailey *et al.*, 1985).

Morus alba is used for hypertension in Spain and as a hypoglycaemic in the Spanish Mediterranean, in Turkey and in Chile (Ríos *et al.*, 1987; Vázquez *et al.*, 1997; Lemus *et al.*, 1999; Yeşilada *et al.*, 1999). The hypoglycaemic activity of a 20% dried leaf infusion of *Morus alba*, was not verified in alloxan and streptozotocin induced hyperglycaemic rats (Lemus *et al.*, 1999). Active principles were thought to be cyanidin, delphinidin glucosides as well as phytosterol glycocides (Oliver Bever, 1986). *Morus alba* leaves contain several flavonoids, two of which exerted significant inhibitory effect on the growth of the human promyelocytic leukaemia cell line and significant free radical scavenging effects (Kim *et al.*, 1999; Kim *et al.*, 2000). P-cresol, phenol and morin were identified in the leaves (Ahmad and Beg, 2001).

Nopalea cochenillifera is used in traditional medicine as a depurative and for inflammations (Duke, 2000)

Ocimum campechianum (syn. *Ocimum micranthum*) is used in Brazil for intestinal disturbances. *Ocimum campechianum* contains 1,8-cineole, alpha-pinene, beta-elemene, gamma-elemene, linalool, sabinene, thymol, eugenol and elemol among others (Vieira and Simon, 2000).

Passiflora quadrangularis is used for hypertension and diabetes in Trinidad (Wong, 1976; Joly *et al.*, 1987). The whole plant contains nor-epinephrine and 5-hydroxytryptamine; a cyclopropane triterpene glycoside (quadranguloside) was isolated from the leaves (Joly *et al.*, 1987). Sixteen flavonoids were isolated from the leaves of *Passiflora sexflora* (Joly *et al.*, 1987).

Persea americana leaves are used for high blood pressure and pains in Jamaica, Panama and Nigeria (Asprey and Thornton, 1953-1955; Adeboye *et al.*, 1999; Caballero-George *et al*, 2001). Intravenous administration of methanol and aqueous extracts of *Persea americana* to anaesthetised normotensive rats produced a fall in mean arterial blood pressure which lasted less than five minutes (Adeboye *et al.*, 1999). The short duration of this effect may indicate rapid metabolism of the active principles (steroid and triterpene glycosides).

Petiveria alliacea has shown a hypoglycemic active principle in the leaves and stems of the plant (Lores and Cires Pujol, 1990). Extracts from leaves and stem powder were found to produce a decrease of blood sugar concentration of more than 60% one hour after oral administration in male Balb/C mice (Lores and Cires Pujol, 1990). Alpha-sitosterol in the plant has antihypercholesesterolemic and antiprostatic activities (Duke, 1989) Clinical trials have demonstrated analgesic effects and the plant has been shown to have anticonvulsant properties (Morton, 1980; Elisabetsky and Wannmacher, 1993).

Phyllanthus urinaria and *Phyllanthus niruri* are used for diabetes and bladder calculus in Trinidad and Tobago in Perú and other countries (Desmarchelier *et al.*, 1996; Guilliford and

Mahabir, 1997; Santos *et al.*, 2000). Some *Phyllanthus* species have shown activity against the hepatitis B virus and HIV type 1 (Rajeshkumar and Kuttan, 2000; Santos *et al.*, 2000).

Spiranthes autumnalis and *Spiranthes diuretica* are used as depuratives, tonics and diuretics (Duke, 2000).

Tamarindus indicus is used ethnomedicinally in Mexico (Duke, 2000). *Tamarindus indicus* aqueous extract presented protective activity against lipid peroxidation (Joyeux *et al.*, 1995).

Tournefortia hirsutissima plant was used in Jamaica and Mexico for diabetes (Steggerda, 1929; Duke, 2000). *Tournefortia hirsutissima* is used in Latin America as a diuretic, for infections, skin problems and venereal diseases (Duke, 2000). Alarcon-Aguilara *et al. (*1998) found that *Tournefortia hirsutissima* had a antihyperglycaemic effect validating its clinical use in diabetes mellitus control.

The plants used for hypertension, jaundice and diabetes that may be safe and justify more formal evaluation are *Annona squamosa, Aloe vera, Apium graveolens, Bidens alba, Carica papaya, Catharanthus roseus, Cecropia peltata, Citrus paradisi, Hibsicus sabdariffa, Momordica charantia, Morus alba, Persea americana, Phyllanthus urinaria, Tamarindus indicus* and *Tournefortia hirsutissima*. Several of the plants are used for more than one condition and further trials should take this into account.

Conclusion

The following plants used for eye problems, headaches, dental problems etc., have been understudied and therefore few claims can be made about their validity: *Lepianthes peltata, Musa species, Ocimum gratissimum, Piper hispidum, Ricinus communis, Senna occidentalis* and *Tagetes patula.* More studies are needed to establish the validity of the following plants for their respective uses: *Acnistus arborescens, Capraria biflora, Chrysobalanus icaco, Citrus nobilis, Cocos nucifera, Crescentia cujete, Kalanchoe pinnata, Rosmarinus officinalis* and *Spondias mombin.* Some of the plants such as *Annona muricata, Aristolochia trilobata, Chrysobalanus icaco,* and *Datura stramonium* may produce minor to serious side effects.
More formal evaluation of the plants used to improve glycaemic control and for hypertension is justified: *Annona squamosa, Aloe vera, Apium graveolens, Bidens alba, Carica papaya, Catharanthus roseus, Cecropia peltata, Citrus paradisi, Hibsicus sabdariffa, Momordica charantia, Morus alba, Persea americana, Phyllanthus urinaria, Tamarindus indicus* and *Tournefortia hirsutissima.*
The use of eggplant extract as a hypocholesterolemic agent has some support but needs more study.
Chamaesyce hirta, Cissus verticillata, Kalanchoe pinnata, Peperomia spp., *Portulaca oleraceae, Scoparia dulcis,* and *Zea mays* have sufficient evidence to support their traditional use for urinary problems, "cooling" and high cholesterol.

Non experimental validation of plants used for skin and stomach problems in Trinidad and Tobago

Plants used for skin problems
Twelve plants are used for skin problems including one for the rash caused by measles plus one for shingles. The thirteen plants belong to nine plant families.

Table 8. Ethnomedicinal plants used for skin problems in Trinidad and Tobago

Scientific name	Family	Common name	Plant part used	Use
Achyranthes indica	Amaranthaceae	Man better man		Skin problems
Acnistus arborescens	Solanaceae	Wild tobacco	Leaves	Bathe babies for eczema
Azadirachta indica	Meliaceae	Neem	Leaves	Measles
Bidens alba / Bidens pilosa	Asteraceae	Needle grass/ Railway daisy	Leafy branch	Bathe children
Cassia alata	Fabaceae-Caesalpiniaceae	Senna	Leaves	Skin problems
Chamaesyce hirta / hypericifolia	Euphorbiaceae	Malomay	Flower	Skin rashes, measles
Croton gossypifolius	Euphorbiaceae	Blood bush/ Bois sang	Leaves	Bathe babies for eczema
Eclipta prostrata	Asteraceae	Congolala		Bathe for children's malnutrition for 9 days & woodlice nest
Manihot esculenta	Euphorbiaceae	Cassava	Leaves	Bathe babies for eczema
Origanum vulgare	Lamiaceae	Majoram		Bathe babies
Sida carpinifolia (syn. *Sida acuta*)	Malvaceae	Garaba broom	Leaf	Eczema
Solanum americanum	Solanaceae	Agouma, gouma	Plant	Bathe for children's malnutrition
Spondias mombin	Anacardiaceae	Hogplum	Leaves	Eczema

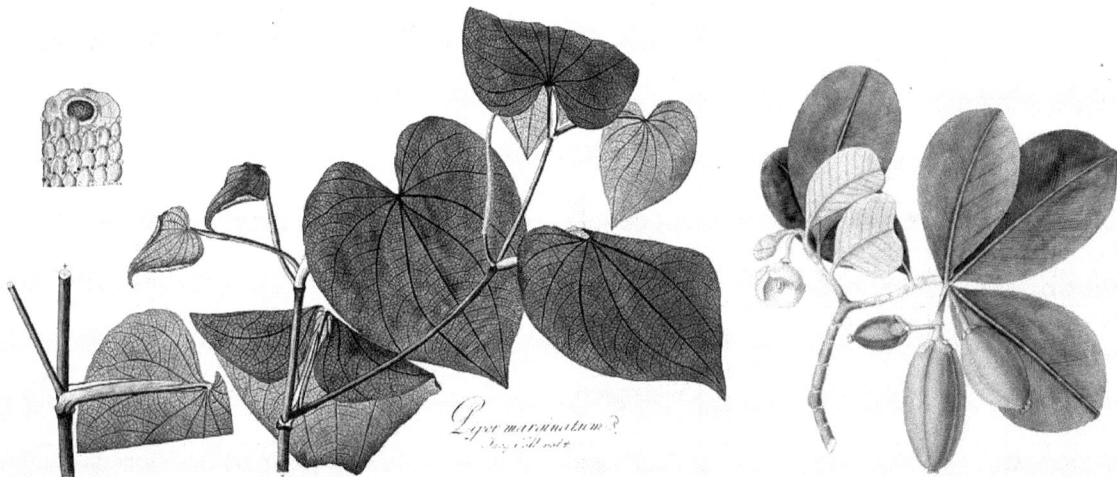

Figure 92. Piper marginatum
Figure 93. Clusia alba

Plants used for stomach problems, pain, internal parasites

The medicinal plants used for stomach problems, injuries, endoparasites, arthritis and bites are combined in Table 9. This grouping partially reflects the analgesic activity of many of the plants used. Eighteen plants are used for stomach problems including diarrhoea. Another fifteen plants are used for various kinds of pain including cuts, bites, sprains and arthritis. Four plants are used as anthelmintics. Other plants in the table are used for dropsy (congestive heart failure?). Twenty-seven plant families are represented in this table.

Table 9. Plants used for stomach problems, pain and internal parasites in Trinidad

Scientific name	Family	Common name	Part used	Use
Abelmoschus moschatus	Malvaceae	Gumbo musque	Seeds	Grind in rum for foot cramp
A. melegueta	Zingiberaceae	Guinea pepper	Seeds	Carminative
Ambrosia cumanenesis	Asteraceae	Altamis	Bark	Stomach pain, 2*3 inch piece bark in urine for 3 days use to wash foot for 3 days for arthritis
A. rugosa, trilobata	Aristolochiaceae	Mat root, anico	Root	Stomach pain, colic, poisoning
B. vulgaris	Poaceae	Bamboo	Leaves	Poultice
Bidens alba / Bidens pilosa	Asteraceae	Needle grass	Leafy branch	Cuts
Bixa orellana	Bixaceae	Roucou	Root	Dropsy
Brownea latifolia	Fabaceae	Cooper hoop	Flower, leaves	Gripe, pain
Cajanus cajan	Fabaceae	Pigeon pea	Leaves	Food poisoning, colic, constipation
C. biflora	Scrophulariaceae	Du thé pays	Leaves	Flavour for purgative
Cecropia peltata	Cecropiaceae	Bois canôt	Stem	3 'Ridges' from inside stem boiled as a carminative
Centropogon cornutus	Campanulaceae	Deer meat, crepe coq	Leaves	Snake, scorpion bite
C. hirta	Euphorbiaceae	Malomay		Diarrhoea
Citharexylum spinosum	Verbenaceae	Bois côtelette	Leaf	Anthelmintic
Cocos nucifera	Arecaceae	Coconut	Root, 7 ins, Shell	Dropsy, Hernia
Cola nitida	Sterculiaceae	Obie seed	Seed	Any kind of pain
Cucurbita maxima	Cucurbitaceae	Pumpkin	Seeds	Anthelmintic
Cucurbita pepo	Cucurbitaceae	Pumpkin		Sprains, breaks
Dorstenia contrayerva	Moraceae	Refriyau		Food poisoning
Eleusine indica	Poaceae	Pied poule		Diarrhoea

Table 9. Plants used for stomach problems, pain and internal parasites in Trinidad (cont.)

Scientific name	Family	Common name	Part used	Use
Eupatorium macrophyllum	Asteraceae	Z'herbe chatte		Pain
Eupatorium triplinerve	Asteraceae	Ayapana, japanned	Leaves	Stomach problems (worms)
Ferula asafoetida	Apiaceae	Asafoetida		Carminative
Jatropha curcas/ gossypifolia	Euphorbiaceae	White/Red Physic Nut	Leaf	Clean sores
Scientific name	Family	Common name	Part used	Use
Momordica charantia	Cucurbitaceae	Caraaili	Vine	Stomach problems
Morinda citrifolia	Rubiaceae	Noni	Leaves	Pains
Neurolaena lobata	Asteraceae	Z'herbe á pique	Leaves	Tincture for arthritis
Nicotiana tabacum	Solanaceae	Tobacco	Leaves	Arthritis
Nopalea cochenillifera	Cactaceae	Rachette	Joint	Snake bites
Peperomia rotundifolia	Piperaceae	Mowon		Diarrhoea
Petiveria alliacea	Phytolaccaceae	Mapourite		Arthritis and rheumatism
Phyllanthus urinaria	Euphorbiaceae	Red seed under leaf	Plant	Diarrhoea
Portulaca oleraceae	Portulacaceae	Pussley	Plant	Anthelmintic
Punica granatum	Punicaceae	Pome-granate	Seeds	Stomach problems
Rosmarinus officinalis	Lamiaceae	Rosemary	Leaf	Arthritis, Snake bites
Scoparia dulcis	Scrophulariaceae	Sweet broom	Root	Diarrhoea
Solanum melongena	Solanaceae	Melongene	Fruit	Breaks
Tagetes patula	Asteraceae	Marigold		Anthelmintic
Tamarindus indicus	Fabaceae	Tamarind		Scorpion bite
Tournefortia hirsutissima	Boraginaceae	Chigger bush	Leaves	Tea, carminative, chiggers[22]

---

[22] "Tis now the vampire's bleak abode, Tis now the apartment of the toad: ' Tis here the painful Chegoe feeds,

Non-experimental validation of plants used for skin problems

Achyranthes aspera leaf paste is applied on cuts, boils and blisters in Uttar Pradesh, India (Singh and Maheshwari, 1994). *Achyranthes bidentata* is a commonly used Chinese medicinal plant and is used in Nepal and in Mauritius and Rodrigues for skin diseases (Gurib-Fakim *et al.*, 1993; Zeng *et al.*, 1994).

Acnistus arborescens in Brazil contains a withanolide (Barata *et al.*, 1970).

Azadirachta indica oil has proved useful for wound healing (Bhargava *et al.*, 1989). Charles and Charles (1992) found that a paste made of *Azadirachta indica* and *Curcuma longa* used to treat 814 people with scabies cured 97% of them within three to five days of treatment.

Bidens pilosa is used as a bath for children (malaise or susto) for high temperatures and is applied externally to cure wounds in Guatemala, Madeira and Porto Santo Islands (Rivera and Obón, 1995; Tan *et al.*, 2000). Infusions of *Bidens aurea* are used in northwest Spain as sedatives (Blanco *et al.*, 1999). Geissberger and Sequin (1991) found that extracts of dried aerial parts of *Bidens pilosa* showed some antimicrobial activity. Similar results were found by Sarg *et al.* (1991), Rabe and van Staden (1997) and Alvarez *et al.* (1996) (*Pseudomonas aeruginosa*, *Trycophyton mentagrophytes*, and *Microsporum gypseum*). Components of the extract such as phenylheptatriyne, linolic acid and linolenic acid have antimicrobial activities (Alvarez *et al.*, 1999).
The triterpenes as well as several flavonoids (aurones, chalcones) are antiinflammatory agents (Alvarez *et al.*, 1999). The chloroform fractions from the roots of *Bidens aurea* caused 86% inhibition of parasite growth *in vitro*.

The constituents of *Bidens pilosa* explain the use of this plant in traditional medicine in the treatment of wounds, against inflammations and against bacterial infections of the gastrointestinal tract (Geissberger and Sequin, 1991). *Bidens pilosa* was screened for prostaglandin-synthesis inhibition and showed a high activity (Jager *et al.*, 1996).

Cassia alata is used for skin problems in the Caribbean, India and the Ivory Coast (West Africa) to treat bacterial infections caused by *Escherichia coli*, and fungal infections caused by *Candida albicans* and dermatophytes (Honychurch, 1986; Murdiati and Manurung, 1991; Crockett *et al.*, 1992). *Cassia alata* has antifungal activity that may be attributed to chrysophanol (Palanichamy and Nagarajan, 1990). When *Cassia alata* extracts were evaluated relative to a standard antibacterial agent chloramphenicol and antifungal agent amphotericin B and found to have therapeutic potential for the treatment of opportunistic infections of AIDS patients (Crockett *et al.*, 1992). A 10-year human study indicated that a *Cassia alata* leaf extract can be reliably used as a herbal medicine to treat *Pityriasis versicolor*. The leaf extract contains anthraquinones, flavonoids, quinones and sterols and had no side-effects (Damodaran and Venkataraman, 1994). An ethanolic extract of *Cassia alata* leaves showed high *in vitro* activity against various species of dermatophytic fungi, but low activity against non-dermatophytic fungi (Ibrahim and Osman, 1995). Bacterial and yeast species showed resistance against *in vitro* treatment with the extract.

Chamaesyce hirta is used in West Bengal for ringworm (Mukhopadhyay *et al.*, 1995).
Antibacterial effects of *Chamaesyce hirta* leaves were found by several investigators (Emele *et al.*, 1998; Vijaya *et al.*, 1995). An aqueous extract of *Chamaesyce hirta*, strongly reduced the release of prostaglandins I2, E2, and D2. Additionally *Chamaesyce hirta* extracts exerted

---

'Tis here the dire Labarri breeds, Conceal'd in ruins, moss, and weeds.' (Waterton, 1973)

an inhibitory effect on platelet aggregation and depressed the formation of carrageenin-induced rat paw oedema.

Barks of *Croton* species produce a red viscous latex which is used in South America for wound healing and is used by the Zapotecs of Oaxaca, Mexico for dermatological conditions (Frei *et al.*, 1998; Pieters *et al.*, 1993). *Croton lechleri* tree sap contains an alkaloid (taspine) which was responsible for cicatrizant activity in mice (Fernández *et al.*, 1997). In Belize *Croton schiedeanus* is used as a bath tonic (Arnason *et al.*, 1980). *Croton guatemalensis* was active against *Candida albicans* (Cáceres *et al.*, 1991b). A biologically active lignan did not stimulate the cell proliferation needed for wound healing but inhibited thymidine incorporation, while protecting cells against degradation in a starvation medium (Pieters *et al.*, 1993). The sap was not cytotoxic but contained simple phenolic compounds and diterpenes which showed potent antibacterial activity (Chen *et al.*, 1994).

Eclipta prostrata contains steroidal alkaloids, resin, sulphur-containing peptides, coumestans, flavonoids, polyacetylenes, antiviral ingredients and tannins (Abdel-Kader *et al.*, 1998; Hudson, 1990; Kapoor, 1990; Melo *et al.*, 1994; Saxena *et al.*, 1993). The hydroalcoholic extract of *Eclipta prostrata* plant showed antinociceptive and antiinflammatory effects (Leal *et al.*, 2000).

The use of *Manihot esculenta* in Trinidad for boils, marasmus and sores has been previously recorded (Wong, 1976).

Sida acuta is used in Oaxaca, Mexico for dermatological conditions (Zamora-Martínez and Nieto de Pascual Pola, 1992; Frei *et al.*, 1998). *Sida rhombifolia* leaf paste is used in Uttar Pradesh India and in Madeira for cuts, open sores and boils (Singh and Maheshwari, 1994; Rivera and Obón, 1995). In previous studies alcoholic leaf extracts of *Sida cordifolia* and *Sida rhombifolia* showed antibacterial and antifungal activity in contrast *Sida acuta* did not show activity in this 1999 study or in previous ones (Oliver Bever, 1986; Perumal Samy *et al.*, 1999). Phytochemical analysis of the leaves of *Sida cordifolia* showed the presence of sympathomimetic amines, ephedrine and pseudoephedrine (a potent vasoconstrictor), and alkaloids (vasocinone and vasicine) (Franzotti *et al.*, 2000). *Sida cordifolia* aqueous extract exerts antiinflammatory and analgesic properties by interfering with the cyclooxygenase pathway (Franzotti *et al.*, 2000). *Sida rhombifolia* contains ascorbic, malvalic and sterculic acids, vasicine, choline, betaine, ephedrine, campesterol, minerals, vitamins and saponin (Dunstan *et al.*, 1997; Duke, 2000).

Solanum americanum is used in refreshing baths in the Caribbean and is used in Latin America against dermatomucosal infections, leucorrhoea and vaginitis (Honychurch, 1986; Cáceres *et al.*, 1998). *Solanum torvum* is used by the Zapotecs of Oaxaca, Mexico for dermatological conditions (Frei *et al.*, 1998). *Solanum nigrescens* extracts were active against *Candida albicans* and dermatophytes. The anti-yeast activity is attributed to spirostanol glucosides (Cáceres *et al.*, 1998; Muñoz *et al.*, 2000a). *Solanum surattense* showed antipyretic activity comparable to aspirin (Vedavathy and Rao, 1991).

Spondias mombin leaf poultice is used to bathe sores by the Caribs (Honychurch, 1986).

Non-experimental validation of plants used for stomach problems, pain and internal parasites

The use of *Abelmoschus moschatus* in Trinidad for rheumatism has been previously recorded (Wong, 1976).

Aframomum melegueta is used in India as a carminative (Duke, 2000). *Aframomum melegueta* contains alkaloids (piperine), essential oils and resins (van Harten, 1970).

Ambrosia hispida has been used traditionally for rheumatism (Duke, 2000). An infusion of *Ambrosia hispida* was used by Caribs for worms and in a tea with absinthe for gripe and stomach aches (Honychurch, 1986). The Jamaican *Ambrosia peruviana* contains sesquiterpene lactones and a sesquiterpene diol (Goldsby and Burke, 1987).

Aristolochia species are used by the Amerindians in western Panama, Brazil, Bolivia, Ecuador and French Guyana for diarrhoea and stomach ailments and as analgesics (Joly *et al.*, 1987; Milliken and Albert, 1996). Aristolochic acid shows enhancement of phagocytosis and was formerly used in Europe for that purpose but it was withdrawn due to suspected carcinogenic effects (Wagner, 1990; Kay, 1996; Frei *et al.*, 1998).

In Nepal *Bidens pilosa* is pounded and the juice is used to check bleeding (Joshi and Joshi, 2000). *Bidens pilosa* is used in Cameroon, Brazil and Venezuela for leg ulcers, wounds and chronic ulcers (Tan *et al.*, 2000). Alvarez *et al.* (1996) found bioactive polyacetylenes in the methanolic extract of *Bidens pilosa* (whole plant). The antiinflammatory effect of aqueous extracts of the three plants *Bidens pilosa* var. minor (Blume) Sherff, *Bidens pilosa* and *Bidens chilensis* DC was significant (Chih *et al.*, 1995). The immunosuppressive activity of *Bidens pilosa* is attributed to the polyacetylene isolated from leaves (Pereira *et al.*, 1999). One new compound showed overgrowing action against normal and transformed human cell lines in culture (Alvarez *et al.*, 1996). Mirvish *et al.* (1985) found that *Bidens pilosa* as eaten in South Africa contributes to the aetiology of human oesophageal cancer. Alvarez *et al.* (1996) found insecticidal activity in *Bidens pilosa*. Brandão *et al.* (1997) found antimalarial activity of *Bidens pilosa* related to the presence of aliphatic acetylene compounds.

Bixa orellana has been used ethnomedicinally for dysentery and malaria (Ankli *et al.*, 1999; Duke, 2000).

Brownea latifolia is used ethnomedicinally in Trinidad (Wong, 1976).

Cajanus indicus leaves are used ethnomedicinally in India. A protein was purified from the leaves and may enhance body immunosurveillance (Datta *et al.*, 1999).

Capraria biflora is used in Cuba and Mexico for indigestion and is used for cooling in Martinique (Morton, 1968b; Honychurch, 1986).

Centropogon cornutus is used for ulcers in the Atlantic forests of Brazil (Voeks, 1996).

Chamaesyce hypericifolia causes vomiting and is considered poisonous in Nicaragua (Barrett, 1994). *Chamaesyce hypericifolia* contains caoutchouc, gallic acid, phorbol esters, resin and tannin (Duke, 2000). *Chamaesyce hirta* plant extracts act as antidiarrhoeic agents by a triple pronounced antibacterial, antiamoebic and antispasmodic action. The flavonoid quercitrin is the active compound (Galvez *et al.*, 1993; Tona *et al.*, 1999). Biological activities of *Chamaesyce hirta* were concentrated in the polyphenolic fraction, and not in the saponin or alkaloid-containing fractions (Tona *et al.*, 2000). *Chamaesyce hirta* whole plant extract inhibited *Entamoeba histolytica*, *Vibrio cholerae* and *Shigella flexneri* and showed inhibition of induced contractions on isolated guinea-pig ileum (Vijaya and Ananthan, 1997; Tona *et al.*, 2000).

Citharexylum spinosum is used in the Caribbean and Mexico (Honychurch, 1986; Duke, 2000). *Verbenoxylum reitzii* (Citharexyleae) leaves contain the viroside (10-hydroxy-iridoid) (Von Poser *et al.*, 1995).

Cocos nucifera root decoction is used as a diuretic in India. The red-hot shell is used as a rubefacient (Kapoor, 1990).

Cola nitida nuts contain primary and secondary amines, polyphenols, tannins and caffeine (Atawodi *et al.*, 1995).

Cucurbita species seeds are used as a vermifuge in Jamaica, Turkey, South America, India and Europe (Asprey and Thornton, 1953-1955; Oliver Bever, 1986; Sezik *et al.*, 1997). Cucurbitine is active on trematodes but not against nematodes and cestodes. Cucurbitine is active against Taenia but a purge is necessary to expel the parasite (Oliver Bever, 1986).

Dorstenia contrayerva is used by the Kuna Indians of Panama, in Mexico, Belize and formerly in Jamaica for snakebites, as an anthelmintic and for muscle aches (Arnason *et al.*, 1980; Sheridan, 1991; Terreaux *et al.*, 1995; Tovar-Miranda *et al.*, 1998). *Dorstenia contrayerva* is used in Jamaica, Guatemala, Costa Rica, Panama and Mexico it is used for digestion, diarrhoea, to 'strengthen the stomach', gastrointestinal cramps, and promote diaphoresis and urine (Hazlett, 1986; Sheridan, 1991; Pöll, 1993; Comerford, 1996; Ankli *et al.*, 1999; Duke, 2000). The dichloromethane extract has antimicrobial activity against *B. subtilis* and yielded two furanocoumarins (Terreau *et al.*, 1995). The roots of *Dorstenia contrajerva* contain dihydrofurocoumarin 1b (Tovar-Miranda *et al.*, 1998). Aerial parts of *D. mannii* in Cameroon yielded prenylated flavanones and flavonoids (Ngadjui *et al.*, 2000).

Eleusine indica ethanol extract showed activity against vesicular stomatitis virus (Ali *et al.*, 1996). The plant is reported to contain hydrocyanic acid (Ahmad and Holdsworth, 1994).

Eupatorium macrophyllum tea is used as a carminative in the Caribbean and for headaches by the Shuar in the Ecuadorian Amazon (Honychurch, 1986; Russo, 1992).

Eupatorium triplinerve leaf infusion is used for burning sensations in the stomach, indigestion, diarrhoea, insomnia, nausea, ulcers, vomiting and for respiratory conditions in Trinidad, Mauritius and Rodrigues (Wong, 1976; van den Berg, 1984; Gurib-Fakim *et al.*, 1993). *Eupatorium triplinerve* ethanol extract and its essential oil were active against *Staphylococcus aureus*, *Aspergillus flavus*, *Penicillium digitatum* and *Aspergillus fumigatus* (Verpoorte and Dihal, 1987; Yadava and Saini, 1990).

Asa-foetida is the resin of the root of *Ferula asa-foetida*. Asa-foetida is considered to be a sedative, carminative, antispasmodic, diuretic, and expectorant in Nepal (Eigner and Scholz, 1999). *Ferula asa-foetida* effects a slight inhibition of the growth of *Staphylococcus aureus* and *Shigella sonnei* (Eigner and Scholz, 1999). *Ferula asa-foetida* oleogum resin contains glucuronic acid, galactose, arabinose, rhamnose, sulphur containing compounds, farnesiferoles, umbelliferone and ferulic acid (Eigner and Scholz, 1999).

Momordia charantia is widely used in the Caribbean for digestive troubles and intestinal worms (Muñoz *et al.*, 2000a). *Momordica charantia* was active against *S. aureus* and *Streptococcus* group A (Martínez *et al.*, 1996b; Facey *et al.*, 1999).

Vincent Yáñes, the captain of the caravel Niña dug up *Morinda citrifolia* in Hispaniola on December 30, 1492 (Morison, 1963). *Morinda citrifolia* is used in Nicaragua and Asian countries for inflammation, swelling, infections and for its antiseptic and antibiotic properties and hypotensive and anticoagulant activities (Barrett, 1994; Farine *et al.*, 1996). The ripe fruit contains carboxylic acids (octanoic, decanoic and hexanoic), alchohols, methyl and ethyl esters, ketones, lactones, coumarins (scopoletin) and other compounds (Farine *et al.*, 1996).

Nopalea cochenillifera is used for inflammations in India (Duke, 2000).

Peperomia rubra is used in Peru for intestinal infections and cholera (Jovel *et al.*, 1996). *Peperomia galioides* H.B.K yielded two prenylated quinones and a prenylated dihydroquinone and prenylphenols (Mahiou *et al.*, 1996). Clusifoliol (a prenylated benzopyran derivative) has been isolated from whole plants of *Peperomia clusiifolia* (Seeram *et al.*, 1998). Proctoriones A - C were isolated from the endemic Jamaican species *Peperomia proctorii* (Seeram *et al.*, 2000). Hydropiperone exhibited significant anti-parasitical activity against three species of *Leishmania* (Mahiou *et al.*, 1996). *Peperomia galioides* showed cicatrizant activity in mice (Fernández *et al.*, 1997).

Petiveria alliacea root macerated in alcohol is used for hip and knee osteoarthritis and for rheumatic pain in Brazil (Ferraz *et al.*, 1991; Muñoz *et al.*, 2000a; Bourdy *et al.*, 2000). de Lima *et al.* (1991) found that *Petiveria alliacea* extract showed an antinociceptive effect which may be responsible for its popular use as an analgesic (de Lima *et al.*, 1991).

Portulaca oleracea is used in St. Lucia, Mexico, Venezuela, China, Iraq and in the Malay peninsula as an anthelmintic (Wong, 1976; Didier *et al.*, 1988; Duke, 2000). Extracts of *Portulaca oleracea* are bactericidal (Jimenez Misas *et al.*, 1979). *Portulaca oleracea* contains alkaloids, coumarins, flavonoids, alkanes, waxy esters, caffeic, ferulic and sinapic acids, beta sitosteryl glucoside, lupeol, flavonoids (quercitrin, kaempferol), phytoecdysones, cardiac and anthraquinone glycosides, and a leucocyanidin (Cambie, 1997). The stem contains the acylated betacyanins, oleracin 1 and oleracin II (Cambie, 1997).

Punica granatum has been used since ancient times as an anthelmintic and astringent drug. *Punica granatum* is used for the digestive system in Palestine, Malaysia, India, Mexico, Spain and Sardinia (Bruni *et al.*, 1997; Vázquez *et al.*, 1997; Ong and Norzalina, 1999; Ankli *et al.*, 1999; Ali-Shtayeh *et al.*, 2000; Ahmad and Beg, 2001). Four yellow-coloured ellagitannins were isolated from the pericarp of *Punica granatum*. Tannins and a ellagitannin (punicafolin) were found in the leaves (Tanaka *et al.*, 1985). *Punica granatum* showed activity against *Staphylococcus aureus*, *Escherichia coli*, *Pseudomonas aeruginosa* and *Candida albicans* (Navarro *et al.*, 1996).

Rosmarinus officinalis (tincture of aerial parts) is used in Almería, Spain for rheumatism (Martínez Lirola *et al.*, 1996).

Solanum torvum and *Solanum mammosum* leaf juice is used for ringworm in Belize (Arnason *et al.*, 1980). *Solanum surrantense* is used for breaks in Pakistan (Shinwari and Khan, 2000). *Solanum americanum* extracts were active against *Microsporum gypseum* and

Cryptococcus neoformans and showed intraperitoneal subacute toxicity in mice (Cáceres *et al.*, 1998; Muñoz *et al.*, 2000a).

Scoparia dulcis is used for diarrhoea in Nicaragua (Barrett, 1994).

Tagetes erecta was used by the Aztecs as a diurectic while *Tagetes patula* is currently used in Mauritius and Rodrigues as a mild laxative (Gurib-Fakim *et al.*, 1993; Peña, 1999). *Tagetes lucida* tincture inhibited five bacteria and was active against *Vibrio cholerae* and *Candida albicans* (Cáceres *et al.*, 1991b; Cáceres *et al.*, 1993a). *Tagetes erecta* and *Tagetes filifolia* inhibited two enterobacteria (Cáceres *et al.*, 1993a).

Tamarindus indicus is used ethnomedicinally for fevers and stomach problems (Duke, 2000)

Tournefortia hirsutissima is used in Central America for stomatitis (Duke, 2000). *Tournefortia hirsutissima* has been used in Latin America as a larvicide (Duke, 2000). *Tournefortia densiflora* is used by the Zapotecs in Oaxaca, Mexico for dermatological conditions (Frei *et al.*, 1998). The plant contains sesquiterpene lactones (tagitinins) with reported antitumour activity (Frei *et al.*, 1998).

Conclusion

Plants used for stomach problems, pain and internal parasites that should take priority in clinical trials are *Bambusa vulgaris*, *Bidens alba*, *Jatropha curcas*, *Neurolaena lobata*, *Peperomia rotundifolia* and *Phyllanthus urinaria*.

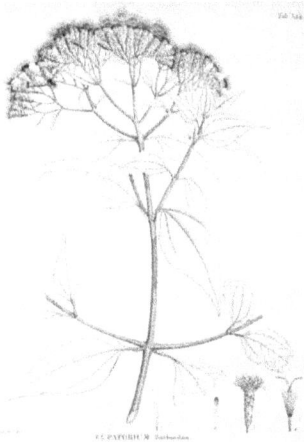

Figure 94. Chromolaena odorata
Figure 95. Curcuma longa
Figure 96. Angostura trifoliata

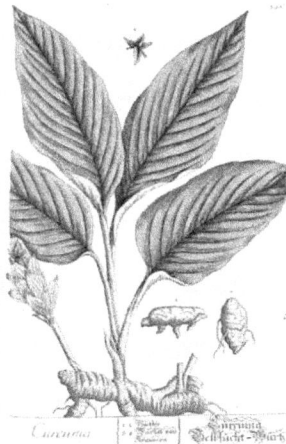

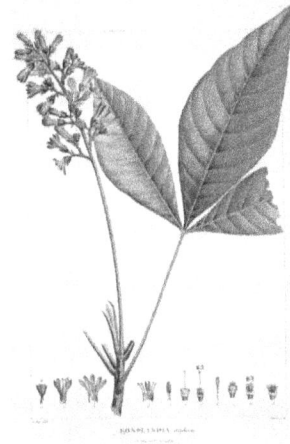

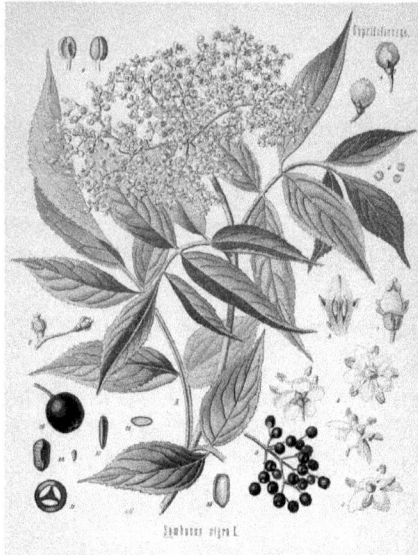

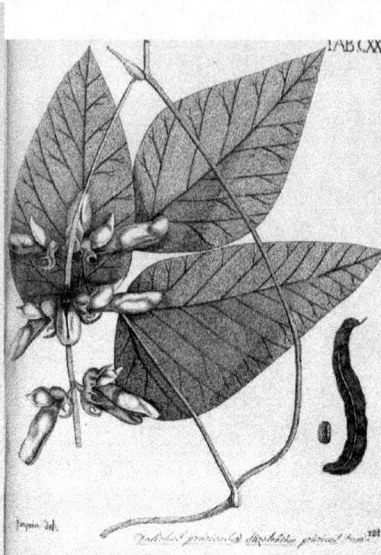

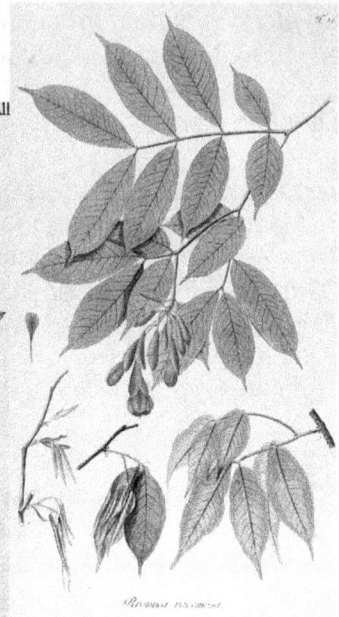

Figure 97. *Sambucus nigra*
Figure 98. *Mucuna pruriens*
Figure 99. *Brownea coccinea*

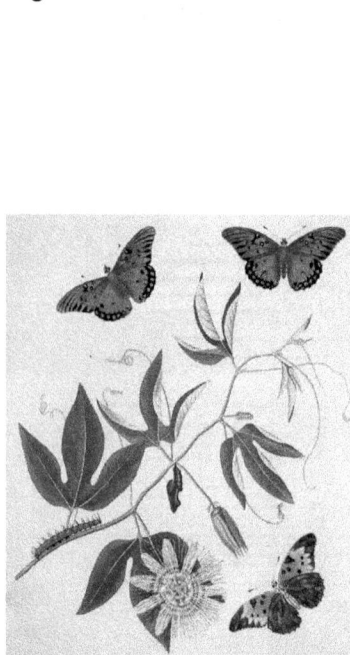

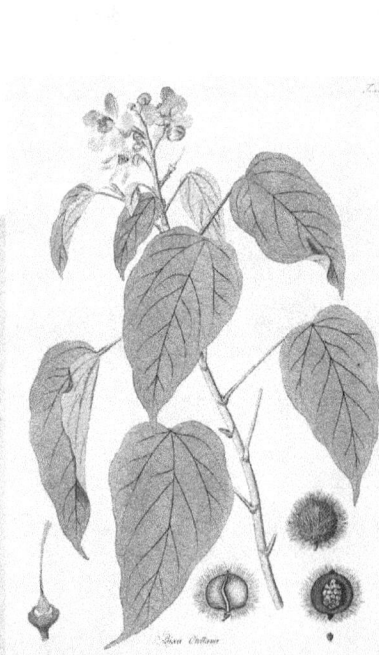

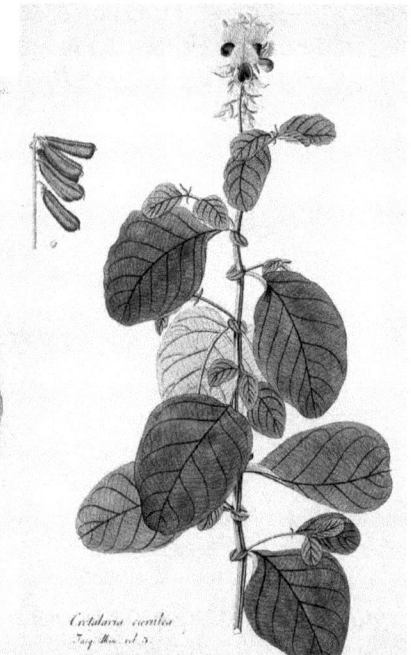

Figure 100. *Papilio passifloræ / Passiflora incarnata*
Figure 101. *Bixa orellana*
Figure 102. *Crotalaria verrucosa*

Ethnomedicines used in Trinidad and Tobago for reproductive problems

Background

Latin American and Caribbean women choose plants for reproductive conditions based on the properties that correspond to the hot-cold valence, irritating action, emmenagogic, oxytocic, anti-implantation and / or abortifacient effects. One cause of infertility is described as "cold in the uterus" and fertility enhancers are considered to be "hot." In Mexico infertility in women is considered a "cold" illness and "hot" remedies are prescribed.

Results

Doctrine of Signatures
The red flowers of forest tree called cooper hook (*Brownea latifolia*) are used for women's menstrual problems, gripes and pain. A decoction of the flowers is red in colour. A male informant whose mother was a midwife used both *Brownea latifolia* and red monkey step vine (*Bauhinia cumanensis / Bauhinia excisa*) to make tisanes for women's problems. He insisted that the vine when cut should not be white in colour but red like blood. This tisane he claimed would clean out women's insides preventing monthly period pain and would also improve fertility. The use of *Brownea latifolia*, in Trinidad for amenorrhea and as an abortifacient has been previously recorded. *Mimosa pudica* was used by one midwife to unwrap the cord from around an unborn baby's neck. Two plant tops were tied crossways, put in a pot and drawn. It was claimed that fifteen minutes after the pregnant woman drank the tisane the baby gave a flip. However a caesarean was still needed because the baby's due date had past.

Plants used for reproductive problems

Forty-two plants from more than twenty plant families are used for reproductive problems of men and women. The term "man's waist pain" was not explained.
Several plants were used for problems of men: *Catharanthus roseus* for "man's disease", *Urena sinuata* and *Clusea rosea* as a bark belt for "man's waist pain"; *Parinari campestris* and *Richeria grandis* for erectile dysfunction; *Scoparia dulcis*, *Ageratum conyzoides*, *Cucurbita pepo*, *Justicia pectoralis*, *Cucurbita maxima* and *Gomphrena globosa* for prostate problems.

Eleven plants were used for "womens' complaints" such as *Commelina elegans*, *Eupatorium macrophyllum*, *Justicia secunda*, *Parthenium hysterophorus*, *Wedelia trilobata*, *Ageratum conyzoides*, *Achyranthes indica*, *Artemisia absinthium*, *Brownea latifolia*, *Eleutherine bulbosa*, *Hibiscus rosa-sinensis* and *Abelmoschus moschatus*.

Nine plants were used for menstrual pain: *Capraria biflora*, *Cordia curassavica*, *Croton gossypifolius*, *Entada polystachya*, *Leonotis nepetaefolia*, *Eryngium foetidum*, *Aristolochia rugosa*, *Aristolochia trilobata* and *Ambrosia cumanenesis*.

Four plants are used for abortion: *Aristolochia rugosa*, *Aristolochia trilobata*, *Cocos nucifera* and *Ambrosia cumanenesis.*

Several plants are used in childbirth, to shorten labour and to remove the placenta: *Mimosa pudica*, *Ruta graveolens, Abelmoschus moschatus*, *Eryngium foetidum*, *Aristolochia rugosa*, *Aristolochia trilobata*, *Coleus aromaticus*, *Laportea aestuans* and *Vetiveria zizanioides.*

Other plants are used for infertility, "cold in womb", and inflammations:
R. graveolens, *Chamaesyce hirta*, *C. nitida*, *Ambrosia cumanenesis* and *Pilea microphylla.*

Nopalea cochenillifera is used for menopause and hot flashes and *Desmodium canum* is used for venereal diseases.

The ethnomedicinal plants used in Trinidad and Tobago for reproductive problems are summarised in Table 10.

Table 10. Ethnomedicinal plants used for reproductive problems in Trinidad and Tobago

Scientific name	Family	Common name	Part used	Use
Abelmoschus moschatus	Malvaceae	Gumbo musque	Leaves, seeds	Female complaints, remove placenta
Achyranthes indica	Amaranthaceae	Man better man		Female complaints
Ageratum conyzoides	Asteraceae	Z'herbe á femme		Prostate, Womens' complaints
Ambrosia cumanenesis	Asteraceae	Altamis	3-inch	Inflammation, abortion, Menstrual pain
Aristolochia rugosa, A. trilobata	Aristolochiaceae	Mat root, anico	Root	Remove placenta, abortion, menstrual pain
Artemisia absinthium	Asteraceae	Wormwood		Female complaints
Brownea latifolia	Fabaceae	Cooper hoop	Flower, leaves	Female complaints
Capraria biflora	Scrophulariaceae	Du thé pays	Leaves	Menstrual pain
Catharanthus roseus	Apocynaceae	White Periwinkle		"Man's disease"
Chamaesyce hirta	Euphorbiaceae	Malomay		Infertility
Clusea rosea	Clusiaceae	Matapal	Bark	Bark belt for "man's waist pain"
Cocos nucifera	Arecaceae	Coconut	Shell	Abortion
Cola nitida	Sterculiaceae	Obie seed	Seed	Infertility
Coleus aromaticus	Lamiaceae	Spanish thyme	Leaves	Shorten labour
C. elegans	Commelinaceae	Water grass	Plant	Douche
C. curassavica	Boraginaceae	Black sage	Leaves	Menstrual pain
C. gossypifolius	Euphorbiaceae	Bois sang	Leaves	Menstrual pain
Cucurbita pepo, C. maxima	Cucurbitaceae	Pumpkin		Prostate problems
Desmodium canum	Fabaceae	Sweet heart bush	Root	Venereal diseases
E. bulbosa	Iridaceae	Dragon blood	Bulb	Female complaints
Entada polystachya	Fabaceae	Mayoc chapelle	Twigs	Menstrual pain
Eryngium foetidum	Apiaceae	Chadron bénée	Leaves	Menstrual pain, remove placenta, shorten labour
Eupatorium macrophyllum	Asteraceae	Z'herbe chatte		Womens' complaints

Table 10. Ethnomedicinal plants used for reproductive problems (cont.)

Scientific name	Family	Common name	Part used	Use
Gomphrena globosa	Amaranthaceae	Bachelor button		Prostate problems
H. rosa-sinensis	Malvaceae	Hibiscus	Flowers	Female complaints
Justicia pectoralis	Acanthaceae	Carpenter grass	Leaves	Prostate problems
Justicia secunda	Acanthaceae	St. John's bush		Womens' complaints
Laportea aestuans	Urticaceae	Red stinging nettle	Leaves	Shorten labour
L. nepetaefolia	Lamiaceae	Shandileer		Menstrual pain
Mimosa pudica	Fabaceae	Mese marie		Childbirth
Nopalea cochenillifera	Cactaceae	Rachette	Joint	Menopause, hot flashes
Parinari campestris	Chrysobalanaceae	Bois bandé	Bark	Erectile dysfunction
Parthenium hysterophorus	Asteraceae	White head broom		Womens' complaints
Pilea microphylla	Urticaceae	Du thé bethelmay	Leaves	Inflammation, womb cleanser
Richeria grandis	Euphorbiaceae	Bois bandé	Bark	Erectile dysfunction
Ruta graveolens	Rutaceae	Ruda	Leaves	Childbirth, carminative, menstrual pain, cold in womb
Scoparia dulcis	Scrophulariaceae	Sweet broom	Leaves	Prostate
Urena sinuata	Malvaceae	Patte chien		"Man's waist pain"
V. zizanioides	Poaceae	Vetivert	Plant	Shorten labour
Wedelia trilobata	Asteraceae	Venven caribe	Leaves	Womens' complaints

Discussion

Non-experimental validation of plants used for reproductive problems

Abelmoschus moschatus plant is used for reproductive purposes in Fiji (Cambie, 1997). *Abelmoschus manihot* is used for menorrhagia in Vanuatu (Bourdy and Walter, 1992).

The use of *Achyranthes indica* for venereal diseases has been previously recorded (Duke, 2000). In Nepal *Achyranthes aspera* is used to facilitate parturition (Bhattarai, 1994). The benzene extract of the stem bark shows abortifacient activity in the rat (Bhattarai, 1994). *Ageratum conyzoides* is used for venereal disease in El Salvador (Hirschhorn, 1982). Sampson *et al.* (2000) found that *Ageratum conyzoides* had activity on the mediation of acute pain in the mammalian central nervous system (Sampson *et al.*, 2000). *Ageratum conyzoides* plant extract inhibited uterine contractions induced by 5-hydroxytryptamine suggesting that the extract exhibited specific antiserotonergic activity on isolated uterus plant extract but had no effect on uterine contractions induced by acetylcholine (Achola and Munenge, 1998; Silva *et al.*, 2000). The results gave support to the popular use of the plant as a spasmolytic. Yamamoto *et al. (*1991) found that oral treatment of rodents with *Ageratum conyzoides* neither reduced the inflammatory edema nor did it decrease the reaction to pain stimuli. Chromenes, benzofurans, polyoxygenated flavones, sesquiterpenes (farnesene derivatives) and daucanolide have been isolated from the plant (Ahmed *et al.*, 1999; Vyas and Mulchandani, 1986).

Wong (1976) recorded the use of *Ambrosia cumanenesis* for women's problems. *Ambrosia cumanenesis* contains 11-hydroxyguaien, altamisin, cumambrin-A, cumambrin-B, cumambrin-C and isoguaiene (Duke, 2000).

Aristolochia species are used in Mexico, western Panama and Guatemala as analgesics, for stomach pain, female disorders, menstrual pain and as contraceptives (Joly *et al.*, 1987; Girón *et al.*, 1991; Ankli *et al.*, 1999). Phytochemical analyses of *Aristolochia* species yielded essential oil, alkaloids, lignans, allantoin, nitrophenanthrenes (including aristolochic acid), aristolactams and phenanthrenes (Frei *et al.*, 1998). The latter group is assumed to have antiinflammatory effects.

Artemisia absinthium is used together with other plants as fertility regulators in western Panama and Paraguay (Arenas and Azorero, 1977; Joly *et al.*, 1987). *Artemisia* species are used similarly by the French, Spanish New Mexicans (emmenagogue) and in Madeira and this use is ancient (Conway and Slocumb, 1979; Weniger *et al.*, 1982; Novaretti and Lemordant, 1990; Rivera and Obón, 1995). *Artemisia absinthium* is used by the Caribs in Guatemala for fever, vaginitis and stomach pains (Girón *et al.*, 1991). In Mauritius and Rodrigues, Tuscany and Sardinia, *Artemisia* species leaf infusion or decoction is used for digestive upsets, and as emmenagogues (Gurib-Fakim *et al.*, 1993; Bruni *et al.*, 1997; Pieroni, 2000). Compounds in *Artemisia* species are sesquiterpene lactones, artemisinin, camphor and 1,8-cineole (Lewis, 1989; Allen *et al.*, 1997). *Artemisia absinthium* contains thujone a terpene that can cause excitation, convulsions that mimic epilepsy, and even permanent brain damage (Arnold, 1988).

Chamaesyce prostrata was used in Barbados prior to 1834 for venereal complaints (Handler and Jacoby, 1993). The water extract of the whole plant of *Chamaesyce hyssopifolia* (Euphorbiaceae) and its active compound corilagin were potent inhibitors of HIV-RT (IC50: 6-8 microg/ml) (Matsuse *et al.*, 1999). The plant contains resin, tannin, gallic acid, phorbol esters (co-carcinogenic compounds) and quercetin among others (Chen, 1991; Duke, 2000). *Chamaesyce hirta* aqueous extract exerted central analgesic properties (Lanhers *et al.*, 1991).

Cocos nucifera shell produces a fluid when hot that is used ethnomedicinally in India (Kapoor, 1990).

Cola nitida nuts contain nitrogen-containing compounds, tannin and 2.5% caffeine (Oliver Bever, 1986; Osim and Udia, 1993). *In vitro* crude extracts of kola nuts depress smooth muscle activity (Osim and Udia, 1993).

The use of *Coleus aromaticus* for menorrhagia in Trinidad has been previously recorded (Wong, 1976). *Coleus barbatus* is used to interrupt pregnancy in Brazil and is used as an emmenagogue in other countries (Almeida and Lemonica, 2000). *Coleus barbatus* showed an anti-implantation effect in the preimplantation period in rats, but after embryo implantation the extract had little effect.

Commelina elliptica is used in a bath by the Alteños Indians in Bolivia to reduce high fevers (Muñoz *et al.*, 2000b). *Commelina pallida* is used as a haemostatic and ecbolic in Mexico (Jiu, 1966).

Cordia alba was used by the Aztecs as a diuretic (Peña, 1999). *Cordia spinescens* is used in Colombia to relieve postpartum pain (Laferriere, 1994).

Cucurbita pepo is used for prostate disorders and urine intermittence in Palestine (Ali-Shtayeh *et al.*, 2000).

Desmodium ganngeticum is used as an antipyretic in India (Oliver Bever, 1986).

Eleutherine bulbosa is used in Columbia for menstrual cramps and in Haiti as an antifertility agent (Weniger *et al.*, 1982; Laferriere, 1994; Fernández *et al.*, 1997). *Eleutherine* species are used in the Malay Peninsula, Bolivia and Peru for vaginal discharge, wounds, dysentery, diarrhoea and anaemia (Ayala Flores, 1984; Fernández *et al.*, 1997; Muñoz *et al.*, 2000a; Duke, 2000). *Eleutherine bulbosa* bulbs contain lipids (n-hentriacontane), triterpene alcohols, sterols, and quinones and the bulb extract showed antifertility and cicatrizant activity and was non toxic (Weniger *et al.*, 1982; Fernández *et al.*, 1997). Eleutherin extracted from the bulb has a weak and transient effect of decreasing the prothrombin time (*in vivo* in rats) and a weak antibacterial activity on *Bacillus subtilis* (*in vitro*) (Bianchi and Ceriotti, 1975).

Eryngium foetidum is used in the Caribbean and South America for the treatment of fevers and antiinflammatory disorders (Robineau, 1991; Muñoz *et al.*, 2000b). *E. foetidum* hexane extract is rich in phytosterols, (95% stigmasterol) (García *et al.*, 1999a).

Eupatorium species are used in South America as contraceptives, abortives and emmenagogues (Elisabetsky and Posey, 1989). Two species of *Eupatorium* were used in Trinidad for menstrual problems in 1893 (Broadway, 1893). The use of *Eupatorium macrophyllum* for amenorrhoea, dysmenorrhea, prolapse and womb problems in Trinidad has been previously recorded (Wong, 1976).

The glycoside isorhamnetin 3-O-beta-robinobioside was found in *Gomphrena boliviana*. Upon inoculation of various doses of 5,6,7-trisubstituted flavones on two murine tumour lines, Sarcoma 180 and Ehrlich's carcinoma, a decrease of tumour growth was observed. An *in vitro* KB cultured cell screen indicated cytotoxicity (Pomilio *et al.*, 1994).

Hibiscus rosa-sinensis flower decoctions are used in folklore medicine in India and Vanuatu as aphrodisiacs, for menorrhagia, uterine haemorrhage and for fertility control (Bourdy and Walter, 1992; Kasture *et al.*, 2000). Flower extracts produced an irregular estrous cycle in mice with prolonged oestrus and metoestrus and other indications of antiovulatory effects, androgenicity and estrogenic activity (Murthy *et al.*, 1997; Prakash *et al.*, 1990; Pakrashi *et al.*, 1986; Pal *et al.*, 1985; Reddy *et al.*, 1997). Flowers contain anthraquinone, quercetin, cyanidin and their glucosides and florachrome B (Cambie, 1997; Kasture *et al.*, 2000).

Justicia pectoralis showed antinociceptive, bronchodilator and antiinflammatory effects (Leal *et al.*, 2000). These activities might be due to the coumarin in the plant (Mills *et al.*, 1986).

Mimosa pudica is used in Nicaragua and Mexico for stomach aches, 'cleaning the womb', as a sedative, to stop menstruation and for gonorrhoea (Asprey and Thornton, 1953-1955; Zamora-Martínez and Nieto de Pascual Pola, 1992; Barrett, 1994).

Nopalea cochenillifera is used for pains and inflammations in India (Duke, 2000).

Parinari species are used for venereal diseases in some African countries (Lee *et al.*, 1996). Two *ent*-kaurene diterpenoids and 15-oxozoapatlin were isolated from the root bark of *Parinari curatellifolia* and fatty acids, flavonoids and their glycosides have been found in *Parinari* species (Lee *et al.*, 1996).

Parthenium hysterophorus is used as a tonic, analgesic, antipyretic, antiperiodic, febrifuge and emmenagogue in Mauritius, Rodrigues, Mexico, Belize and India (Gurib-Fakim *et al.*, 1993; Arnason *et al.*, 1980; Duke, 2000). Analgesic properties have been found in *Parthenium hysterophorus* (Duke, 2000). Vijayalakshmi *et al. (*1999) found depolarizing neuromuscular junctional blocking action of *Parthenium hysterophorus* leaf extracts in the rat. The plant contains pseudoguaianolides, sesquiterpene lactones, flavonoids, and a lignan ((+)-syringaresinol) among others (Sethi *et al.*, 1987; Das *et al.*, 1999; Lomniczi de Upton *et al.*, 1999; Duke, 2000). *Parthenium hysterophorus* has antibacterial activity against *Staphylococcus* species, *Bacillus subtilis*, *Escherichia coli*, *Klebsiella pneumoniae*, *Pseudomonas aeruginosa*, *Salmonella* species and *Serratia* species (Facey *et al.*, 1999; Feresin *et al.*, 2000). *Parthenium hysterophorus* has antiamoebic activity against *Entamoeba histolytica* comparable to the standard drug metronidazole (Sharma and Bhutani, 1988).

Pilea microphylla is used ethnomedicinally in Asia and Tropical America (Hirschhorn, 1983; Duke, 2000). The entire plant is given to women in labour in Jamaica (Duke, 2000). *Pilea microphylla* was active against *Staphyloccocus aureus* (Facey *et al.*, 1999).

The use of *Richeria grandis* (syn. *Guarania ramiflora*) as an aphrodisiac has been recorded by Uphof (1968). *Roupala montana* is also used in Trinidad and was documented as a nervine by Uphof (1968).

Ruta graveolens and closely related species are used as emmenagogues, abortives, antispasmodics, sudorifics and anthelmintics in France, Spain, Brazil, Paraguay, New Mexico, Italy, Madeira and in other cultures and the antifertility uses were documented by Galen and Pliny the Elder (Arenas and Azorero, 1977; Conway and Slocumb, 1979; van den Berg, 1984; Novaretti and Lemordant, 1990; Riddle, 1991; Rivera and Obón, 1995; Martínez-Lirola *et al.*, 1996; Vázquez *et al.*, 1997; Guarrera, 1999; Bonet *et al.*, 1999). *Ruta* species contain different alkaloids and furanocoumarins and may show toxic side effects when used as abortifacients (Morton, 1975; Ankli *et al.*, 1999). *Ruta graveolens* has shown weak activity *in vitro* on excised uterine muscle (Conway and Slocumb, 1979). The antimicrobial activity of the plant is possibly due to the essential oils or flavonoids (Ojala *et al.*, 2000).

Scoparia dulcis is used in Nicaragua for belly pain and to 'clean the blood, kidney and system' (Barrett, 1994). Antitumour-promoting compounds and antiviral agents were found in *Scoparia dulcis* (Nishino *et al.* 1993; Hayashi *et al.* 1988, 1990). Betulinic acid in the plant has antiinflammatory properties (Duke, 2000).

Urena sinuata plant is used for reproductive purposes in the Pacific, Trinidad, China and India (Wong, 1976; Cambie, 1997). In Mauritius and Rodrigues *Urena lobata* is used against intestinal inflammation and is emmollient (Gurib-Fakim *et al.*, 1993). The plant contains beta-sitosterol, stigmasterol and alkanes (Cambie, 1997). *Urena lobata* is a fibre plant and is sometimes substituted for jute (Heinrich et al. 2005).

Vetiveria zizanioides is used in Pakistan as an emmenagogue and stimulant and is used by the Caribs in Guatemala for stomach pains (Girón *et al.*, 1991; Shinwari and Khan, 2000).

The use of *Wedelia trilobata* for amenorrhea in Trinidad has been recorded by Wong (1976). *Wedelia paludosa* and *Wedelia trilobata* contain a diterpene (kaurenoic acid), eudesmanolide lactones and luteolin (in leaves and stems) (Block *et al.*, 1998a&b; Bohlmann *et al.*, 1981). Kaurenoic acid has antibacterial, larvicidal and tripanocidal activity; it is also a potent stimulator of uterine contractions (Block *et al.*, 1998b). Luteolin exerts antitumoural, mutagenic and antioxidant effects, has depressant action on smooth muscles and a stimulant action on isolated guinea pig heart (Block *et al.*, 1998b). Kaurenoic acid and luteolin in *Wedelia paludosa* showed antinociceptive action more potent than the standard analgesic drugs (acetyl salicylic acid, acetaminophen, dipyrone and indomethacin). The root was the most potent part while the flower showed weak activity. Kaurenoic acid was 2 - 4 fold and luteolin was 8 - 16 fold more potent than acetyl salicylic acid, acetaminophen, dipyrone and indomethacin (some well-known analgesic drugs) (Block *et al.*, 1998b).

No data was found to support the use of the following plants: *Justicia pectoralis*, and *Vetiveria zizanioides*. The following plants have established analgesic or sedative effects: *Capraria biflora* and *Chamaesyce hirta*.
The plants used for reproductive problems have some support. *Chamaesyce hirta* has scientific support but as a diuretic.
Other plants with level 3 validity are: *Achyranthes indica*, *Coleus aromaticus*, *Hibiscus rosa-sinesis*, *Parthenium hysterophorus* and *Ruta graveolens*. Plants that have limited support are: *Abelmoschus moschatus*, *Ageratum conyzoides*. *Ambrosia cumanenesis*, *Aristolochia rugosa*, *Aristolochia trilobata*, *Artemisia absinthium*, *Cocos nucifera*, *Commelina elegans*, *Cordia curassavica*, *Croton gossypifolius*, *Cucurbita pepo*, *Cucurbita maxima*, *Desmodium canum*, *Eleutherine bulbosa*, *Eupatorium macrophyllum*, *Justicia pectoralis*, *Justicia secunda*, *Mimosa pudica*, *Nopalea cochenillifera*, *Parinari campestris*, *Pilea microphylla*, *Richeria grandis*, *Scoparia dulcis*, *Urena sinuata*, *Vetiveria zizanioides*, and *Wedelia trilobata*. Plants that have little research data are: *Brownea latifolia*, *Capraria biflora*, *Catharanthus roseus*, *Clusea rosea*, *Cola nitida*, *Entada polystachya*, *Eryngium foetidum*, *Gomphrena globosa*, *Laportea aestuans*, and *Leonotis nepetaefolia*.

Creolization with western medicine

Creolization with Western medicine is seen in Trinidad, the Caribbean and South America in the combination of western drugs with folk medicines (see also Coe and Anderson, 1996a). Rubbing alcohol, aspirin, spices, Vicks, Negasunt™, petroleum products and other products are used. More on these is given in the list below.

List 1: Pharmaceutical and non-plant ingredients and their uses

1. Arrow root flour mixed with water and drunk for diarrhoea. Soda water is mixed with a tablespoon of arrowroot flour and used for dysentry.
2. Babash/mountain dew is illegally-produced rum. It is used for menstrual period pain. It is also used with z'herbe á pique (*Neurolaena lobata*) for colds/fever.
3. Sour milk / Dahi is used for calf diarrhoea, for purges and for fevers.
4. Disinfectant is used on inflamed hooves, wounds, myiasis and to replace iodine.
5. The brine from pickled meat is used for external injuries and warts.
6. Fiery Jack™ balm was used to irritate horses to make them run faster but is now a banned substance.

7. Garlic and coals from fireside cooking is used for snake bites on dogs.
8. Ashes from fireside cooking are used on wounds, maggots, pip, sore hoofs, diarrhoea, as a charcoal substitute and to wash gumboils. Charcoal is used on wounds.
9. Gas/kerosene is used for maggots and mange.
10. Used engine oil is put on horses hooves to make them pliable and is also used for maggots and mange.
11. Sugar is used for respiratory problems in chickens, as an antidote to poison, and the osmotic gradient is put to use for prolapse and eye infections.
12. Vicks™ is used for respiratory problems in horses.
13. Salted butter is used on prolapses and for udder problems.
14. Blue stone (copper sulphate) is used on stone bruises.
15. Blue soap is used on chicken pox and for fleas.
16. Epsom salts is used for tendon injuries on horses, as a purge, for ground itch and on animal's hooves.
17. Cobwebs are used on broken horns and to seal cuts, similarly to Turkey (Sezik *et al.*, 1997).
18. Ants nests are used for mastitis.
19. A piece of termite nest is lit and put in a bucket attached to a horse's halter. The smoke from the nest is said to help with lung problems in horses. An infusion of a piece of termite nest (couloubois) is drunk for high blood pressure
20. Soft candle is used for colds, to poison goats and for abscesses.
21. Stout/ Guinness is drunk hot with various plants two days before the menstrual period, to remove the blood clots responsible for the pain. Hot stout is also used for retained placenta and as an abortifacient. B) Boiled stout was combined with one common fowl egg, a handful of bamboo leaves and put in a bottle. This decoction was given to the cow in first quarter moon phase. Three days before the full moon the cow would be ready to be bred.
22. Camphor (*Camphora offinarum*) with coconut oil was used as a replacement for Negasunt™, for the umbilicus of neonates. Three veterinarians accepted and used/recommended this substitute. Camphor is also used for respiratory problems in horses.
23. Sugar of lead or lead acetate is used for sores on the shoulders of draft animal. It is also used for tete worm, ground itch, men's genital problems and burns.
24. Vaseline is used for wounds, sores and eye problems. Yellow tanner grease is rubbed on cows skin.
25. Coal tar is put on broken horns, used for ground itch and for hoof care.
26. Jack spaniard[23][24] (wasp) stings are used to make dogs aggressive and for arthritis.

---

[23] In 1886, U. S. Marshal William Irvin was taking Felix Griffin to Ft. Smith to be tried for horse stealing. Jack Spaniard a half-Chickamauga (British-supporting Cherokee) and a friend, Frank Palmer ambushed and killed the officer near Pheasant's Bluff. They killed Griffin and released Griffin then they rode away, not noticing that Spaniard's dog stayed behind with the body. Spaniard and Palmer had been seen soon after they left the scene without the dog. This fact along with the appearance of the animal at the place of Irvin's murder and the testimony of men who had seen the dog in Spaniard and Palmer's company previous to the murder linked them to the crime.

"When Wes Harris and I was given the warrant and ordered to go after the dog, we spent some time looking for the dog. We at last located him in Mrs. Griffin's yard, about 10 miles northeast of Webber's Falls. I was acquainted with Mrs. Griffin but she did not know I was a Marshal. It was about noon and I asked if dinner was ready; she answered that it would not be long and for us to come in. When dinner was ready Wes just ate a few bites, excused himself, went out and got a chain from the saddle bag and caught the dog. I gave him what I thought was enough time, then I left the table. Mrs. Griffin came to the door with me, and seeing we had the dog, she asked: "What the hell are you doing with my dog?" I told her were U. S. Marshals and had a warrant for the dog. She ran back into the house, got a Winchester rifle, but we were out of sight when she returned. http://oklahombres.org/eve/ubb.x/a/tpc/f/5176036794/m/79410032511

The dog was kept at the jail for months, held as a witness. He was brought into the courtroom during Spaniard's trial and the dog went directly to Spaniard. This led to the conviction. Felix Griffin was shot in 1887 trying to steal another horse. Palmer was never captured. http://www.usgennet.org/usa/ok/county/muskogee/cemeteries/griffin/griffinlist.htm

[24] Jack Spaniard is also a character in Daniel Defoe's "The further adventures of Robinson Crusoe." Man Friday was supposed

27. Lime Ca(oh)^2 is put on walls to repel ticks.
28. Linseed oil is drunk for retained placenta.
29. Castor oil and lamp oil are used as a purge, colds and for colic.
30. Shark oil, cod liver oil or peppermint oil are used to 'clean out' horses or as diet additives.
31. Mustard oil was put into the dog's drinking water for distemper.
32. Coconut oil is used on neonate navels, warts, fever, joints, and for cows with headaches.
33. Alum (a double sulphate of aluminium and potassium) (2 or 3 ounces) is mixed with water in a bucket. Ruminant hooves are put in the bucket. This practice keeps the hoof solid. Alum is also used for shaking teeth and for oestrous induction.
34. Snails are rubbed on warts.
35. Molasses is used for oestrous induction, to improve appetite, for milk production, as a purge, as a tonic, as a component in poultices, for colic and for retained placenta.
36. Salted fish is used to induce oestrous.
37. Asafoetida (tatajab) is used to repel insects, deworm children, keep away spirits, bathe guns for hunting and as a carminative.
38. Salted beef is used for 'loss of cud'.
39. A hair from a cow's tail is used to remove warts.
40. Gentian violet (*Gentiana lutea*) is rubbed on dogs for mange.
41. The penis of the leatherback turtle is used to increase the effectiveness of hunting dogs.
42. Canadian healing oil is used for many purposes including healing horses' tendons.

Non-experimental validation of snake oils, etc

In Nepal, crushed snails are used to treat skin diseases with the root powder of *Achyranthes bidentata* (Joshi and Joshi, 2000). Researchers at the University of Wisconsin Medical School discovered that dark beer like Guinness contains large amounts of flavonoids which have an antioxidant effect, absorbing the free radicals of cholesterol which cause blood platelets to stick together and clog up arteries. Guinness was given to new mothers in Irish hospitals until the 1970s for nutritional reasons (M. Hanrahan, Dept. Communication and Innovation Studies, WUR, pers. comm. 2001). Pugliese *et al.*, 1998 claim that shark liver oil has been used for over 40 years as both a therapeutic and preventive agent. Shark liver is a major natural source of alkylglycerols, which have no known side effects in dosages of 100 mg three times a day. Alkylglycerols may be used both as an adjunct therapy in the treatment of neoplastic disorders and as an immune booster in infectious diseases (Pugliese *et al.*, 1998). Boa constrictor fat (BCF) significantly (p less than 0.0001) inhibited the *in vitro* growth of both keloid and normal dermal fibroblasts. Fatty acids. the main constituents of the oil, may be responsible (Datubo-Brown and Blight, 1990).

Conclusion

Those plants with very few ethnomedicinal references are perhaps the true 'indigenous [to Trinidad] knowledge'; or perhaps the relevant ethnomedicinal references were not found or are still unpublished. These 'indigenous' ethnomedicinal plants are *Antigonon leptopus*, *Justicia secunda*, *Microtea debilis*, *Eupatorium macrophyllum*, *Centropogon cornutus*, *Bontia daphnoides*, *Brownea latifolia*, *Richeria grandis*, *Roupala montana*, *Eupatorium triplinerve*, *Persea americana* and *Hippobroma longifolia*.

---

to be an Amerindian.

...coarse-grained, wide-meshed intellectual conceptions cannot grasp a more finely woven Nature' (Steiner 1924).

Caribbean Epistemology? Critical sociology, Creole remedies and scientific actor-networks

The Creoles, in general, have only precarious medical attendance, because of their own unwillingness to renumerate a regular practitioner; in lieu of this, they prefer the assistance of a class of imposters, both male and female, who unite the practice of Obeahism and quackery, exact little from their patients but are commonly satisfied with the amount and mode of renumeration tendered for the nostrums they administer, and the incantations they perform (L.A.A. de Verteuil, 1884)

10. Caribbean epistemology? Critical sociology, Creole remedies and scientific actor-networks

Abstract

Caribbean women are the repositories of oral history and folk medicine. This chapter uses moderate constructivism and Actor Network analysis to determine why women's folk knowledge is considered non-scientific. Social interests and negotiations shaped scientific decisions. Additionally Trinidad and Tobago is said to have a triple patriarchy based on ethnicity. Within this triple patriarchal structure, folk medicine may be considered too close to[25] the marginalized female status to be considered appropriate knowledge for modern medicine.

Introduction

The term feminist epistemology is used to refer to the ways in which gender influences what we accept as knowledge (Anderson, 1995). Actor-network theory (ANT) has its origins in post structuralism-influenced science studies and the sociology of medicine. An actor network is best described as the totality of social, political, economic, technological and other relationships between humans and non-humans that shape science, technology, knowledge production and society (Law, 1991). Actor-network theory (ANT) addresses the deadlock between constructionism and realism and in this chapter like others before it, examines the ontological question of how knowledge comes into being. Rather than engage in the theoretical debates over the range and solidity of ANT, for the purposes of this chapter I utilize ANT as a coherent theory and adopt its utilization of 'ordinary language' so that my findings can be understood by a variety of audiences and perhaps used to make a difference. In the Caribbean mothers, great aunts and grandmothers have long been recognized as the repositories of oral history and folk medicine (Price and Price, 1997). This chapter will use the framework of moderate constructivism and Actor Network analysis to determine why women's knowledge of folk medicine has been left out of scientific and folk knowledge networks. Moderate constructivism allows for a study of science and technology that addresses issues of science policy, appropriate technology and science-and-technology created dependency (Baber, 1992).

Star (1991) claims that there is "nothing inevitable about the marginalization of indigenous or traditional knowledge by some scientists" and "that it might have been otherwise." The marginalization takes place because non-scientific events and circumstances such as social interests and negotiations shape scientific knowledge (Code, 1993). These are: the influence of social factors on knowledge production; who gets to participate in theoretical inquiry; who listens to whom; the relative prestige of different styles and fields of knowledge; the influence of socially constructed conceptions and norms of gender; and the gender-specific interests and experiences on the production of knowledge. The chapter also introduces Mohammed's (1995) concept of triple patriarchy to the field of feminist epistemology. This focus on patriarchy accepts that view that feminist research should not focus exclusively on women's lives but should also investigate men and their power.

Scientific knowledge lays its claim to superiority on the basis of universal validity, since its methodologies are said to be applicable across time and space (Raedeke and Rikoon, 1997). This conception of science leads to an understanding of the world that exists outside of cultural and social contexts and ignores the origin of western science from very specific scientific and knowledge networks in scientific and other specialized institutions at specific times (Raedeke and Rikoon, 1997). Allopathic medicine can transfer almost intact from western countries because of its reference to the natural science paradigm and its standardized jargon and procedures (Brodwin, 1998). Allopathic medicine is similar to other formal institutions such as schools or churches in which people must negotiate the discourse and social norms of western powers while failing or succeeding in holding on to local beliefs (Brodwin, 1998). However the local medical beliefs continue to be used in localized pockets due to the cost of drugs, distance from centralized state hospitals, or dissatisfaction with hospital conditions and staff treatment. Many scientists assume that "if the[ir] science is good, it will serve the people" (Star, 1991). But some feminists have pointed out that no one is responsible for ensuring that science does serve the people. If we accept that scientific and technical truths and indigenous knowledge are partial we are still faced with the problem of distinguishing what knowledge is helpful and which is not (Longino, 1993; Nelson, 1993). It was in this context of determining whether women's folk medicinal knowledge was helpful in instances when allopathic medicine was either unavailable or unaffordable that a recent study of ethnoveterinary medicine in the Caribbean nation of Trinidad and Tobago was undertaken (Lans, 2001). This study revealed that the majority of the 180 plant-based folk remedies identified during the fieldwork were being used for what scientists would call "rational reasons."

This chapter is organized in the following manner: the first section defines ethnoveterinary research in relation to science and the data collection process. In the second section extracts from the interviews are presented to illustrate the attitudes of professionals towards folk medicine and the strategies and struggles of folk medicine practitioners. In the third and fourth sections the process through which folk knowledge is being marginalized and the complexities of the process are presented in Matrices that link the various practices to terms of ANT. For the purposes of this chapter the most relevant definition of science is that it is a human performance or human enterprise (Goodwin and Tangum, 1998). As part of this human enterprise the boundaries and contents of science are continually negotiated and re-negotiated rather than being only pre-existing entities needing to be discovered and revealed (Goodwin and Tangum, 1998; Code, 1993). Truth claims are then the result rather than the cause of agreement within a scientific community (Nelson, 1993). Therefore scientists cannot claim that they are accountable only to their evidence since scientists act as epistemic agents and their evidence is selected and not found (Nelson, 1993; Code, 1993; Deichmann and Müller-Hill, 1998).

The five-year research study into ethnoveterinary medicine revealed an on-going tension between western-trained scientists and practitioners of ethnoveterinary knowledge (Lans,

2001). Extracts from the interviews conducted with practitioners of ethnoveterinary medicine, AHAs, EOs and veterinarians contained themes related to the unscientific and un-validated nature of folk and ethnoveterinary medicine. These views were heard repeatedly throughout the fieldwork. These interview extracts are built into the matrices presented in the body of the chapter and are used to illustrate how the less powerful actor-network of folk medicine is kept in marginalized parallel to the more powerful actor-network of western science. Newspaper clippings and one example are also utilized to show how scientific debates can shape which knowledge is accepted and which not. This combination of approaches is used to reflect the heterogeneous nature of an actor-network. No claim is made that traditional knowledge should replace scientific knowledge but that each has its merits and flaws.

The interview extracts are taken from group and individual interviews that were held in 1995 with officials from the Ministry of Agriculture Land and Marine Resources (MALMR).Participant observation took place from 1996 - 2000 at the School of Veterinary Medicine. These interactions were used to confirm the initial observations in 1995. In 1997 the author also initiated an organizing committee that planned to host an herbal medicine workshop in 1998. Extensive participant observation of nine meetings of this organizing committee was conducted in the last quarter of 1997. Data from these meetings, the resulting Herbal conference, and the formation of the scientific association called the Caribbean Association of Researchers and Herbal Practitioners (CARAPA) are used to illustrate the operations of a newly created actor-network based on alternative knowledge.

Negative media coverage of folk medicine is also presented to show how this impacts on the survival of folk medicine. The media-related secondary source material was obtained from the daily newspapers existing in Trinidad and Tobago --- the Trinidad Guardian, Newsday and the Express. Three library collections of media clippings on folk medicine were examined in 1995 and twelve articles dating from 1984 to 1994 were copied. Media clippings from 1996 – 1999 were taken from the authors' personal collections. Herbalists wrote eight of these articles and recommended folk medicine. Four articles were written by two doctors and a chemist and recommended caution. The last was an obituary for a well-known herbalist. Three extracts from these newspaper clippings are used as texts to show how the struggle and conflict over the control of knowledge is conducted in the media and how emphases are placed on risks or benefits.

Folk medicine versus Science

Many of the professionals interviewed had personal knowledge of ethnoveterinary medicines, which were often identical to the folk medicines used for human illnesses. For example during a follow-up interview with veterinarian Churaman[26] to obtain more details on the ethnoveterinary practices that he knew, Churaman called his mother to obtain the name of a medicinal plant that he had forgotten. Churaman claimed to be actively involved in collecting ethnoveterinary practices used for ruminants from the older villagers that he met in rural areas. He said that he used some of these practices with poorer rural clients. The following interview extracts will provide a richer picture of the socio-economic environment in which folk medicine exists. Veterinarian Ivan who was formerly in charge of the PSU notes how folk knowledge dies with its holder-practitioners:

My old aunt was a walking encyclopedia but she died. I wasn't willing to listen until I was in university and it was too late then. Folk medicine used to be recognized as real knowledge, but not by the modern generation. Plus their parents don't use it anymore. Where do you get folk

---

[26] All names are pseudonyms except for Chadband.

medicine now? You cannot ask anymore. The old aunts used to say pick two leaves of this, four leaves of that.

The emphasis given to import substitution in manufacturing in the 1950s and 1960s led to shoddy manufactured goods. The perception that everything foreign is automatically better is seen in this interview extract:

Old people used to know more about folk medicine but now everyone goes to the doctor. It is more convenient to go to the doctor around the corner. The doctors are wise enough to get medication from herbs. They can work out a dosage while we will just take two leaves and boil it. Foreign herbs are packaged. Foreigners are better salesmen. The herbs we use (for racing pigeons] are not manufactured locally. I don't know if they are available here. I see the success stories in foreign magazines. These stories encourage you to go and buy the same medication as that mentioned. Everything outside, foreign, is always better. It is substandard locally with funny labels on it. Some around the corner herbalists don't know the Latin names of the plants, they are just selling.

Harry's ideas are one actor's views on the acculturation process referred to in the ethnomedicinal literature which is always in evolution since it is always open to new ideas, discarding the ineffective and incorporating the latest remedies (Laguerre, 1987).
The western system produces curing and pain relief while simultaneously reproducing trust, authority and control or dominance (Pappas, 1990). Through the respect and authority that doctors get from their helping activities they are also able to reinforce status hierarchy (Pappas, 1990). Opportunity hoarding in professions sometimes results when other knowledges are subordinated as inferior (Gilbert, 1998). For example Trinidad and Tobago doctors trained abroad in the "mother country", and reproducing the privileged and ethnocentric standpoint of their white male professional tutors, discouraged the use of folk medicinal practices because "they smack of pagan Africa, and are no longer necessary in the light of Trinidad's medical progress" (Mischel, 1959; Laguerre, 1987). Krumeich (1994) documented a similar negotiation of professional roles and renunciation of traditional knowledge in Dominica. Dominican dispensary nurses denigrated women's traditional healing expertise with folk medicine; although historically, untrained midwives were highly esteemed for their empirical knowledge. Goodwin and Tangum (1998) show that some of the scientific resistance to new ideas arises when "outsiders" to the particular discipline in question act as "usurpers" by attempting to cross over to higher status professions. Scientific resistance to "usurpers" acting as "popularizers" who take their message directly to the public still exists as can be seen in the interview extract below from Scientist Guardia:

Duke like Farnsworth[27] and Awang tend to popularize, and challenge the system. Duke is a hard scientist, but he is fooling around, popularizing. Scientists should know what they are doing when they popularize [they are] acting like novelists. [Duke, Farnsworth and Awang] can't get into the scientific literature so [they] have started popular magazines to establish guidelines on standardization for adoption by countries. Readers might assume it's [the standardization] happening already. They are challenging the system by making connections in the World Health Organization (WHO). WHO can't discuss "Health for all", unless the Ministries strive through primary health care to legalize herbal medicine.

---

27 Dr. James A. Duke, Economic Botanist, USDA (Ret.), Dr. Dennis Awang, Medi-Plant Ltd., Canada, Dr. Norman Farnsworth, University of Illinois at Chicago.

After 100 years of British rule the newly emerging coloured middle class assimilated Victorian values, and respectability was achieved through education and entering the professions. A quote from a speech given in 1910 by L.O. Inniss, the head of the Pharmacological society in Trinidad and Tobago, shows how this new middle class disassociated itself from its background in traditional medicine in its quest for social mobility and acceptance.

Creole Remedies. Paper read before the pharmaceutical society by the President L.O. Inniss. ....One wonders what those Creole remedies are, which succeed, when duly diplomaed scions of AEsculapius have signally failed and I have often tried to investigate some of the cases so as to find out these famous remedies -generally of the bush persuasion.... Every druggist is familiar with those pieces of paper, written in the most barbarous French, fearfully and wonderfully spelled in which roots and barks and leaves are all jumbled up with alcali, lavande rouge, vinaigre, quart voleurs and beaume tranquille and there is no doubt that those archaic and delphic remedies have been credited with more cures, than the most skilful and learned doctors have achieved. Let me say just here, that the Creole manner of diagnosing any disease is so simple that any one could pass as an MD after a few minutes explanation of the process. The sole and solitary cause of all diseases that Creole flesh is heir to is a cold---pleurisy is a severe cold, rheumatism is a cold in the blood, dysentery a cold in the bowels, asthma a cold on the chest, phthisis a cold on the lungs, influenza a fresh cold, etc, etc... There can be no doubt that many of our native herbs have good medicinal properties and it is well that people should know and use them, especially in the country parts where doctors and pharmacies are few and far between, (emphasis added) but I have always been induced to discount the value of these bush remedies, on account of the vague information their votaries seem to possess as to the dosage of them. Having been trained as a druggist and having had to pass many hours before my examination, learning the doses of medicine, I can't understand the fast and loose way in which these Creole remedies are prescribed. The only quantity mentioned is 'some'. If no one is ever killed by these Creole remedies, it must be because their virtues are very mild indeed.

There are also on-going negotiations as to who can be recognized as an actor with "visibility", and a "voice." An extract from a newspaper advertisement taken out by the late self-described research herbalist Chadband is reproduced below. Chadband claims that in his network of relationships (as an experienced elder) he is recognized as an authority. However when he tries to enter a more professional network several strategies are employed to prevent this:

The names of the people worldwide I have helped are on record. I have the help of God. Every disease that is said to have no cure comes here. All I know is that I was called in by one of the Dateline Program [TV show] officers, and was told that there was a meeting of the Dental Association and those who were called "quacks" were invited, and someone asked where I should be placed whether among the quacks? So, he was advised to ask me to present my papers, which I immediately did. Two months have since passed, and each time I make inquiries, I am told that they are very busy. (Chadband, 1987)

Chadband's claim that he was called a quack is one of two published in advertisements by Chadband and was also referred to in his eulogy published by one of the media houses. According to Latour (1988) some forms of knowledge are "higher" than others because "the superior have used their power to raise themselves with the connivance of the inferior." Power is one aspect of relationships and is visible in the use of resources or "using your strategies and skills to get others to do what you want" (Pappas, 1990). Power is then based on successful use and is present in all interpersonal interactions.
Powerful professions can protect their task domain and professional boundaries from perceived encroachment (Gilbert, 1998). The irony is that herbalists have been the ones to

see their boundaries encroached and their practices made illegal or sanctioned by professional medicine through what Tilly (1998) refers to as opportunity hoarding. Continuous access to and control of scientific resources requires the maintenance of distinctions between insiders like doctors and non-group members like herbalists and quacks or between insiders and non-true scholars (Douglas, 1995; Tilly, 1998).

Maintenance of group control and guaranteeing continuity and the status quo can be obtained using gatekeeping tactics such as querying the credentials of traditional medicinal practitioners and writing a letter to the editor expressing caution over non-scientific knowledge. Professional monopolization of knowledge can involve calling a committee to investigate a new topic or a science-created problem, issuing a news release, or other everyday recurrent practices that maintain or modify the positions of the scientists vs. the uniformed layperson (Tilly, 1998). Group control also occurs when "big men" at the height of their professional careers (or even more likely just past their peak), control ceremonies, select neophytes, exclude deviants and prioritize research topics (Douglas, 1995). These professional boundaries can become locked into place, making them habitual and necessary to both insiders and outsiders (Tilly, 1998; Gilbert, 1998). When science as a whole and all associated professional associations adopt the same categorical distinctions, these distinctions become more omnipresent and deep-rooted (Tilly, 1998).

The term professional gatekeeping is familiar to those involved in conventional science trying to incorporate new insights or paradigms into a discipline when those insights contradict well-established theories (Goodwin and Tangum, 1998). Professional gatekeeping can include political ritual or exerting social authority. Other gatekeeping practices are hosting a conference to establish a new subject area, or calling for more research before action on a specific area can be taken. As Longino (1993) has claimed, power is not located [only] in texts, but exercised through texts by those who rule. The newspaper extract that follows shows an individual act of gatekeeping. A middle-aged male heart specialist Kenroy, through the intermediary of a letter to the editor, uses denunciating language against the 'uninformed laypersons':

I wish to comment on material contained in an article in the Trinidad Guardian under the headline Ayurveda Prevention Center uses local herbs to fight disease. With reference to the advised usage of local medicinal plants to 'cure' a wide range of illnesses, I wish to warn: much research requires to be done on this subject before attributing properties to certain plants. The fact that a particular plant might have customarily been used for a particular illness is no proof whatsoever as to the medicinal efficacy of that plant. [Lists 7 doubtful uses then says] The situation could be considered mildly amusing if only minor illnesses were involved in this herbarium brew. However, when one begins to discuss diabetes, cancer, hypertension, and leprosy, as being possible indications for the use of unproven herbal medicine, we are letting ourselves in for a great deal of trouble, and risking lives. This is dangerous tomfoolery, and the proposed practice should not be allowed to go unchallenged, especially when traditional medicine has so many proven means of management of these illnesses [ ]. I fear the Greeks even when they bring gifts. Let this be a warning [Mentions a book on medicinal plants written by an academic]. The research goes on [ ]. In the meantime, let us be careful and do not make fools of ourselves by dispassionately imbibing without forethought any form of witches' brew, that might be inflicted on us by any charlatans, who might suddenly appear out of the blue. (Trinidad Guardian 1988).

The research referred to in the letter above was conducted prior to 1988 in Trinidad and Tobago and it was minimal, concentrated on "poisonous" plants, and was not written in a way that made it accessible to the lay public (Lans, 1996). Despite this the lay public is being cautioned not to bypass it. This heart specialist wrote a similar letter in 1999 published in two newspapers (Express July 3, 1999; Newsday July 5, 1999 pg. 24), repeating his warnings against vague and unproven remedies and added brief accounts of three patients who were adversely affected by taking the herbalist's advice instead of his own, one of whom died. This letter in turn generated two feature articles in the Express newspaper (Express July 18, 1999 pg. 7; Express July 20, pg. 21) in which the up-and-coming male writer(s) claimed that:

....many [ ] remain adamant that herbalists are little more than charlatans promising their patients miracle remedies. One of these is [Kenroy] who has noted a marked increase in the use of alternative forms by his patients'. (Express July 18, 1999 pg. 7)… an Arima-based herbal company has accused [Kenroy] of doing a hatchet job on the (herbal) industry….[the owner of this company claims that] 'Government [is] looking at the implementation of complementary medicine within the National Drug Policy. In the interim doctors like Kenroy were hiding behind the laws of the country which give doctors a monopoly on health care[28] (Express July 20, 1999, pg. 21).

If Kenroy has noted a marked increase in the use of alternative forms by his patients, this might be related to recent findings of high levels of patient dissatisfaction related to inadequate communication of information by doctors to their female patients, and an apparent insensitivity to the patients' condition (Phillips, 1996). High levels of professional dominance were noted in a sample of obstetric and gynecology wards in four of Trinidad and Tobago's public hospitals and there was also evidence of negligence, incompetence, malpractice and evasive practices (Phillips, 1996).

Actor Network Theory and Ethnoveterinary Medicine

In the next section the process through which folk knowledge is being marginalized through micro-practices of power and the beneficiaries and losers of this marginalization process are presented in Matrices.

Actor-networks such as universities and research institutions grow by enrolling other entities like students, other scientists and their institutions. The heads of these actor networks are successful based on their translating the projects and purposes of these other entities, and establishing themselves as the spokesmen of those who are being associated (Callon, 1987). The core translator can make the enrolment either desirable or unavoidable from the standpoint of the peripheral entity being enrolled, using research and development funds for example (Callon, 1987; Alatas, 1993). Scientific objectivity can be described as a translation that the dominant group uses to deny other people access to power, political power or fact-making power (Hubbard, 1988).

Matrix 1 below uses a moderate form of constructivism (Henry, 1998) and the Actor Network theory, and links these to science and technology.

Actors in the matrix are portrayed in two dimensions, as a set of strategies that exercise power and as a set of materials that are the end results of those strategies (Law, 1991).

---

[28] British law in the Commonwealth forbids the sale of bush teas as medicines.

Matrix 1. Science,Technology and Society (STS), and Lans (2001)

Term	Meaning in STS	Illustration
Maintenance	Maintaining power by constituting a set of relations and holding these in place. This set of relationships becomes the actor-network	Retention of scientific objectivity and standard dosage as norms makes it difficult for alternatives to take shape
Distribution	A set of relations is constituted between elements of the network. The original actor network is enlarged by enrolling others and maintaining the structure	Pioneers bring IK into normal science they give it respectability and so are able to enroll others
Circuits	Patterns in the network are circuits that reproduce themselves and their distributive effects. Another form of maintenance	Conferences and newsletters are circuits. So are regional institutes that are set up worldwide to investigate, document and share information
Social Relations	The distribution goes on to regulate the relations between elements. Through social relations norms are maintained and left unchallenged to become self-evident	Farmers are not considered to be information producers in normal science.

Source: Law (1991) and Henry (1998).

The term circuits in Matrix 1 is best illustrated by the history of the First International Workshop on Herbal Medicine in the Caribbean (FIWHMC). It was hosted in 1998 by the School of Veterinary Medicine of the University, a local NGO-- the Caribbean Network for Integrated Rural Development (CNIRD), and a regional organization the Inter-American Institute for Co-operation in Agriculture (IICA). The original idea was to have a participatory workshop similar to the one that resulted in the publication Ethnoveterinary medicine in Asia: An information kit on traditional animal health care practices (IIRR, 1994). The originator of the workshop idea started a small working committee with the African-born then head of the School of Veterinary Medicine, who had none of the West Indian professional disdain towards folk medicine. He in turn invited other scientists to join while the originator invited the head of CNIRD because this NGO had headquarters in Trinidad but managed Caribbean-wide projects. CNIRD's mandate is integrated rural development and in certain circumstances CNIRD has acted as a mediator between marginalized actors in the informal economy as it either sought benefits for them from the post-colonial state or provided state-denied benefits using external donor funding.

It was felt that the involvement of the female-headed CNIRD would help focus the workshop committee on the original goal of a participatory workshop that would ultimately benefit small-scale herbalists and farmers. CNIRD quickly recognized that its client group of micro-entrepreneurs involved in herbal medicines could be helped with a medicinal plant-based project. CNIRD also recognized the skepticism that exists about available non-standardized herbal products. However after numerous committee meetings and the involvement of the "big men" in the Inter-American Institute for Co-operation on Agriculture (IICA), the coalitions in the committee and the focus for the conference shifted. The result was a conference held with great fanfare at the Holiday Inn Hotel in Trinidad in April 1998 with the main presenters being scientists (field notes and various Minutes of the FIWHMC Organizing Committee). A participatory idea could not stand up against the prestigious occasion sought by IICA and university scientists, nor were the traditional female herbalists present at the Holiday Inn to challenge the professional prestige of the scientists or present their own alternative knowledge of medicinal plants.

At this conference an umbrella organization the Caribbean Association of Researchers and Herbal Practitioners (CARAPA)[29] was formed. The Trinidad and Tobago Steering Committee of CARAPA comprised six scientists and one herbalist with a B.Sc. in Botany. The Caribbean island and South American mainland representatives of CARAPA-Trinidad, CARAPA-Jamaica and CARAPA-St. Lucia were again scientists. This was to be expected since scientists were the main participants of the first Conference (Lans, unpublished).

This means that successful translation has taken place since the original committee grew into an actor network by enrolling other entities and shaped the second annual conference in the U.S. Virgin Islands (UVI) on June 14 - 16, 1999 as seen in the extract below:

The [CARAPA] meeting agreed with the [UVI representative] that attendance at the technical sessions of the [UVI] conference should be restricted to serious herbalists, producers and students while other sessions could be available to the interested public... The meeting also agreed that pharmaceutical companies and business interests should be invited to participate in the conference since their business and marketing expertise was needed (CARAPA minutes April 7th 1999).

The extensive discussion sessions of the first conference were reproduced at the end of the proceedings[30] (print and CD-ROM versions) to "prove that the conference had been participatory." The problem of bringing folk medicine into science was then solved based on previous experience of how conferences are organized and on proven ways of creating networks (Hatten et al., 2000). The term social relations is then clearly demonstrated: since these are Conferences organized by scientists in venues like the Holiday Inn Trinidad and Hotel on the Cay U.S. Virgin Islands, the typical practitioners of folk medicine (grannies and great aunts) are represented only by the data they have reported to those presenting research papers.

Scientists commanded data from female herbalists from which they drew significantly increased returns by co-ordinating the lifetime effort of the herbalists into presented papers while excluding the herbalists from conference participation and societal recognition by hosting the conference and subsequent annual conferences in such formal venues and in such formal ways (Tilly, 1998). No disrespect is intended to the distinguished personnel who addressed any of the annual meetings. For example the 2001 4th International Symposium on Herbal Medicines in the Caribbean held in St. Lucia, was addressed by the Honorable Minister of Health of St Lucia, the Governor General and the Head of Health Sector Reform. In fact CARAPA should be commended for organizing subsequent meetings in St Croix, Jamaica, St Lucia, Suriname and most recently in Trinidad, thus spanning the geographical boundaries of the Caribbean and raising the awareness of medicinal plants among policy makers. However this example shows that while scientists can be enrolled into a newly created actor-network based on alternative knowledge, previous relationships built on hierarchy, professional norms and bureaucracy have great influence over the direction of the new network and the creation of durable materials[31] (Law, 1991). Added to this is the complication of what Mohammed (1995) calls the triple patriarchal system operational in Trinidad.

---

[29] The Caribbean Association of Researchers and Herbal Practitioners (CARAPA) promotes responsible bioprospecting and the appropriate use of indigenous Caribbean herbs, based on sound information about their properties and their therapeutic effectiveness. CARAPA is the Amerindian name of the indigenous evergreen Caribbean tree *Carapa guianensis*.
CARAPA's mission's goals and objectives can be seen at the following website: http://www.uwi.tt/carapa/ .
[30] Herbal Medicine in the Caribbean: to restore a Caribbean heritage. Proc. First International Workshop, Port of Spain, Trinidad and Tobago, 6 - 8 April, 1998, CNIRD.
[31] One very useful 'durable material' was the compilation of all the resources available on herbal medicine in the UWI library that was prepared for and made available at this 'First International Workshop'.

Matrix 2. Terms and theories of the actor-network concept

Terms and Meaning in STS	Application
An actor is any entity able to define and build a world filled with other entities and intermediaries (Callon, 1991).	Intermediaries are texts, funding, instruments and drugs and they evolve and describe their networks (Callon, 1991).
A network is a set of relations of heterogeneous elements. This is constituted and held in place (Callon, 1987). Scientists' networks have conventions of use about materials, goods and standards. It is costly professionally speaking to practice outside these conventions (Star, 1991). Publishing, foreign labs, scientific articles and prestigious journals are networks with standards. Hiring, promotion and tenure are linked to the network.	Because of the network structure agricultural scientists have sought to control nature in order to be regarded as conventional scientists. Scientists think it is normal to concentrate on locality neutral, standardized agriculture, seeking generalizable solutions to problems by testing hypotheses under controlled and replicable conditions (Molnar et al., 1992), farmers who do the opposite do not fit the norm. Those farmers who resist conventional technology are termed laggards (Flora, 1992).
Translation is the process in which actor networks grow by enrolling other entities. It generates a shared space. Stable relationships in the network come by disciplining or maintaining that translation, so that there is no deviation from accepted theories (Star, 1991). Invisible colleges are informal networks of eminent scientists and groups of lesser or younger scientists propagating their ideas, without deviating (Dolby, 1979).	Professional gatekeeping practices prevent alternative research from appearing in mainstream channels (Spender, 1981). Agency is the conversion of synergy into resources and resources into networks (Foucault, 1979). These networks can suppress research findings or persecute dissidents or deny tenure (Molnar et al., 1992). Dominant research traditions reduce other perspectives to the status of 'craft' or folk wisdom.
Convergence is a measure of agreement and has two aspects, alignment and co-ordination (Callon, 1991). By using alignment and co-ordination the network becomes an indispensable, irreversible passageway of constraining norms through which all the other entities that make up its world must pass. Definitions, problematization, codification and publishing in the right journals are some of these strategies. Translation depends on the capacity of the actor-network to work together and to define and enroll those entities, which might challenge the dominant ideas and theories. Successful translation makes a theory self-evident and buries the debates of the initial theory formation stage (Callon, 1991).	There are scientific conventions about who may speak on behalf of whom (Callon, 1991). If scientists invest with agribusiness and entities at the cutting edge of science and technology they are recognized as standard setters (Star, 1991). Junior scientists enroll in standardized technologies and organized scientific programs, which are influenced by industry to benefit from the privileges attached to the network (Star, 1991), rather than branch off into uncharted territory. Social interests and these individual actions shape science. There are structures of dependency like access to funding and equipment that link developed world and Third World scientists which affects their research choices (Alatas, 1993).
Weak convergence and partial commitments mean that the translations were not durable or robust but unsuccessful. One actor cannot speak for the others. The experts' status is questioned. The expert finds it hard to mobilize other parts of the network like research funds and government support (Callon, 1991).	Those who are non-members of the community of practice, or standard network, suffer (Star, 1991). For example researchers who have no access to labs, funds and equipment cannot take part in the standardization process. The network as a whole cannot focus its efforts.

This system consisted of the dominant white system which (until 1962) controlled state power (colonialism); the Creole patriarchy of mixed race and Afro-Trindadians functioning in and emerging from the white group (and struggling to obtain and maintain middle class status), and the East Indian form which in the beginning was at the bottom (brought to do the labor that the emancipated slaves refused) but through state or Christian-provided education

125

and hard work is now claiming equal rights to state power (Munasinghe, 2001). In this triple patriarchal system the association of folk medicine with the denigrated female role may have been extremely difficult to overcome.

Matrix 2 demonstrates the routine ways in which the categories of science and folk medicine are constituted. As in Matrix 1 the terms and definitions are taken from (Law, 1991). Each row in Matrix 2 has a term, its definition and the real world or scientific world application of the term and definition.

The usefulness of the term convergence in Matrix 2 is best illustrated by the debate over dosages in folk medicine. The scientific dichotomy of objectivity vs. subjectivity underpins scientists' claims to status by emphasizing the distinctiveness of their working practices from those that they characterize as ordinary understanding.
One of the strategies by which the scientific actor-network renders itself indispensable and suppresses dissent is by convergence, which involves co-ordination and alignment. The strategies of alignment and co-ordination are constraining norms that make the scientific actor-network an almost indispensable, irreversible passageway through which all other knowledge must pass. For example, clinical anthropologists are sometimes encouraged to participate in medical discourse and drop their anthropological insights, which are considered an inappropriate incursion of political ideology into the domain of scientific medicine (Baer, 1993).

The call for standardized dosages is one of these constraining norms as can be seen in the following interview extract. Male veterinarian Nunes claims that a disadvantage of folk medicine is the vagueness of the dosages:

There is some truth in it, but you need to find out what the active ingredient is. I don't believe in 'bush'. There is some truth, but the problem is dosage. In Cotton leaf, [Gossypium species] there must be some active ingredient; no one has ever tried to formulate it. I tell my clients if you boil three leaves, how do you know the season, the health of the plant, you can't control the dose[32]. The majority of dogs are still full of worms. Cotton bush might be good for roundworms. Pea pod (Cajanus cajan) for worms, that is a recent one; they boil it up.

The consequence of this scientific attitude is that folk medicine remains unproven due to its un-standardized dosages and it needs scientific validation as claimed by male veterinarian Singh: "Before selling folk medicine you have to validate it with some company."

Another consequence of this attitude is that potent (but perhaps problematic) leads for the development of antidepressive therapeutics and other medicines have not been used (Hasrat et al, 1997b). To show that Trinidad and Tobago scientists are as similarly constrained by the actor-network as their foreign counterparts an extract from an editorial written by western scientists is presented below:

Alternative medicine [has] an ideology that ignores biologic mechanisms, often disparages modern science, and relies on [ ] purported [ ] ancient practice[s] and natural remedies (which are seen as somehow being simultaneously more potent and less toxic than conventional medicine). Accordingly, herbs or mixtures of herbs are considered superior to the active compounds isolated in the laboratory. And healing methods [ ] are

---

[32] Passreiter and Medinilla Aldana (1998) found that sesquiterpene lactones in *Neurolaena lobata* cultivated in Guatemala differed quantitatively from those in natural populations.

126

fervently promoted despite not only the lack of good clinical evidence of effectiveness, but the presence of a rationale that violates fundamental scientific laws ...surely a circumstance that requires more, rather than less, evidence [ ]Therapeutic successes with botanicals came at great human cost. The indications for using a given botanical were ill defined, dosage was arbitrary because the concentrations of the active ingredient were unknown [ ] Now with increased interest in alternative medicine, we see a reversion to irrational approaches to medical practice, even while scientific medicine is making some of its most dramatic advances [ ]. It is time for the scientific community to stop giving alternative medicine a free ride. (Angell and Kassirer, 1998)

This extract from Angell and Kassirer (1998) reflects the political processes and the technological "pushes" that determine what knowledge is considered relevant by the dominant knowledge makers. It is also a good example of how stable relationships in the scientific actor-network come by "disciplining or maintaining translations" so that there are no deviations from accepted theories (Law 1991; Callon, 1991).

The rhetorical task of upholding one's own construction of science seems to necessitate undermining or ignoring alternative interpretations (Foucault, 1980; Goodwin and Tangum, 1998). Scientific medicine is currently based on evidence-based medicine, which means that a therapy has been shown to improve well-defined patient outcomes by well-designed, appropriately powered, randomized, controlled clinical trials (Dalen, 1998). All drugs that have been approved by the American Food and Drug Administration (FDA) since the 1960s have met this standard, however many therapies introduced before the 1960s do not (Dalen, 1998). Three of the major antithrombotic agents prescribed by western-trained physicians were introduced prior to the randomized clinical trial; these are wafarin, aspirin and heparin and up to 1998 were still not evidence based (Dalen, 1998). Other medicinal practices adopted before they were subjected to clinical trials according to Dalen (1998) are coronary artery bypass grafts--the efficacy of this procedure based on early reports was described as "self-evident." Percutaneous transluminal coronary angioplasty was performed in hundreds of thousands of patients from 1979 until 1992 when the first randomized clinical trial demonstrating efficacy was conducted (Dalen, 1998).
Bedside pulmonary artery catheterization has been performed millions of times since 1970 and until 1998 was still devoid of "good clinical evidence of effectiveness" (Dalen, 1998). None of these non-evidence based practices or others like them are described as unconventional or quackery because they were introduced from the mainstream of western medicine (Dalen, 1998).

Complicated realities and weak convergence

Donna Haraway (1988 in Weasel, 2001) has outlined a post modern feminist theory that "insists on the multiple fractured identities of knowers (race, class, sexuality, gender) and upon the contextual, situated position of persons occupying multiply overlapping and contradictory categories". The analysis above shows that the local scientists' "split and contradictory self" within triple patriarchy did not give them a strong enough base to accept the knowledge of female healers without validation by allopathic medicine. These men are located in a political situation in which Afro-Trinidadian and Indo-Trinidadian men are struggling to control state power (Munasinghe, 2001). In this context they accept without question the dictates of the external western man; be he IMF-man, the World Bank-man or male western scientist.

Matrices 1 and 2 demonstrate that networks incorporate many social and economic factors that shape and guide knowledge and actors. Folk knowledge exists in (marginalized) parallel to western science (Laguerre, 1987; Lans, 1996). Allopathic practitioners have legal rights but other practitioners are free to work as long as they do not claim to be doctors. The limits placed on who is recognized as a valid health practitioner is one factor that preserves the unequal status between western trained and empirically trained health providers. Extracts from interviews conducted with the veterinarians are used below to illustrate how well-established actor-networks seem to insist on annihilating personal experience; instead Star (1991) claims that scientists behave as if the standardized science network is the only valued reality there is, like male veterinarians Ames, Singh and Maynard quoted below:

Ames: The Folk claims are not valid, they are psychological. Seventy-five percent would have healed anyway. They have a false sense of security, clients might bring the animal to the vet too late, after they first mis-diagnose it.

Singh: Maybe if we find that the use of folk medicine seems to have efficacy, we could do trials to see how it works. The use of folk medicine doesn't affect veterinarians. I am not aware that there has been any demonstrated efficacy of folk medicine. Even if they use it, if they are in trouble they call the veterinarian, especially modern farmers. Hindu pundits' jharay animals (conduct a religious ritual for them) then the farmer will call the veterinarian. But I tell them don't call the veterinarian so late, call the pundit after the veterinarian, don't wait so long.

Maynard: Science requires years of research, hard work, man has to pay and work. Periwinkle (Catharanthus roseus) extracts weren't discovered by accident, Periwinkle was tested by biochemists for years[33]. Drugs are made so patients don't absorb alkaloids when they are ingested, that is why science is important to unlock chemicals and synthesize drugs..... My granny knows about Kojo root (Petiveria alliacea). She puts it in the chicken's nests, it is a potent insecticide, it smells very bad and it keeps away snakes. I swear by this folk medicine.

   In the interview extract above, the veterinarian Maynard showed the dichotomy of having a cultural base in folk medicine and a professional standing in science. Actors and actor-networks are hybrid groups always prone to dissension and internal crises (Callon, 1991).

Matrix 3 builds on Matrices 1 and 2 and shows how the international scientific actor-network impacts on Trinidad and Tobago's scientists and professionals (Lans, 1996).
The struggle over science versus traditional is more complex than can be depicted in Matrix 3. The term knowledge community like Actor Networks theory describes the dynamic network of actors, processes of negotiation and the diverse ways in which knowledge is constructed and performed (Raeder and Rikoon, 1997). The term communities is used in recognition that individuals may participate in and utilize several knowledge communities. Finally the word community also reveals the poroous boundaries between knowledge groups; with knowledge communities influencing science and folk medicine more than others. My account goes further than that of Raeder and Rikoon (1997) who did not discuss the power dynamics of the different knowledge communities in their account.
Ramlal echoes the financial and other constraints reflected in the Ministry of Food and Marine Exploitation Annual Report 1990. His views also illustrate the term in Matrix 3 called weak convergence:

---

[33] Periwinkle was being used traditionally to treat diabetes and became useful to treat cancers. Barsh (1997) points out that no ethnography was done to establish that this property of *C. roseus* was previously unknown.

There is no money here to do research. There is no Pharmacology Department, only Chemistry. CARIRI[34] will only do work if paid, but few can pay. Foreign research is misapplied in the Caribbean.

Matrix 3. The Trinidad and Tobago scientific and societal actor network

Terms and Meaning in STS	Scientist/public response	Illustration
A stabilized network is only stable for those members who form/use/maintain it. Network users who are non-members of the community of practice suffer (Star, 1991). Scientist-communities of practice, have conventions of use.	Scientists often take sabbaticals to do research in other countries so they can publish. Scientific texts are networks for the in-crowd. Social management of trust moves from herbalist to professionals.	Trinidad and Tobago scientists sign on to the standardized technologies in order to gain from already established external scientific networks. This is a network with established norms.
The Gatekeeper standpoint the strategies by which an actor-network becomes indispensable and maintains itself. Eminent scientists become gatekeepers. Gatekeeping influences topic selection and research funding for most scientists.	Folk medicine is not modern, or progressive. Research is done on poisonous plants, and weed control.	Peer review and publishing in the right journals excludes folk medicine from animal health science.
An intermediary is anything passing between actors, which defines the relationship between them. Intermediaries describe their networks; they compose them by giving them order and form. Knowledge and funding, scientific articles, drugs, instruments and software are intermediaries (Callon, 1991).	Foreign science is more profitable career-wise. Agro-chemical shops and Pharmacies sell drugs to farmers without prescriptions leading to abuse of drugs. There is no monitoring of drug residues at the abattoir.	Uncertain folk medicine discarded in favor of certain imported drugs. Discarding of local knowledge as folklore. Foreign technology becomes embedded in local social networks. Institutionalization.
Every enrolment entails both a failure to enroll and a partial destruction of the world of the non-enrolled (Star, 1991).	Rejection of folk medicine as an actor since some involved in the conventional drug industry are afraid of loss of sales if farmers use their own plant-based solutions.	The joint creation / nullification of knowledge: Farmers and herbalists want to gain some autonomy and prestige for their own knowledge, but are actively discouraged.
Partial signings-on and commitments, no intermediaries, no standardized package, all lead to a Weakly convergent network.	Under-funded actors in the Ministry of Agriculture find their status is constantly in question and it is difficult to mobilize other parts of the network.	Veterinarians do not get sufficient resources from Government.Without money vets have less power so farmers use their own strategies.

An interview quote from scientist Guardia who has conducted research into poisonous plants demonstrates Weak convergence and the structures of dependency between developing world and developed world scientists:

[We do] Research here in chemical synthesis with no water, no chemicals, no electrical power, and the chemicals are very expensive or toxic. Others do their chemistry in another place; they

---

34 CARIRI is the acronym of the Caribbean Research Institute, based at the University of the West Indies, Trinidad and Tobago

go and spend 3 months in the USA, and pay for the facilities to do Chemistry. For [my work in] poisonous plants the first necessary step was to get other people to do the tests. Further tests were done in the United Kingdom. I also have University of Toronto connections. I spent two summers in Toronto, so I had money and equipment.

Real world conditions constrain the attempts of the professionals to marginalize other healers. These real world conditions result in partial enrolment and a weakly convergent network. Clients and livestock keepers continuously challenge the Trinidad and Tobago veterinarian's claims to be the sole source of animal health knowledge. This is illustrated by quotes from farmers Ganesh and Haskell presented below. These farmers were treating their own animals after the veterinarian had failed to provide solutions. They were confident of their own solutions under certain circumstances.

Genesh: My cow got away, it had a sore that remained for two years. The cow was tied by the horn so that it couldn't lick the sore. The veterinarian said to shoot it. I used a poultice of rachette (*Nopalea cochenillifera*), flour and water. It recovered.]

Haskell: My first cow in 1968 gave trouble to make young. The veterinarian said to put it on the table [slaughter it]. My neighbor told me to use Epsom salts and *Aloe vera*. I have had many offspring from that cow since. I have 7 cows now and I gave some to relatives.

Conclusion

Arnold (1994) suggests that certain Caribbean intellectuals think cultural production is solely a masculine activity. In the struggle for recognition between Caribbean males and western males folk medicine may be too closely associated with the denigrated female role to be considered a suitable inclusion into modern development. The agency and power of western science lies in the interlocking interests that make up the "Old Boy" networks of relationships that exist in science (Callon, 1991; Deichmann and Müller-Hill, 1998). Actors in these relationships can be resistant to new ideas that may require a loss of, or at least re-negotiation of existing scientific networks and interests (Goodwin and Tangum, 1998; Law, 1991). The debates between science and non-science presented in this chapter reveal an underlying structure in which the actors position themselves. The matrices, clippings and interviews showed the different actors trying to define legitimate health services and health providers, and then trying to persuade others to subscribe to those definitions. The temporarily stabilized outcome of these negotiations is the preservation of unequal relations of power for professionals versus herbalists.

The scientific actor-network offers the security of a valued social identity, which is perhaps what some herbalists are seeking. There seemed to be a limited range of socially valued knowledge positions available. To seek entry into existing scientific networks, maintain their status in them, or prevent entry to these knowledge positions, scientific actors invented and re-invented their personal and professional histories and made references to terms such as: efficacy, validation and dosages which were used in self-validating ways. Science is increasingly seen as a social process of making narratives where meanings are contested and stabilized for a time through the productive relations of power (Morawski, 1988). This means that the epistemological paradox of using political enterprises like feminism to achieve a more accurate, coherent and less masculinist science, that would include alternative medicine, can be resolved through the reconsideration and alteration of existing social relations of power (Morawski, 1988). Researchers self-reflexivity involves a realistic appraisal of the limits of research as a locus for authentic political activity (Glucksman,

1994). However that does not mean that researchers should not strive for an outcome of greater awareness that leads to social change (Mies, 1983).

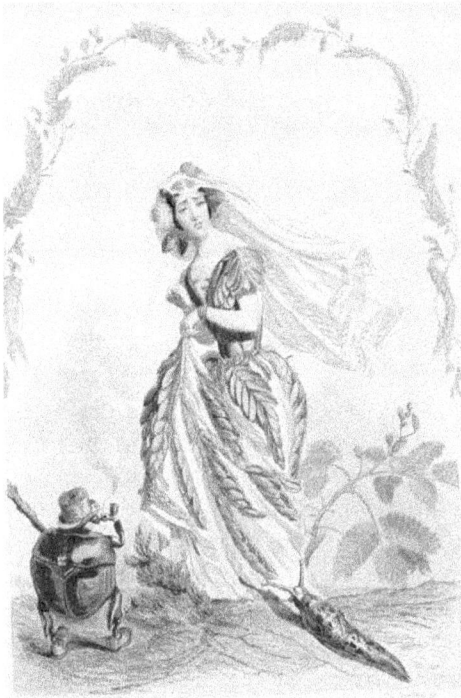

Figure 103. Mimosa pudica
Figure 104. Nicotiana tabacum

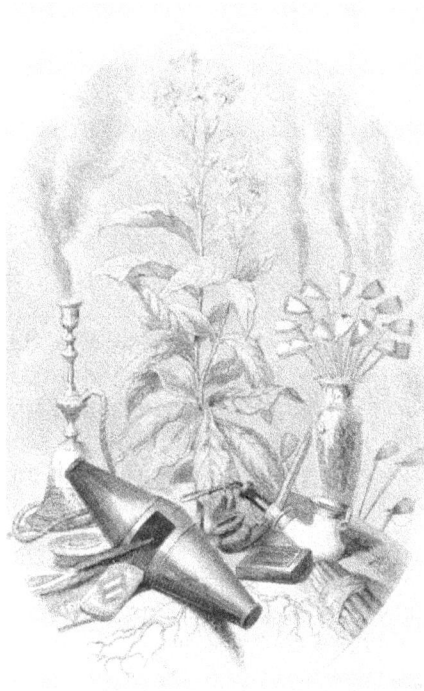

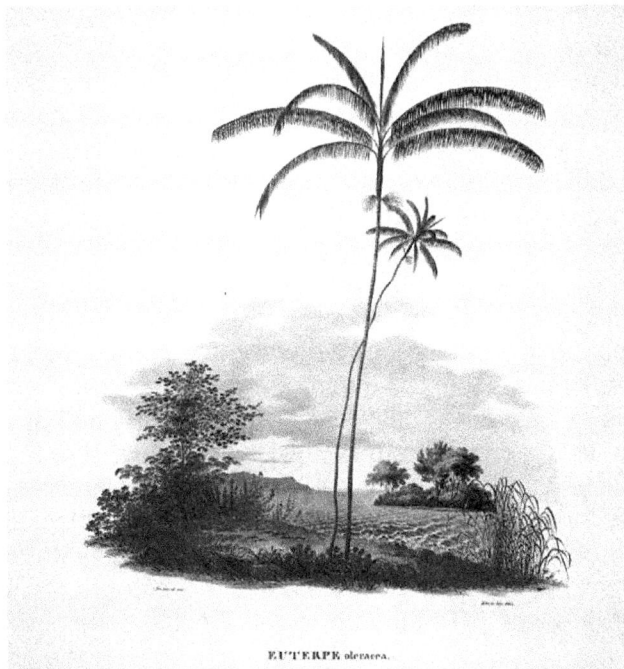

Figure 105. Euterpe oleracea

Becoming Creole

It is certainly dubious sense to write as if all peoples equally desired to have their own history intact (whatever that might mean). People may prefer to live in the present or to skip bits of their history. It is usually wise to leave bygones to be bygones. If doing without history is the path of forgiveness, it is also true that forgetting on one's own behalf is easier than forgetting injuries done to the dead (Douglas, 1995).

11. Becoming Creole[35]

Introduction

This chapter addresses the research question of whether Trinbagonian folk medicinal knowledge fits a theory of [ethnomedicinal] agrarian creolization. First the historical past is described to give the societal setting for folk medicine. Then the concepts Creolization, hybridity and passing will be discussed, and these will be applied to folk medicine. In Trinidad and Tobago like in other modern societies cultural meanings are volatile, plural and fragmented. New knowledge in all knowledge cultures is always (re) interpreted in terms of the available frames of reference of the cultural system. This cultural system is in turn porous, and as such influenced by the borrowings from external influences especially transcultural scientific knowledge (national health care services, school education, etc.) and the international mass media (Stewart, 1999). The domination of privileged discourses like western science and medicine, amplified by mass media houses, silences other discourses but they are not speechless yet.

The struggles described in Chapter 12 between scientists and herbalists illustrated by heart specialist Kenroy making warnings in the newspapers against vague and unproven [herbal] remedies (Express July 3, 1999; Newsday July 5, 1999 pg. 24), and the discussion that this generated (Express July 18, 1999 pg. 7; Express July 20, pg. 21) is only partly about science versus 'nonsense'. The deeper issue is the desire to forget all history and leave the colonial past behind[36]. The Caribbean was colonised by western powers for more than five centuries. This history has produced a dilemma in that progress is associated with the colonisers but is still considered desirable. The languages spoken belong to the West and the historical past is difficult to face (Price and Price, 1997).

The historical past

Under the Cédula de Población 1783, local people of all races were granted certain rights. Under the Articles of Surrender of 1797, the British accepted these rights, which allowed all people to inherit property, hold commissions in the local forces, practice professions, to have exemption from certain taxes, and to apply to the crown for grants of land. Article 5 of the Cedula gave all settlers citizenship after five years of residence and it made few distinctions between whites and coloureds, which was unique to Trinidad. The Cédula de Población 1783 offered incentives to all settlers. The free blacks and coloureds received free grants of land: 16 acres for each man, woman and child and half of that for each slave brought. This was about half the grant of a white settler (Joseph, 1837). Due to the Cédula some free

---

[35] 'Creole Remedies' is a local term with a literal historical, 'local parlance', pre-academic meaning. The term is reclaimed as a positive force, with strong female elements (grandmothers, old aunts). Throughout the book European and Amerindian elements of the folk culture are included alongside and equal to those of Africa and India as a validation of the Creole past which can be seen as a quilt of diverse patterns.

[36] Farage (2003) claims that the Wapishana in Guyana have a saying: "you cannot see *kotuanao* [the old, the dead] with your eyes." Farage says that the main attribute of the dead and its ghost (*ma'chai*) is that of putrefaction which can spread among the living who are still grieving. Therefore forgetting is the ideal attitude towards the dead and the past.

blacks were slave-owning proprietors of large sugar estates. They had come to Trinidad from Martinique, Guadeloupe, Ste. Domingue, Grenada and St. Lucia as educated and professional people or military men. They developed a black middle class. Sometimes their sons were educated in Europe or took the grand tour of Europe and they adopted the style of European élite's of equal education and wealth. Some young sons had blood ties to titled people of a previous generation, which provided some mobility in the social stratification system[37]. The snobbishness of the times are illustrated in this local rhyme:

> "and this was sweet old Trinidad, land of the sugarcane and the cocoa pod, where the Ganteaumes spoke only to the de Verteuils, and the de Verteuils spoke only to God" (Besson, 2000).

However these free blacks did not enjoy their prosperity for long. The new British Governor Sir Ralph Woodford felt that the non-white Creoles were upstarts not in their 'proper place' who had been given too much freedom and privileges by the former Spanish government. The local whites were also foreign to Woodford (French, Irish, German and Spanish). Woodford, the first civilian governor decided to civilise all of Trinidad's 'disorder[38]' which came from the vicarious origins of its people by replacing military force with the institutionalisation of a settled society graduated in terms of social rank, which paralleled racial stratification (Besson, 2000). In the 1820s Woodford started to put social pressure on the free blacks and he prevented their advancement wherever he could. Local white Creoles changed their former cordial attitudes and adopted Woodford's prejudices to enhance their own social standing because as 'inferior colonials' they were excluded from the top administrative posts which were reserved for British expatriates (Barnes, 1998; Besson, 2000). After 1876, the English monopoly over government came to an end but the English influence continued (Besson, 2000). The racial and social stratification in Trinidad lasted in modified form until the 1970 Black Power movement forced social changes.

Despite the efforts of Woodford and others to prevent the advancement of the coloured population, agriculture played a role in shaping the society. By the 1950s cocoa had become a staple in Trinidad's export market (Besson, 2000). Whereas sugar cane is only viable with vast acreage's, people with small plots of land were able to participate in cocoa cultivation so the middle classes of all races became comfortable between the 1860s and the 1920s. The French Creoles had become both cocoa planters and exporters-importers (Besson, 2000). The Hispanic-Amerindian population (cocoa panyols) was the poor but hospitable backbone of the cocoa economy, clearing the forest and cultivating the cocoa fields. Many families of the coloured lower and middle classes alongside the Madeirian, Chinese, Syrian, Lebanese and East Indian immigrants were able to own small cocoa estates, own/operate small and medium-sized businesses, live comfortably, and educate their children to become professionals (Mohammed, 1995; Besson, 2000).
These new middle classes strove to maintain the values and morals of the colonial society (Besson, 2000).

Gender roles: Man better man

The historical dilemmas of slavery and colonialism have produced anticolonial counter discourses like antillanité and Négritude. These discourses have masculinist overtones; only male talent and pursuits are permitted and anything with female overtones like folk medicine is pushed into the background (Arnold, 1994). The underpinnings of these anticolonial discourses are that western imperial discourse had feminised those cultures,

---

[37] Maryse Condé explores the quest for identity of the 'fatherless bastards' of elite men and domestic servants (Rosello, 1995).
[38] Trinidad was a British crown colony, with a French-speaking population and Spanish laws (Besson, 2000). Moore-Gilbert (1997) claims that colonials used the existing hybridity in their colonies as an excuse to impose central power as a unifying force.

which it had subjugated, in order to justify that subjugation. This feminisation process is intolerable to all colonised men since the role of the real productive man is occupied by the European or American white man (Arnold, 1994). One theorised reaction to this dilemma was the early anticolonial discourse of Négritude which established the ideological dogma that only African contributions to Caribbean culture could be counted[39] and held the escaped slave or Maroon as the super male but absent hero (Arnold, 1994). The absence of the hero was important because of the real presence or role occupation of the western man. Négritude inverted the racist stereotype but left the underlying racist structure intact (Arnold, 1994).

The newer discourse of créolité created by Jean Bernabé, Patrick Chamoiseau and Raphaël Confiant shifted the theoretical focus to the plantation and the joint Afro-Creole culture of cultural and biological métissage between white masters and black female slaves. In this account the black man still has no creative or procreative role in society but is a male story teller, a docile slave trusted by the master who uses words to spread a subversive message similar to that of the calypsonian[40] of today (Price and Price, 1997). What both discourses have in common is the absence of women. This is more important in the discourse of créolité since it silences the grandmothers, great aunts and village midwives who are recognised by most others as the transmitters of folk tales, folk medicines and oral culture (Herskovits and Herskovits, 1947; Weniger *et al.*, 1982; Kainer and Duryea, 1992; Milliken and Albert, 1996). Arnold (1994) suggests that intellectuals who think that cultural production is solely a masculine activity created the masculinist anticolonial discourses. In the struggle for recognition between Caribbean males and western males folk medicine may be too closely associated with the denigrated female role to be considered a suitable inclusion into modern development.

The dilemmas of history, language and western-derived gender roles that are said to be not economically realistic have shaped a continuous struggle over origins and whether Creolization is preferable to maintaining separate ethnic identities. It has been claimed that Creole subjectivity is dependent on the structures and ideology of European colonialism and becomes unravelled in a postcolonial Caribbean (Barnes, 1998). Added to this is the pull between the colonisers Eurocentrism and the colonized's Afrocentrism. Price and Price (1997) criticise the French West Indian intellectuals Bernabé, Chamoiseau and Confiant for understating the diversity of the African origins of the French West Indian islands. The West Indians are also criticised for tracing links from the Martiniquan Creole language to the French language of 1652 in Normandy and Anjou. Price and Price claimed that France was pushing this ideology of European linkages to hasten the assimilation of the French West Indies into the metropole.

This assimilation process is an indication that the French West Indian islands are perhaps more actively fathered than the former and current British West Indian islands assuming that the Caribbean islands and their populations are what Latour calls 'hybrids' (Elam, 1999). These hybrids are the mongrel miscegenations of the West, the creations, 'outside children', the responsibilities of the West (still to some extent) (Elam, 1999). The West may not give these mongrel hybrids enough love and attention, but has not abandoned them either. When Indo-Trinidadians accuse Afro-Trinidadians (the academic élite of whom they call Afro-Saxons) of attempting to Afro-Creolize all Trinidadian culture the implication is 1) that they are trying to take over the role of the original 'bad Western fathers' and trying to create more

---

[39] In Brathwaite's concept of creolization the Asian contributions are considered secondary because they are more recent arrivals than the planters and slaves (Moore-Gilbert, 1997).
[40] Latour assumes this subversive storyteller role and claims that he is seeking 'weaker explanations and accounts that could defeat the strong scientific ones (Elam, 1999). Latour's storyteller role like that of créolité can only be occupied by a few specially gifted men 'all-seeing' men (Elam, 1999).

134

'mongrel' children (Afro-Indo mixtures are called 'dougla') and, 2) that they are showing racial self-contempt by wanting mixed-race children. Indo-Trinidadians in return are accused of clinging to their traditions and refusing to Creolize[41]. Underlying the debate is which ethnic group should assume the role that the Western colonising male previously occupied. Mohammed (1995) has claimed that in 1917, Trinidad and Tobago had three co-existing and competing patriarchal systems. These were the dominant white system which in those days controlled state power, the 'creole' patriarchy of mixed race and Afro-Trinidadians functioning in and emerging from the white group and the Indian form which was at the bottom (brought to do the labour the emancipated slaves refused) (Mohammed, 1995). As stated above, the discourse of créolité silenced the female healers in the struggle for recognition between Afro-Caribbean males and western males. In the triple patriarchal system of Trinidad and Tobago the association of folk medicine with the denigrated female role may have been even more difficult to overcome.

Trinidad is a complex society where authority and values have traditionally been contested. Also playing a role was the competition for economic, social and political power among the three patriarchal groups. Colonialism and the first post-Independent governments were based on Christian values. The predominantly Hindu current government does not accept these values as the norm[42]. This reassertion of Hindu values was a surprise to those long accustomed through school and work relationships to the élite sub-group of westernised, Christianised middle class Indians. It has now become apparent that some in this sub-group had only temporarily jettisoned their Hindu traditions in order to gain political and social power through state education, and that the ones who remained Christian did not represent the larger Hindu group. This larger group consisted of Indo-Trinidadians who had reconstituted their institutions and culture in rural villages and have historically been represented by religious leaders (Mohammed, 1995). In an ironic twist this argumentative Trinidad and Tobago[43] resembles what Elam (1999) calls the Victorian definition of hybridity: different races continue to live separate lives and promote diverse cultural identities within the body of the hybrid state in a form of internal apartheid.

Many musical forms have been Creolized. The Spanish Catholic and religious Parang has been Creolized into Soca-Parang with profane themes. Likewise Indian chutney music formerly the domain of women before marriage ceremonies has become a more public Creolized Chutney-Soca in a comparatively natural and generative way. The development of Chutney-Soca troubled the conservative Hindu leaders who did not want these formerly private sensual dances exposed to the male Creole gaze. Cultural hybridity is generative and fertilising (like Chutney Soca) or disruptive, anxiety producing and transgressive depending on the view of the audiences (Friedman, 1999; Werbner, 2001).

Ethnicity implies the maintenance of social boundaries (Friedman, 1999). Ethnic identity seems to require socio-cultural contrast for its validation (Hastrup and Elsass, 1990). This contrast is sometimes artificially created especially in the 'silly season' between 'Indian Arrival Day' in May and 'Emancipation Day' in August. A few examples of this are given. These examples were taken from newspaper debates that generated numerous letters to the editor and comments on radio talk shows. The belief that Carnival in Trinidad has roots in France and Spain and includes African-based additions among others was called Eurocentric. Carnival's 'true' roots were traced to West Africa and the European Carnival tradition was traced to Egyptian fertility rituals (Gilkes, 1999). Serious attempts are being

---

[41] Brathwaite (1971) leaves East Indians outside of Creolization processes in Jamaica. His reasoning could be linked to their small population in Jamaica.
[42] Respecting the principle of cultural difference generates problems and issues for discussion (Moore-Gilbert, 1997).
[43] One long standing and respected journalist calls this bickering "The guava season of our discontent" (Pantin, 1999).

made to have a Park in an élite residential area turned into a memorial for slaves based on the contentious claim that slaves were buried there. Slaves were obviously buried all over the country. No one taking part in the debate over the Park contested the need for a memorial, the choice of site is the discussion point[44] (Anthony, 1999; Shah, 1999). The small brick enclosure left behind after a Port of Spain store was looted and burned in the 1990 coup was labelled as a slave cell and a ceremony was conducted. The enclosure was built and used as a safe by the Portuguese-origin storeowners (Besson, 2000). These struggles can be interpreted sympathetically as 'dramatised' rituals or transgressive performances in which the performers' aims are to get the blessings of the community (Werbner, 2001). A less sympathetic interpretation is that the performers' unconscious or conscious strategy is to create hyper-Creolized forms in the expectation that these hyper-forms may eventually become accepted as correct (Jackson, 1989).

'Retentions, adaptations and so on'

Brathwaite[45] (1971) writes in his chapter 'The 'Folk' Culture of the Slaves' that he does not intend to enter the argument about African 'survivals', 'retentions', 'adaptations' and so on. He then quotes slave customs that are very similar to Amerindian traditions. M.G.Smith (1957) critiques the theoretical claims of Herskovits and Herskovits (1947). Mintz (1974) claims that social scientists attribute African origins to traditions because they are frustrated by the painstaking and inconclusive research required in order for origins to be traced. Mintz also claims that survivals are considered interesting because they reflect the resilience of the human spirit even under slavery. The ubiquitous Caribbean dish of rice and peas is not so interesting because as a creole cultural form arising from slavery it is treated as cultural defeat rather than capacity. Brathwaite (1971) claims that there was a tendency for Caribbean people to depend on the mother countries for normative value-references rather than using residential Creole traditions and the Amerindian heritage has been poorly documented.

Subaltern politics

Culture[46] has become a site where an attempt is being made to establishment a new set of values and ideologies over the existing colonial and black Creole values (Dissanayake, 1992). Indo-Trinidadians claim that black Creole culture was pushed as national culture after national independence in a hegemonic way and Indians (self-described social and cultural subalterns) who did not play along were called the "recalcitrant minority" by the first Prime Minister Dr. Eric Williams (Ryan, 1999; Ryan, 2001). Controversy erupted when May 31, 1999 was created as a new public holiday called 'Indian Arrival Day' since other ethnic groups made counter claims that all Trinidad and Tobago's ethnic groups 'arrived'. There are two vocal camps[47] pushing what they call African and Indian culture. Ryan (1999) claims that both of these identities are built on half-forgotten collective memories or myths spun or resuscitated by political and cultural interest-seekers who are using them to bolster their political, social or economic agendas... political ethnicity. The debates centre on whether the so-called African-based cultural forms are given more state financial support than those considered Indian-based, and the debates are part of a wider discussion on what it means to be Trinidadian (Munasinghe, 2001). The debate centres on

---

[44] Previously existing sites are renamed rather than new sites being created.

[45] Edward Brathwaite, *The Development of Creole Society in Jamaica 1770-1820*, Clarendon Press, Oxford.

[46] The Ministry of Culture and Gender Affairs was called the Ministry of Black Culture and Gender Affairs by Indo-Trinidadian spokesman Kamal Persad as part of a larger claim that Indo-Trinidad festivals are underfunded and that Carnival is not truly national but gets the largest amount of funding (Persad, 1999).

[47] "A cacophonous din of spoilers and dividers.. opportunistic carrion crows…[responsible for] a hysteria of racial and religious bigotry spreading like maljo" (Pantin, 1999).

which group can claim to represent the nation and thus legitimise their control over the state (Williams, 1989). The contestation over which culture is funded (dance, music, Carnival, and other 'feathers and flourishes') means a neglect of un-funded culture (folk medicine, patois).

These ethnic 'pushes' along with the rush to 'modernity and the determination to forget everything associated with the colonised past are perhaps strategic. These strategies are undertaken in recognition that culture does not exist in and of itself but evolves through borrowings, appropriations and inventions (Werbner, 2001). If 'forgetting' is a strategic amnesia, if the 'real' history is erased, then another historical narrative[48] can be created. In one of these new narratives the dead slave becomes the absent hero, venerated in a public park strategically located in an élite residential area, and the élite location perhaps represents another attempt to occupy the role of the western man (King George V Park) by the Afro-Creole man (Emancipation Park).

Cultural integration

Assimilative cultural integration exists when acceptors take the values of the giving culture as a point of departure. Incorporative cultural integration exists when the acceptors' own system of values is the point of departure (Tan, 1989). Assimilative cultural change describes the newly emerging coloured middle class. After 100 years of British rule they had assimilated English Victorian - values (Christianity, politeness and respectability) (Besson, 2000). The original ties to France and Spain had been lost by this time so instead of the tour of Europe, some middle class sons became scholarship winners at the best universities in England and Scotland. Many became professionals, lawyers and doctors, schoolteachers and civil servants. Others, like L.O. Inniss, owned pharmacies (Besson, 2000). In 1910 L.O. Inniss was the head of the pharmacological society in Trinidad and Tobago. It is in the context of the move away from the lower classes towards a professional life style embued with British values that one can re-read the address Inniss made to the Pharmacological society in 1910:

> ....One wonders what those Creole remedies are, which succeed, when duly diplomaed scions of AEsculapius have signally failed... Having been trained as a druggist and having had to pass many hours before my examination, learning the doses of medicine, I can't understand the fast and loose way in which these Creole remedies are prescribed (Inniss, 1910).

The expanding middle class fuelled by education and desirous of social mobility and acceptance, disassociated itself from its background in agriculture and traditional medicine (Rollocks, 1991). This disassociation was then reinforced in and by the British-based educational system which reinforced transcultural scientific knowledge and did not teach alternative approaches at either the Eastern Caribbean Institute of Agriculture and Forestry (ECIAF) or at the University of the West Indies (UWI). Wilson (1961) alluded to the minimal prestige agriculture had (still has) as an academic subject, this reflects the marginal position of agriculture in the economy, but it also reinforces that very marginality.

Trinidadian doctors trained abroad in the 'mother country', discouraged the use of folk medicinal practices[49] because they "smack of pagan Africa, and are no longer necessary in the light of Trinidad's medical progress" (Mischel, 1959; Laguerre, 1987). Dispensary nurses in Dominica still denigrate women's traditional healing expertise with bush teas and Obeah (Krumeich, 1994). These attitudes were also present in academia as in the UWI sociologist quoted by Pereira (1969) who claimed that 'a study of folk medicine has no sociological significance'.

---

[48] 'One of the past's greatest strengths is its power to change' (Shannon, 1998).
[49] Part of the development discourse was to remove populations from the domain of folk wisdom, domestic remedies and non-modern healers (Nandy and Visvanathan, 1990).

Despite the social aspirations of the early pharmacists, doctors and nurses, folk medicine was resorted to for emergencies. For example large quantities of *Momordica charantia* were harvested and sold during the severe influenza epidemic in Barbados in 1938 and even pharmacists bottled and sold infusions (Bayley, 1949). In the 1930s the impact of western medicine was that of a dominant paradigm that was not totally accepted, but which offered elements that were selectively appropriated in a process of indigenization. The concepts of 'structural superiority' and 'functional strength' imply that western medicine acquired élite status because of its ability to control diseases (or suppress symptoms), while the folk medicinal system retained functional strength because it was more accessible and available to those isolated communities that existed well into the twentieth century (Brereton, 1981).

Diachronic and synchronic analyses can be used to explore transactions in social networks which help to explain how one explanatory model, like western medicine, becomes dominant in a medical system (Tan, 1989). In the Cayman Islands folk medicine was once a robustly functioning set of beliefs and practices that served the social and physical needs of the community (Buchler, 1964). In the 1960s Caymanians believed that liquids (like tisanes) were more potent than pills. Inaccurate prognoses and occasional deaths were explained in terms of the system and rarely resulted in a questioning of the basic axioms of the system. However, increased educational opportunities, economic mobility and the expansion of communication networks left Caymanians stranded between folk medicine which is increasingly ridiculed and western medicine (Buchler, 1964). A parallel system developed in Dominica where women eagerly accept modern biomedical services for their children. Culturally women are solely responsible for their children, including their health, so women try to master a range of therapeutic skills. High technology biomedical care is appropriated as a missing element from women's own repertoires of herbal and religious healing (Brodwin, 1998).

In the Spanish-speaking Caribbean Cuba's medical diplomacy and investment in biotechnology generates symbolic capital: intangible qualities (like honour, prestige, and reputation) which appear opposed to strictly economic interests, are in fact convertible back into material capital (Brodwin, 1998). The Cuban policy is to demonstrate that its socialist state can provide a modern health care system and need not settle for small-scale technologies or China's barefoot doctors (Brodwin, 1998). Cuba's biomedical service with its massive ideological weight may be considered a modernising vanguard that undercuts local therapies and conceptions of illness and suffering (Brodwin, 1998). When a modernising vanguard like biomedicine is introduced into a rural or poor community, its clients are forced to adopt certain perspectives and learn new scientific phrases (Brodwin, 1998). People then detach themselves from or modify local contexts of meaning when they accept western-derived biomedical treatments (Brodwin, 1998).

One instance of this process was seen in one interview in northern Trinidad. The respondent whose puppies had parvovirus used aloes (*Aloe vera*) to purge her dogs for the first day. Then she used store-bought golden seal and myrrh (*Commiphora myrrha*) and gave this for five days. The respondent interpreted the western-derived golden seal in both western and Creole terms: "golden seal is a kind of antibiotic, a blood purifier."

Colonially derived attitudes are also seen in non-academics as depicted in a Jamaica study of 125 pregnant women (Landman and Hall, 1983). Eight-two percent of the women reported drinking bush teas during their pregnancy (Landman and Hall, 1983). These women claimed that drinking *Momordica charantia* would make their babies' skin attractive (brown, fair, and clear). Patricia Mohammed (2000) has described how 'brown' skin has become stereotyped and coded as more desirable. The colonial bourgeois cultural model, and social aspiration are also seen in the phenomenon that a preferred item, usually imported and more expensive, replaces cheaper, more traditional, locally-produced foods when funds are available (Mintz, 1983; Purcell, 1983). As mentioned before the emphasis given to import substitution in manufacturing in the 1950s and 1960s led to shoddy manufactured goods and to the perception that everything foreign is automatically better.

This perception is manifested in the tendency to label local medicine 'bush' and imported medicines 'herbs', these latter are considered superior and consumers ask for them[50] (Express Newspaper April 1986; Express Newspaper June 1986). The interaction of folk medicine with formal medicine in Trinidad and Tobago can be described as tolerant scepticism, it is 'less than' western medicine (Laguerre, 1987). Allopathic practitioners have legal rights, but other practitioners are free to work as long as they do not claim to be doctors. Tolerant scepticism leads many Caribbean people to rely on the more progressive 'foreign market' for answers. In this context one respondent told a story about Canadian healing oil, a joint/limb healing ointment that is produced in Guyana but is called Canadian Healing Oil because "the people know their market"... "one woman I know sent all over Canada for it, but they never heard of it over there."

These attitudes towards folk medicine fit the concept of ethnic ideology (Serbin, 1981). A series of colonially derived, diffuse ethnic ideologies were developed about the dominant European group and the other subordinated ethnic groups. These ideologies were generated from various factors: the survival of ties in the colonial society and the impact of the dominant ideology and culture on the pattern of each group's differing process of acculturation. These ideologies then gel to become what Balutansky (1997) has described as the Caribbean colonial bourgeois cultural model with its distinct dualisms of head/body/reason/instinct: intellectuals don't play sports, scholarship winners don't read for discovery only to pass examinations. Creolization is then personified as the West Indian love for the vitality of Caribbean life coupled with the need to leave the Caribbean; to be trained in the classics yet argue for socialism, and to refuse to replace the colonisers Eurocentrism with the colonised's Afrocentrism (Balutansky, 1997).

Crab antics

Wilson (1969) has drawn parallels between Mediterranean concepts of 'honour' and 'shame' in his theorisation of Caribbean concepts of 'reputation' and 'respectability'. Respectability or 'social worth' can only be obtained by adhering to the Eurocentric colonial system of social stratification based on class, colour, education, and propriety based on church-going and marriage (Besson, 1993). Wilson claims that Caribbean women value respectability. Reputation is derived in opposition to the values of respectability and is based on 'personal' worth and is valued by young Caribbean men. Groups of men meet in bars and recreate their reputations based on their recounted boasting of sexual conquests, fathering many children, being able to use words impressively in arguments or debates, participating in Rastafarianism, and having skills like music, hunting, healing, Obeah, etc. As men age and become less able to compete on 'reputation' and more concerned with careers and the after-life they become more interested in 'respectability' (Besson, 1993). The reputation/respectability dialectic is indigenous to the Caribbean in the form that it takes and the long-term implications of the everyday practices.

---

[50] Most of the Trinidad and Tobago herbal shops sell foreign herbs in conjunction with Kloss's book, (Kloss, J. 1992. *Back to Eden*, 2nd Ed, Back to Eden Books Publishing Co. Loma Linda, California). Plants discussed have similar common names to local plants but are different botanically. Several of the respondents referred to this book or showed the book during the interviews in the first phase of the research.

Wilson's concepts are important because folk medicine, village midwives and Obeahmen are firmly lodged in the 'reputation' realm, while medicine and pharmacy are located in the 'respectability' realm. This dialectic may have influenced the formality of the first and succeeding international workshops on herbal medicine which sought to pull folk medicine into the realm of 'respectability'. The veterinarians' response to their homeopathic colleague first raised in Chapter 13 can also be analysed in terms of reputation and respectability. It may be that scientists involved in controversial research at the research frontiers, [like Homeopathy], are expected to be located in 'Ivy League Universities', and not struggling in, or re-migrating to Third World countries (Collins, 1981). 'Emigrated crabs' once out are not expected (or welcomed) to return and compete economically with the crabs who stayed behind. The dialectic between reputation and respectability is manifested in 'crab antics' behaviours which are designed as status levellers (Wilson, 1973). If one crab is placed in a bucket it climbs out and escapes easily. If there are many crabs in the bucket each one will prevent the others from escaping 'in order to retain a community of the impoverished' (Lewis, 1998). Ridicule and gossip are everyday 'crab antics' (Besson, 1993). 'Crab antics' are also found in medicine and agriculture in that pharmacists are accused of altering veterinary prescriptions so that they can obtain drugs to sell without prescriptions. Agrochemical shops are accused of selling the wrong drugs with sometimes fatal effects to livestock and pets. When veterinarians complain about these practices: "we get threats about interfering with a man's ability to earn a living."

Veterinarians were accused similarly by agricultural officers: "[if you tell farmers to use 'bush'], veterinarians take you up on it…. they cannot make money if bush medicine is being used, they say that you are encroaching on a man's power to make a living." Praedial larceny of crops and livestock are 'crab antics' that undermine the viability of the agricultural sector, while petty business thefts and deliberate unproductivity undermine the small business and entrepreneurial sectors. The irony is that these two sectors if vibrant, could provide the lifestyles desired by those engaged in 'crab antics'. Crab antics can manifest itself as the 'politics of disappearance of local knowledge' (Shiva, 1993). As stated in chapter 12 the scientific actor-network offers the security of a valued social identity and some herbalists are seeking to occupy this privileged space. A seminar (see Box 1) was planned that can be seen as an attempt at legitimisation in two ways. A recently departed and well-known herbalist C.H.B. Chadband was being honoured, and a Canadian expert (a local boy made good) had been invited to speak. As the time for the evening seminar to begin approached, the Police came from their section of the building to tell the public to leave because there had been an early morning phone call about a bomb. The police and the public (exercise classes and other activities) had been in the building for the whole day but the police had not yet checked the building. The alleged bomb had not been an issue prior to the seminar however. The speaker returned to Canada without sharing his views. The crabs who sought legitimisation were pulled back down into the bucket.

Box 1: Information control in folk medicine

Director: Francis K. Morean,　　　H.E.R.B.S　　　　　　　B.Sc. Botany/Zoology Herbal, Educational, Recreational and Biological Services in conjunction with the family of the late CHB Chadband cordially invites the Public to the Inaugural CHB Chadband Memorial Lecture At City Hall, Port-of-Spain on Thursday August 17, 1995 at 7.00 p.m. **Feature Speaker: Dr. Dennis C.V. Awang** **Topic: The Potential of Traditional Medicinal Plants Preparation**
For further information contact: MR FRANCIS MOREAN. TEL/FAX:667-1889/2115

There are other ways of creating 'disappearance'. Power can be used strategically over women and their subjugated [traditional] knowledges through researchers defining objective knowledge as superior to personal experience[51] (Holland and Ramazanoglu, 1994). One veterinarian for example knew of ethnoveterinary practices but when pressed for details claimed that they were 'anecdotes that were more amusing than factual'. One more detailed example of this strategy is given below; the scientist involved is one of the few publicly known Trinidad scientists involved in medicinal plants.

Scientist D: "Pavy's book should never have been published. Her heart was in the right place, left alone she would not have written a book. I am not a healer; I am interested in useful knowledge. From Pavy's writings there was no clear set of statements, she doesn't know how the human body works that some parts are frailer than others. There are misleading and harmful things in the book. I read to get news, information, and how to treat illnesses. The book fails on all three counts. Pavy's book should not get as much publicity as mine. One good thing about Pavy's book is that it is of great interest to see how folklore is established and proliferated. Jethro Kloss' book, *Back to Eden*, is full of garbage, it is most misleading. Our common names are poisonous plants, but these names are similar to the foreign plants in *Back to Eden*. *Back to Eden* is pseudo-pharmacognosy, it is about promoting without criticism the use of herbs."

A critique of this scientific attitude is found in Lave (1996). Foucault (1980) claims that those who declare, 'I who conduct this discourse am conducting a scientific discourse, and I am a scientist', diminish other subjects of experience and knowledge. The exact circumstances are not known but perhaps the changes put in place by Woodford could be seen as the unleashing of 'crab antics' .

Hybridity

Hybridity has been suggested as a useful postmodern tool for this study. It has been claimed that postmodern theorists stave off their anxiety that the ground is beginning to shift below their feet by questioning the basis of truths that they are losing the privilege to define (Mascia-Lees *et al.*, 1989). Hybridity has its origins in a 'post' ideology that Williams (1997) claims has been 'relegated to the warehouse of unclaimed mail with all the other post[ ]isms'. The legitimacy of the term has been questioned: 'an intellectual labelling device for sophisticated cosmopolitans (postmodern tourists who accumulate difference) to define the current state of globalisation and nomadism' (Friedman, 1999).

Hybridity suggests a greater academic consciousness of mixing rather than a greater quantity of mixing which has always existed (Friedman, 1999). Hybridity has conceptual force only if there are non-hybrid cultures (Moore-Gilbert, 1997). The idea that hybridity (as cultural flows coming together in a given place) is new and that cultures were previously whole entities with no passing back and forth suggests unfamiliarity with history. The oldest known sale of *Aframomum melegueta* as a spice from Africa to Lyons was in 1245 AD (van Harten, 1970). Plants introduced to Spain before the seventh century were sugar cane (*Saccharum officinarum*), citron (*Citrus medica*), mulberry (*Morus* species), cotton (*Gossypium* species), ginger (*Zingiber officinale*) and purslane (*Portulaca oleracea*) (Hernández-Bermejo and García Sánchez, 1998). Columbus claimed to have seen purslane and *Amaranthus spinosus* on Cuba in 1492 (Morison, 1963). All of the important Old World food crops had been introduced into the Americas by 1600 (Bennett and Prance, 2000). Spanish colonists introduced crops like *Musa* species and *Citrus* species to the West Indies,

---

[51] In a fertility survey (Anderson and Cleland, 1984) women who said they used herbs as contraceptives (93.5 % of women in Bangladesh) were placed in the category 'not using'.

while British colonists introduced food crops like breadfruit (*Artocarpus altilis*), dasheen (*Colocasia esculenta*) and Mango (*Mangifera indica*) (Mintz, 1974). The trade in food and spices was responsible for the development of several Creole languages (Richards, 1996). A definition of hybridity that goes beyond cross cultural mixing is that it is the situation of being neither inside or outside a culture, but in a third space on the borderline, where one [in terms of social identities and affiliations] is inside and outside at the same time (Friedman, 1999). This inbetween state will be examined but using the term 'passing' rather than hybridity.

Passing

The terms 'passing' and 'role occupation' are terms and phenomena that can be easily recognised by Trinbagonians. Passing as someone you are not carries the constant danger of being caught out, the constant feeling of being inauthentic, and the real danger of becoming confused (Ahmed, 1999). Feeling that you are not adequately filling the role that you are trying to assume often implies that you have unrealistic projections about the role you are trying to occupy. What a 'real man' is for example. Passing as white, or 'passing as foreign' implies renouncing blackness, or being Trinidadian and everything associated with being black or local (like folk medicine). Passing is not confined to blacks. The white Creoles renounced their coloured counterparts in order to 'pass' as the equivalents to the British expatriates. Passing can be an offshoot of the colonising mission which assumes that the colonised-hybrid subject can reflect back the values and practices of the coloniser without ever assuming the colonisers role (mimic men[52]) (Moore-Gilbert, 1997; Ahmed, 1999). As part of the colonising mission, institutional structures like schools and universities, and key actors like scientists and other professionals played a role in the process of colonial cultural construction. It may be that the British origins and early teachings of UWI succeeded in alienating some staff and students from local traditions and culture. This alienation was increased when Britain relinquished control of newly-independent countries to the colonised-hybrid-mimic-men, who chose to prove themselves up to the task in western terms. A post-independence UWI, though somewhat alienated from the colonial institute still operates within its traditions because the passing subject desires to become like the other (Ahmad, 1999). Perhaps demonstrated in the caricature one UWI-staff member painted of fellow UWI staff:

> "I have been here since 1963 and they [UWI staff] haven't changed their attitude. England in the tropics... University in the West Indies Not University of the West Indies, the institution is used as a transit point. There is an identity problem, a lack of self-confidence to handle situations. One UWI Registrar went 'home' to Britain after retirement, he was born in Barbados."

Creolization in folk medicine

The term Creole has become a metaphor for Caribbean peoples, language, habits, cuisine and culture (Mohammed, 1998). Creolization distils the degrading experiences of Caribbean history into a self-consciously de-centred, subversive and transformative creative Caribbean identity (Balutansky, 1997). Local indigenous agricultural practices derived from Creolization are context-specific improvisational capacities, in which successful use and indigenous theory-based logic, conditions belief (Giarelli, 1996; Escobar, 1999; Richards, 1993). Creolization in folk medicine takes place in practice when culturally based cures are shared between neighbours of different ethnic groups (Niehoff and Niehoff, 1960). Perhaps

---

[52] Naipaul's concept of mimic men means the loss of an inner self due to colonialism, hence you adopt whatever role is imposed upon you from the outside (Rohlehr, 1980).

Creolization based on the ethnomedicinal data would include the story of Gokool, an Indo-Trinidadian, with a Hindu temple and the plants used in religious ceremonies (*Ocimum sanctum, Datur stramonium*) in his yard. Gokool has a black polished stone[53] called a 'Belgian black stone' that is used as a snake bite cure. The stone belonged to his grandfather who lived in Arima and carried fresh milk and 'wildmeat' for the Catholic nuns stationed close by. These nuns gave his grandfather the stone. The stone sticks to the bitten spot 'like a magnet' and comes off when it has drawn out the poison. It is then washed in milk and replaced in its container.

Creolization is a difficult analytical tool to use because the fish does not normally analyse the water. There are two perceptions about Creolization. In the first perception 'new' Creolized technologies like folk medicine develop from the synergy between the local knowledge of the Amerindian population and the external knowledge of the immigrants (Richards, 1996). Applying this idea to folk medicine is problematic since the majority of the plants and their uses can be traced backwards to Africa, Europe, India and South America. This implies that the main outcome or synergy in folk medicine is that all the knowledge is available to all ethnic groups in a kind of 'melting pot'. An example of the melting pot would be the slave gardens/provision grounds that became the peasant gardens of today (Mintz, 1974; Tobin, 1999). African crops like pigeon peas (*Cajanus cajan*) and okro (*Abelmoschus esculentus*) were grown together with native American crops like corn (*Zea mays*), cashew (*Anacardium occidentale*), cassava (*Manihot esculenta*), avocado (*Persea americana*) guava (*Psidium gaujava*), sweet potatoes, tomatoes (*Lycopersicon esculentum*) starches like *Xanthosoma* species and possibly African yams such as *Dioscorea rotundata* and *Dioscorea cayenensis*. Also grown were European vegetables and Asian plants like yams (*Dioscorea alata, D. esculenta*, sugar cane (*Saccharum officinarum* and fruits (*Mangifera indica, Citrus* species, *Musa* species and *Tamarindus indica*) (Sanderson, 2005). There was also a native cushcush yam (*Dioscorea trifida)* that may have originated on the borders of Brazil and Guyana. The medicinal use of Guava was recorded for the Aztecs of the 16th century (Heinrich et al., 2005).

The second perception is that Creolization in folk medicine is similar but different to Creolization in languages. In languages the Creole form is a transitional phase in which a new generation assimilates a second, reduced language (Patois), as a first language. Patois has a complexity and a range of meanings (*double entendre*) only available to insiders who shared the lived experience of the country (Mohammed, 1998). Patois has its allotted space in neighbourhood life and is used when deemed appropriate to the social context (Burton, 1993; Friedman, 1999). The social place of Patois in relation to French was thus similar to the relationship of folk medicine with allopathic medicine in Trinidad and Tobago, 'less than'. Another parallel between medicine and Patois is the ability of the Caribbean population to shift back and forth between the official and the unofficial forms. In this idea of Creolization the question is whether a coherent body of Creolized Caribbean folk knowledge was created that was structured and ordered and passed on to subsequent generations as such. There are indications that this has been the case (with limitations). For example the names of plants are sometimes related to their use. An unidentified plant named dégonfler has an ethnomedicinal use for stomach problems. In patois a bloated stomach is called gonflé. The plant used to alleviate the problem is therefore dégonfler. *Xiphidium caeruleum* leaves are rubbed on the feet and knees of children learning to walk. The local name of this plant is walkfast or corrimiento (Spanish correr, to run). Ewen (1896) refers to *Ageratum conyzoides* as 'herbe chatte' and *Eupatorium ayapana* as 'z'herbe à femme'. A name change in the last

---

[53] Whitehead (1997:57) claims that Ralegh endorsed the curative power of Amerindian greenstone *takua* (spleen stones or *piedras hijadas* - liver stones).

century may have occurred because of the use of *Ageratum conyzoides* then and currently (given to women after childbirth and to promote menstruation).

Several plants have been used in Latin America and the Caribbean for at least one hundred and fifty years, suggesting successful generational transmission. *Cordia curassavica* has been used to control ticks in the Caribbean since the 1800s or before (Ewen, 1896). *Justicia pectoralis* is used for muscle fatigue in South America and for bathing and as a beneficial mouth wash in Venezuela (Morton, 1975; Wilbert, 1996). These uses and the use for internal bruises were found in pre-1834 Barbados (Handler and Jacoby, 1993). Wong (1976) has recorded the use of *Desmodium adscendens* and *Desmodium canum* in Trinidad as a depurative, for oliguria, and kidney and venereal diseases. These uses are also current in Colombia, Mexico, Nicaragua and in Barbados where the ethnomedicinal use existed pre-1834 (Zamora-Martínez and Nieto de Pascual Pola, 1992; Handler and Jacoby, 1993; Barrett, 1994; Laferriere, 1994). *Scoparia dulcis* was used in Barbados as a diuretic prior to 1834 (Handler and Jacoby, 1993). *Chamaesyce prostrata* was used in Barbados prior to 1834 for venereal complaints (Handler and Jacoby, 1993).

The unexpected results of experiments are explained in terms of the Creole folk medicine system. A farmer in Tobago had given his cows lime skins as a supplemental feed. An unexpected benefit from these lime skins was explained in terms of the folk medicinal system: "There was a change in their appearance, they put on weight, it was more than a coincidence. The skins were still fresh, they still had lime oil, the oil was a repulsive thing to worms. My father reminded me that long time grannies used to give lime peel tea for stomach problems. So the internal parasites in the gut no longer enjoyed living in the stomach. The cows got the peels for six months out of the year. Also the parasite eggs life cycle in the pasture had an effect, I was rotating the pastures so it was a combination of two things." There were other indications that experiments are taking place which refines the folk knowledge rather than the knowledge being simply handed down or passed on:

One respondent claimed that: "I used to try things as a small boy. When my fowls were sick I gave them lime juice, Canadian oil, and a pinch of salt. If it was good for them it was good for me and vice versa."

Respondent 2: "I learn by experiments, the young they are lazy to do it, they don't know how, it takes time. I use the quantity five [as a dosage] because there are five fingers on each hand, and five senses, each man has his own science, you have to offer and pray over it, and let the sickness go along with the sun when it is setting."

There were also rules of thumb on dosages" Respondent 3: "Take a reasonable handful, with 'bush' you sometimes overdose sometimes underdose."

Respondent 4: "First you have to get the animal accustomed to it. There are alkaloids in 'bush'. You could poison yourself if you take the full dose right away, so take one leaf the first day, two leaves the 2nd day, until the full dose at 9 days. Goats get diarrhoea from juicy things, this is not a medicinal cure, but bamboo is a dry thing, dry breadfruit, give these to the goat. The bacteria will be destroyed by not having enough water. I experiment on many things. People taught me from long time. I am 77, when I am sick I ask people, I do research. I figured out the principle myself. Others did not know why it worked."

However the clearest example of this idea of Creolization as a coherent body of knowledge that was structured and ordered and passed on to subsequent generations as such is seen in the chapter on hunting dogs. A 'reduced' body of knowledge (practising the rituals without knowing the underlying belief-system) was passed from the Amerindian hunters in the 1800s or before to their Creole co-hunters who then passed on this knowledge to family and friends. Unlike some of the other respondents the hunters never assigned their knowledge to Africa or India.

Cultural codes

There are certain instances in which cultural codes transfer from one continent to another with migrants but the original meaning, plant use, or plant used, or belief system is lost or modified in the transfer process. The following section lists and discusses a few of these cultural codes that have undergone a process of Creolization. One unexplained code or practice is given first: "After eating the roast corn, cut the cob into rings and make holes in them, put these on a string and tie it around the dog's neck. This cures kennel cough."

In Paramin, ruda (*Ruta graveolens*) was said to be a spiritual bush, and harvesters had to have clean hands to touch it, and could not be perspiring. The plant could not be told that it smelt funny or it would die. It could not be planted too close to people. "No evil meddles with it." It had to be paid or 'mounted' which means burying a few silver coins near to the plant in exchange for special favours. A similar belief was expressed about hog tannia (*Xanthosoma brasiliense, Xanthosoma undipes*) in Mayaro at the other end of Trinidad. It had to be planted away from people since unclean people caused it to wither. Moodie (1982) describes special plants that are a source of strength, good luck, and success in hunting and cock fighting and protect people and their homes. These 'mounted' plants are planted in holes sprinkled with the blood of a dove or chicken, on Good Friday or the first Friday in Lent, and the roots are sprinkled with milk (Moodie, 1982). The mounted plants whistle to their owners to warn them of danger. This belief is similar to that of the Miskito of Eastern Nicaragua where plants are given symbolic payments if they are considered to have supernatural owners who require such payment (Dennis, 1988).

Guinea pepper (*Aframomum melegueta*) seeds had the reputation of causing quarrels if the seeds were scattered on the ground or if they were thrown into someone's yard. "How you getting on so, like they throw guinea pepper or what"? The reputation for causing quarrels may have come from the ethnomedicinal practice in Liberia. The seeds also caused quarrels among the Europeans with several powers trying to break the 14th century Venetian monopoly of black pepper by using these grains as a substitute (Pickersgill, 2005). *Aframomum melegueta* grains are mixed with rum or brandy to which it bestows a fiery pungency and it is then used as a sexual stimulant (van Harten, 1970). The use of obie seed (*Cola nitida*) is also recognised as an African tradition. Imported seeds are sold in the market, but one respondent had a tree. The seeds are used for a wide range of medicinal purposes while in Nigeria the seeds are often used as a stimulant. These traditions have passed down through the generations in a Creolized form.

Before electric lights were widespread some people put jumbie bead seeds (*Abrus precatorius*, Fabaceae) in the lamp oil with garlic. It was said that no witch / soucouyant[54] could come into the house at night when the lamp was lit. Evidence of a soucouyant was a blue / black mark on the skin. "If you didn't get a lash it had to be a witch." Similar beliefs about witches leaving blue bruises are found in Nepal (Eigner and Scholz, 1999). The Yucatec Maya in Mexico use *Abrus precatorius* baths against evil eye (Ankli *et al.*, 1999).

---

[54] Even the soucouyant is said to be 'Creole' a syncretism of the European vampire and the African complement (Besson, 2000)

Days of the week/ phases of the moon

Rules of thumb about Good Friday may have Spanish origins (Martínez-Lirola *et al.*, 1996). A Talparo respondent claimed that *Bixa orellana* root was to be cut on a Wednesday or Friday for dropsy, 'this was a secret not Obeah, but for jaundice it could be cut at any time'. Seasoning makers in Paramin spoke of a religious-based belief that on Good Friday if someone dug up a clump of fowl foot grass (*Eleusine indica*) they would get a piece of coal below the roots. White/red physic nut (*Jatropha curcas / gossypifolia*, Euphorbiaceae), if cut on Good Friday would produce the blood of Jesus.

According to Bayley (1949) plants which have associations with Obeah can only be cut at certain times of the moon and it is thought that brews which are left overnight in the dew acquire maximum efficacy (Bayley, 1949). These practices were seen in a few instances. Children suffering from marasmi (malnutrition) were bathed for eight or nine days with congo lala (*Eclipta prostrata*). This was to be put in the dew for four days before use. A tisane for colds consisted of kojo root (*Petiveria alliacea*), urine of a young boy, camphor and rosemary (*Rosmarinus officinalis*). This was put in the dew for nine days before external application. A decoction of *Capraria biflora* used as an eyewash is also put in the dew over night before use.

Folk beliefs

G.P. Murdock has developed a global typology of causal theories of illness (Green, 1998). Murdock has a binary classification of natural and supernatural and subdivides the latter into mystical causation (impersonal, contagion), animistic causation (spirit aggression) and magical causation (sorcery and witchcraft). Mystical causation occurs when someone comes into contact with a polluting object, substance or person.. e.g women's reproductive fluids. Mystical causation beliefs still exist in Trinidad. One respondent was bitten by a spider, and fell three times before he reached to the back of his house. When his wife called him he could not answer because before treating himself he had to: "Keep to yourself don't go by too much woman, if you see a pregnant woman you can't survive." He chewed three tref (*Aristolochia trilobata*) leaves found at the back of the house and recovered. Then he spoke to his wife.

A few of the female respondents claimed that pregnant or menstruating women should not climb over a rope tethering an animal or sit cross-legged or on a doorstep where people would cross over them[55]. Landman and Hall (1983) report similar beliefs in Jamaica. Women also should not untie or tie hunting dogs, step over them or could not climb trees during their menstrual cycle. However if a hunting dog was 'tied' by another jealous hunter, a woman was supposed to 'loose' it by bathing it a river. Taylor (1950) claims that Dominica Caribs did not allow 'heaty' women (pregnant or menstruating) to eat hunted meat, handle dogs or guns since this would make the hunter's dogs 'spoiled' or slow and heavy.

If someone crushed another person's foot by accident the hurt person was supposed to return the action otherwise some unknown pain of the 'hurter' might transfer itself to the 'hurt'. Likewise if a woman had painful menstruation she should kick a banana tree and then turn away without looking back. She should also not tell anyone about her actions or condition. There is a widespread local belief in Barbados, also found in Trinidad that *Carica papaya* trees planted to the windward of a house have harmful effects, particularly to women (Gooding, 1940). Gooding claims that it is unlikely that this belief is of African origin.

---

[55] Among the Apache it wasa forbidden to step over a person who was sitting or lying down (Opler, 1965).

146

Mayoc chapelle (*Entada polystachya*, Fabaceae) used for cooling was said to be only for women as it would cut men's 'nature'. It was also said that Lani bois (*Lepianthes peltata*) should be put in all cooling for men otherwise 'they would get like a watchman'. Some people pass a comb over the udder for mastitis. "It is a secret business, nobody must see or hear you do it." ...."When the breast has too much milk, get a basin and comb the breast. The pain and the hardness go; it softens the milk. It is a horse comb, light grey with one-sided teeth, and long like your hand. I don't know why it is called a horse comb."

Transmission through time and space

This body of Creolized Caribbean folk knowledge was organised, made systematic and schematic and taught and learned in an organised form across time and space in the absence of writing (Mathias and McCorkle, 1997; Goodenough, 1996). This was accomplished by recall involving ceremonial and ritual events such as the folk media reported below. In the following section two examples of the oral tradition are given. The first is a calypso that gives an accurate description of the folk knowledge, its uses and the oral tradition from grandparents to the young. Calypsonians can be regarded as the folk socio-cultural historians of Trinidad and Tobago and Calypso has been described as the redemptive potential of Caribbean folk wisdom (Price and Price, 1997). The second is a description of the Tobago Play 'Man better Man'. This play has parallels to the struggle between 'science' and 'non-science' where both are claiming to be the 'better man', rather than 'an equivalent man'. The play gives a description of knowledge as a source of power for its holders. Only those who are accepted by the community as 'knowledgeable' can market this knowledge.

A Calypso: Long Time Remedy by Willard Harris, (Lord Relator) 1971. Verse 1
Nowadays if you sick you in plenty pain, Because it ain't have good medicine again
Nowadays people does be sick for a week, Long time, one day you sick, next day you on your feet, I living at my granny, so I bound to know, You can't beat a remedy of long ago
Long ago, if the cold giving you trouble, 'bois canoe, black sage tea, or some soft candle, vervine, christmas bush or shado beni, bound to pass the cold immediately, It is my belief, you could settle yourself with soursop leaf, I say we have a right to take example, and try to live like the old people, because, as a youngster, I realise, de old people way of living is really wise. It's only recently, look I find it strange, old people used to live to a hundred and change, 'cause anything gone wrong with their body, they could find a suitable remedy (Rollocks, 1991).

Man Better Man: A play for the Tobago Heritage Festival 1990.

The show was entitled 'Man-better-Man' after one of the more efficacious herbs used by the islands' folk practitioners. The play was woven around two 'medicine men', each of who was trying to prove himself more efficient, skilful and powerful, than the other. In other words, they were engaged in battle of 'Man-better-Man'. At the end of this battle which was fiercely fought with ants, nimbles, puncheon rum, 'compelling oil', red lavender, man-better-man, wonder of the world, ruckshun, and verses of Psalm 37 and 59, the 'better-man' surfaced, as master over his opponent. In proving his efficacy as a 'medicine-man' the 'better-man' won the admiration and recognition of the crowd. As the 'better-man', he was able to foil all the tricks of his opponent. The practitioner needs to prove himself efficient as a healer to claim the title (Rollocks, 1991).

Legitimatisation

Indigenous knowledge exists in parallel to Western science. The process of legitimisation in Indigenous Knowledge takes place in a similar manner to what takes place in the scientific world, through culturally esteemed opinion leaders in a community. In folk medicine there are three domains that legitimise the healer: the subjective reality of the healer; the objective reality as measured by his clientele based on his successful cures; and the belief systems of the community [locally and globally influenced] which impacts on the first two (Laguerre, 1987). Laguerre (1987) claims that rejected knowledge [like some types of indigenous knowledge] has three types of adherents. Those born and socialised in it who would be permanent advocates, temporary advocates who turn to it in crisis times, and those who only believe in specific aspects, not in the totality. There are also three types of transmission of indigenous knowledge: the society and community, the family, and the individual (dreams).

Cultural legitimisation

In parallel to the scientific world, actors in traditional medicine use a process of legitimisation in that healers need to be or become culturally esteemed opinion leaders in a community as described in the play above. Cultural esteem is linked to the social standing of the healer. Herbalists and religious healers claim to have the power to effect cures. The gift is regarded as given to be of service to others and if it is not used in this way, it will be lost. These specialists, both Indian and Creole, do not share their knowledge with this researcher or with others because they claim it is 'a gift from God'. Some herbalists ('bush' doctors) view knowledge as a private good and thus a source of revenue and power. Some have learnt about plants through dreams or revelations. Some respondents die with their gifts while others feel compelled to pass on their knowledge at their deathbeds so that they can rest in peace. One respondent had gained her knowledge from a dying healer and claimed that the cock that flew into her kitchen the day after the healer died was a sign from beyond the grave. Trinidad has Indo-cultural specialists such as 'vein pullers' and masseurs who may be consulted for sick animals. One vein puller interviewed in the first research phase is quoted below:

"I know more than them [the Vets]. I treat people as well as animals. I am the eldest son, a vein puller. When doctors 'band' a sprain, I will pull it. If neighbours animals have trouble giving birth I will go. But if the 'young' dies and the animal's belly is swollen I call Dr.G. I can push back a prolapse so that it never comes out again. My father taught me. I can't read, so I watch pictures in books. I asked a doctor for his book of human medicine with lots of pictures. When my animals are sick I buy medicine, and if Dr G. comes to treat them he doesn't charge."

One anecdote related to the objective reality/validation tells of an American tourist who had serious medical problems on a popular beach related to his high blood pressure. A food vendor (shark and baked bread) boiled a tea of *Ocimum* species for him. The story goes that he felt better and rewarded the vendor with a trip to New York.

The social [de]-construction of knowledge

A few scientists were honest enough to admit that they rejected folk medicine based on negative childhood experiences. These negative childhood experiences and the female aspect of folk medicine are described in the excerpt from a short story[56] given below:

My grandmother was regarded by the community around us in Tunapuna as a nurse and a midwife. I rather suspect that she had acquired that reputation by her practical experience and knowledge, and from skills which were handed down. I may be wrong but I do not believe that she had any formal training as a nurse, but her vitality her fund of knowledge on the merits of the different grasses, bushes and shrubs which were always to hand, and her success with confinement cases, had over

---

[56] Quote taken from "Nostalgia" an unpublished short story by Kenneth Lans.

148

the years, built up the respect and the faith in her prowess and they are the two essentials in the healing process. She had delivered all of us, my cousins included, and our health and our vitality bore living witness to her ability.

She was the one to whom we were sent whenever we felt out of sorts, and at the beginning of the school holidays. Castor oil, senna, fever grass, shining bush and all the other mixtures fashionable in those days were inflicted on us with the admonition that they were good for us. Castor oil was usually given during the first week of the holidays. What we got was a foul-smelling, un-refined oil which she had extracted by means unknown to us, from a tree which she nurtured in her yard. She was not one to indulge in the purchase of medicines when all the necessary ingredients were easily to hand either in her yard or in that of the many solicitous neighbours'.

I had a particular loathing for that castor tree, and that dislike extended to a physic nut tree which grew in our own yard. They epitomized the violence done on our persons, both internally and externally. Swallowing that awful tasting thick foul-smelling spoonful of oil was only the prelude to the glass of Epsom's Salts which had to be taken the following day. The salts were given to us by our mother. We were never quite sure which we hated the more, the oil or the salts. The oil was only a spoonful, but we felt the taste in our mouths whenever we burped, while the long glass of the bitter-tasting salts took an eternity to go down, and to our minds only aggravated an already bad situation.

We were all given our doses on the same day, and this created a logistical problem, for there was only one out-house. There were five young busy bodies vying for the offensive relief that it only temporarily gave, and chamber pots were pressed into service….Those first days were traumatically busy, and we soon learnt to develop a pale listless look which was interpreted by the adults as the medicine 'taking hold'. Once that was out of the way, we were considered to be immune to almost everything. The exception was growing fever. 'Growing fever' was any type of ailment which induced a temperature and which did not readily lend itself to any other diagnosis after careful scrutiny by the medicine maker of the family. Remedies for that malady were limited only by the imagination, for readily available within easy reach was a formidable array of herbs, leaves, and other bushes which had proved effective in the past. Confronted by such diversity, volume, and absolute faith, no self-respecting virus - a modern word - would stay around long enough to hamper any child's holiday. Armed with the immunity of the purges, the bush teas, and fortified by the equally effective coolings and tonics, together with the love and patience of all those good people, we were free to conquer the world in any way we chose. So long as we did not get into 'trouble'.

Recapturing European and Amerindian plant knowledge

Stephen Jay Gould wrote in one of his essays that we are all compellingly drawn to the subject of beginnings and we construct myths when we do not have data or suppress data in favour of legend when a truth strikes us as too trite. The psychic need for origin myths for Caribbean folk medicine is particularly strong because oral knowledge does not become 'universalized and immortalized' like written, public knowledge, which is revised, tested and challenged by others and is not lost to future generations (Ingold, 1996, Laguerre, 1987). Unfortunately culturally encoded indigenous knowledge is lost through several negative impacts: the death of knowledgeable individuals, lack of verbal transfers to the next generation and acculturation (Longuefosse and Nossin, 1996). The end result is that there is rarely a systematic body of cultural representations (Ingold, 1996, Maturana and Varela, 1987). This is especially true for Amerindian plant knowledge, which has been poorly documented.

However several plants have been used in Latin America and the Caribbean for at least one hundred and fifty years, suggesting successful generational transmission (Handler and Jacoby, 1993). For example worm grass (*Chenopodium ambrosioides*) is an effective and well-known anti-parasitic remedy used for dogs and farm animals and its use may also lie in ancient Amerindian knowledge (Lans, 2001). *Cordia curassavica* is still used to control ticks

(Lans, 2001). *Justicia pectoralis* is used for muscle fatigue in South America and for bathing and as a beneficial mouthwash in Venezuela (Morton, 1975; Wilbert, 1996). These uses and the use for internal bruises were found in pre-1834 Barbados (Handler and Jacoby, 1993). *Desmodium adscendens* and *Desmodium canum* have been used in Trinidad as depuratives, for oliguria, and kidney and venereal diseases (Wong, 1976). These uses are also current in Colombia, Mexico, and Nicaragua and in Barbados where the ethnomedicinal use existed pre-1834 (Handler and Jacoby, 1993; Lans, 2001). *Scoparia dulcis* has a long-term use in Barbados as a diuretic and *Chamaesyce prostrata* has been used for venereal complaints (Handler and Jacoby, 1993).

A brief history

When Cristòbal Còlon 'discovered' Trinidad in 1498 there were several Amerindian tribes; these were the Aruaca, Garini, Nepuyo, Shebaio and Yaio. These Meso Indians (population 10,000 - 40,000) lived in coastal and riverine villages and were fishermen, hunters and gatherers (Borde, 1876). During the 1700s, Trinidad belonged as an island province to the vice royalty of New Spain along with modern Mexico and Central America (Besson, 2000). The Dutch and the Courlanders had established themselves in Tobago in the 16th and 17th centuries and produced tobacco and cotton. However Trinidad in this period was still mainly forest, populated by a few Spaniards with their handful of slaves and a few thousand Amerindians (Besson, 2000).

Amerindians brought domesticates like guinea pigs and dogs to the Caribbean (Siegel, 1991). Douglas Taylor (1950) and Honychurch (1986) recorded the influence of the Amerindians on Caribbean folk medicine. For example the Dominican Caribs used plants to excite dogs to hunt. Wilbert (1983: 358) wrote that *Warao*[57] navigators traded with Trinidad and that the island was included in *Warao* cosmogony (origin belief). This was previously recorded by Lovén (1935; 29) who claimed that the Orinoco tribes in the lowlands southeast of the river's middle course told the Spaniards that they had left Guiana and settled in Trinidad (*Kaieri* = island). The *Warao* travelled across the Columbus Channel on their way to South Trinidad (Boomert 2000). They paddled from the Caño Mariusa, a branch of the Orinoco to Erin Bay leaving before sunrise and arriving before sunset. The Caño Capure and Caño Macareo[58] were also used to land in Erin Bay or Icacos Bay (Islote).

The Guiana current moves from the south Atlantic along the coast of the Guiana meeting the outflow from the Orinoco. The current carries objects like floating mats of vegetation, reptiles and canoes from the Guianas as well as from the Amazon (Boomert, 2000). The current bifurcates with one stream going through the Columbus channel to the Gulf of Paria and the other going north to Trinidad's east coast and then through the Galleons' passage or around Tobago and then to Grenada. Boomert claims that a 17th century sailing ship went from Tobago to Grenada in eight hours due to the strength of the current. Lovén (1935) [quoting Roth] reported that *Warraus* obtained their tobacco from the Antilles, exchanging their carpentry for it (Whitehead, 1997: 78). He also wrote that Amerindians from Guiana carried on a trade of cassava with the Spaniards on the dry island of Margarita and Cubagua passing the Boca del Drago on the way. According to Boomert (2000) this trip was easy from north Trinidad to Margarita but difficult in the reverse against the current. This trade was especially important during the period 1571 to 1575 when Trinidad had been abandoned by the Spanish (Lovén, 1935: 31). In eastern Trinidad they traded conch-shell trumpets, pears,

---

[57] Other groups in the Guiana Highlands went by the tribal names or nicknames of Patamuna, Makushi, Wapishana, Akawaio, Arecuna and Waiwai (Riley, 2003).
[58] The Caño Macareo was the mythical route taken by the *Warao* hero Haburi who fled from the Delta to Naparima hill with his sister-mothers (Boomert, 2000) *Warao* also consider Naparima hill to be a petrified tree that is the home of the butterfly grandfather *Warowaro*.

salt and axes. Another researcher claims that these Amerindians were *Cumanágoto* and *Araucas* and further states that the trade started in 1512; some 80 years before Ralegh's arrival in the region (Whitehead, 1997).

Boomert (2000) conducted an archaeological study of what he calls the *Orinoco Interaction Sphere*. This consists of the Orinoco valley and delta, the Paria peninsula and the west coast of the Gulf of Paria in northeast Venezuela and the northwest part of the coastal zone of the Guianas with cultural, mythological, political and geographical commonalities and continuities. He claimed that there was frequent exchange among the Barrancoid and Saladoid peoples of Trinidad, Tobago and the Lower Orinoco in goods such as ceremonial items and in oral history. Boomert claims that the Dutch name *Kano baij* for Tobago's canoe bay means that it was a landing place for travellers from Trinidad possibly from Salybia (chaléibe) in northeast Trinidad.

The intoxication of fish before capture as described by Im Thurn (1883: 233) is a noted Amerindian tradition and has been documented by others (Borde, 1876; Lizarralde et al. 1987; Rostlund, 1952). The use of lignum vitae (*Guaiacum officinale*) for women's problems and sexually transmitted diseases may have Amerindian origins (Lawrence, 1998). Lignum-vitae was heavily harvested in the 16th century because its resin was used as a panacea. Other Amerindian survivals are rituals that include *Nicotiana tabacum*, the throwing of alcohol in strategic places to bless a new house and the significance attached to dreams (Butt Colson and de Armellada, 1983; Roth, 1915: 230). This latter is not specific to any one culture.

Commonalities in ethnomedicine are partly derived from the movement of peoples and plants from place to place. For example Reeves (1992) claims that *Aloe vera* and *Punica granatum* were introduced to ancient Egypt from Eastern Africa and South - West Asia respectively. Bennett and Prance (2000) conducted research on the European influence on folk medicine. There are 216 introduced species that are used by populations in northern South America (Brazil, Colombia, Ecuador and Peru). Twenty-one percent of these plants are of European origin, fourteen percent are from Eurasia and seventeen percent are of Mediterranean origin. Two plants can serve as examples. *Ambrosia cumanenesis* and *Ambrosia hispida* are used for colds in Trinidad and in Paraguay (Wong, 1976; Lans, 2001). *Artemisia absinthium* is used together with other plants to regulate fertility in western Panama and Paraguay. *Artemisia* species are used similarly by the French, Spanish New Mexicans and in Madeira and this use is ancient. The Caribs in Guatemala use *Artemisia absinthium* for fever, vaginitis and stomach pains. In Mauritius and Rodrigues, Tuscany and Sardinia, *Artemisia* species leaf infusion or decoction is used for digestive upsets, and as emmenagogues.

"French and Spanish Creoles"

Religious orders such as the Dominicans, Franciscans and Augustinians, Capuchins, tried to establish themselves in Trinidad from 1591 (Besson, 2000). The last Aragon Capuchin came to Trinidad in 1758 (Besson, 2000). The friars organized missions at several areas that are still the major villages and towns in Trinidad (Besson, 2000). In the late 1700s, settlers began coming to Puerto d'España. The conquering British drove French plantation owners and their slaves and families from their estates in Grenada, Martinique and Guadeloupe. Some were French royalists who fled from the French Revolution in France and its aftermath in the Caribbean; others were serving with the British forces in the Caribbean. Amongst these were the Count of Lopinot and his four sons, Chevalier de Verteuil, Chevalier de Bruny, Marquis de Montrichard and Vicomte de Bragelonne (Besson, 2000). These

Chevaliers had a profound influence on social attitudes. The French did not discover or conquer Trinidad but they constituted a large proportion of the population (twenty Frenchmen to every Spaniard) and as the élite they influenced the culture of the society. French words are still part of the local dialect of Trinidad, often as "Patois." The term "French Creole" should but does not always include the free people of colour, the children of the French planters of the early times with their African slaves, and later, their mulatto, quadroon and octoroon mistresses. These locally born people passed on the French share of the creolised culture to their descendants (Besson, 2000).

Spanish traditions were handed down from the original colonial heritage but are reinforced by visits and migrants escaping the turbulent politics of Venezuela. The use of the stigma and styles of corn (*Zea mays*) as a diuretic is found only in those parts of Italy where the Spanish influence was strong. This ethnomedicinal use is also found in Trinidad and in Latin America and is still found in Spain (Lans, 2001). Multiple plant mixtures are used in Caribbean folk medicine especially in 'lochs' for respiratory problems. A similar practice is seen in Murcia and Cartagena, Spain where the guiding principle is: 'the more plants used, the more the medicinal properties are increased' (Lans, 2001). Hispanic prayers are used in Latin America for healing and against mal yeux. These Spanish-Romanic prayers, like the 'oracion' prayer are used during 'santowah' (santigual), which is the Spanish equivalent of the Hindu spiritual healing called jharay. This involves praying on the sick person [or animal] or on the food eaten by him/her. The ceremony includes sweet broom (*Scoparia dulcis*), which is used to sprinkle holy water (Lans, 2001). Some of the prayers kept secret in Trinidad can be found for sale in Cuban shops in Miami (S. Moodie-Kublalsingh, Institute of Languages, University of The West Indies, pers. comm. August, 2000). Moodie (1982) claims that these prayers are magic rather than religion and came to the New World with the conquistadors. In Almería Spain, folk magical plant therapy for warts, evil eye, hepatic ailments or swellings consists of a ritual in which an incantation ("prayer") is recited and a plant (*Malva* species, *Marrubium* species, etc.) is used (Martínez-Lirola et al., 1996). In Tuscany the concept of the evil eye exists and *Foeniculum vulgare* is put into a red cloth and hung on the animal (Lans, 2001). Red cloths are also used in Trinidad and Tobago.

The name semen contra now used in the West Indies as the Creole name for the Amerindian plant *Chenopodium ambrosioides* was originally one of the names of the drug Santonica derived from the introduced European plant *Artemesia cina* B. *Artemesia* was also used as an anthelmintic but perhaps less effectively. Some 'French Creoles' were amateur naturalists and one, T.W. Carr, compared the native *Parthenium hysterophorus* to the European *Artemisia* in appearance and smell, calling it 'country wormwood' or 'absinthe bâtarde des antilles' in his flora. In Trinidad rashes are bathed with St. John's bush (*Justicia secunda*, Acanthaceae). It is claimed that this plant imparts a red colour to the bath water. In Europe the red pigment from crushed flowers of St. John's wort (*Hypericum perforatum*) represents the blood of St. John at his beheading, because the herb is in full flower on June 24th, St. John's Day. Other European influences can be seen in the plants used in cock fighting. The early Spanish and/or French colonists probably introduced cock fighting to Trinidad (Moodie-Kublalsingh, 1994). It is presently an illegal sport and has been an illegal activity for at least the last century although keeping gamecocks is not an illegal. Eyebright (not yet identified) and planten (*Plantago major*) leaves are used for injuries to the eyes (Lans, 2001). Eyebright is the name of the ancient herb *Euphrasia officinalis*. *Plantago major* fresh leaf juice or bath is used for ophthalmic injuries in Venezuela, France, Madeira and Mauritius and Pliny and Erasmus recorded these plant uses. Leaves of ruda (*Ruta graveolens*) are used for childbirth, as a carminative, for menstrual pain and cold in the womb. *Ruta graveolens* and closely related species are used as emmenagogues, abortives, antispasmodics, sudorifics and anthelmintics in France, Spain, Brazil, Paraguay, New Mexico, Italy, Madeira and in other cultures and Galen and Pliny the Elder documented these antifertility uses. Turmeric was called "Indian saffron" in Europe and is called saffron in Trinidad (Pickersgill, 2005). A frothy solution is obtained by crushing the leaves of syrio (*Sambucus simpsonii*) in water. This is used to rub dogs with mange (Lans, 2001). Those interviewed claimed that when the dog licks its skin, this medicine would also work internally. Infusions of *Sambucus nigra* inflorescence are used in baths as emollients in northwest Spain. *Sambucus lanceolata* flower decoction is used for open sores and leaves are used in poultices on bruises, wounds and sores in France, Turkey, Madeira and Porto Santo. *Sambucus species* were recorded in Egyptian papyri as being of ancient use (Kay, 1996). Unfortunately it was not possible to find similar comparisons of plant uses with Egypt and as explained below this was not due to the erased African heritage.

"Survivals" and so on

Mintz (1974) claims that African 'survivals' are considered interesting because they reflect the resilience of the human spirit even under slavery. There has been some effort made to reclaim the erased African heritage of the Caribbean peoples and this is necessary work. However as claimed by Haslip-Viera et al. (1997) this historical restoration has to be accurate and should not detract from the contributions of other groups. McClure (1982) claims that slaves transported *Abrus precatorius* from Africa to the Americas 'because it had potential against evil spirits to be encountered in new lands.' No indication is given of how slaves knew they would be transported or how (manacled and stripped) they were able to carry anything with them. Two other plants McClure reports were carried to the Americas by slaves are *Ricinus communis* and *Citrus aurantifolia*. McClure admits that Arab traders took both *Citrus aurantifolia* and *Abrus precatorius* from Asia to Africa before 1454 and that the uses in Africa are similar to those in Asia.

How then can one be sure that there is parallel usage of medicinal plants by Africans and their Caribbean descendants when Asians also live in the Caribbean?
An example of the syncretism that took place in Trinidad with *Abrus precatorius* and possible links to Amerindian and Asian culture follows. Before electric lights were widespread some people put jumbie bead seeds (*Abrus precatorius*) in the lamp oil with garlic. It was said that no witch / soucouyant[59] could come into the house at night when the lamp was lit. Evidence of a soucouyant was a blue / black mark on the skin. Respondents claimed, "if you didn't get a lash it had to be a witch" (Lans 2001). Similar beliefs about witches leaving blue bruises are found in Nepal; while the Yucatec Maya in Mexico use Abrus precatorius baths against evil eye (Ankli et al. 1999: 149; Eigner and Scholz 1999). Similar beliefs may exist in West Africa, but these were not obtained during my research. In 1997 a pharmacologist resident in Trinidad began research to trace the linkages between the folk medicine in Trinidad and Tobago and in her native Nigeria. She was told to include the stately silk cotton tree (*Ceiba pentandra*) in her list of African 'survivals'. It is widely known that African slaves revered these huge trees, that blood[60] was found on them, and that ceremonies were held before they were cut down. There is a legend in Tobago of Gang Gang Sara, a powerful old female slave who climbed up a silk cotton tree in Les Coteaux in a failed attempt to fly back to Africa. However Roth (1915: 229) pointed out that the presumption of transmission of this superstition from Africa to Latin America is incorrect.[61] *Ceiba pentandra* was the sacred tree of the Mayan people. Mayans believed that 'souls ascend to heaven by rising up a mythical silk cotton tree whose branches are heaven itself' (Kricher 1989: 88: Roth 1915: 229). Comparable beliefs are found in Bolivia where the Tacana believe that malevolent spirits

---

[59] The soucouyant is said to be a syncretism of the European vampire and the African complement (Besson, 2000)

[60] Vampire bats (*Desmodus rotundus*) are probably responsible for the blood.

[61] Boomert (2000) raises another objection. He claims that the Island Caribs never ate salt or fat associating it with a dangerous anaconda spirit. Therefore the taboos against salt in certain cultural practices in Trinidad and Tobago and the linking of abstention against salt by slaves to flying back to Africa have an Amerindian basis.

dwell in canopy trees such as *Dipteryx odorata* and *Ceiba samauma* and that walking by them or cutting them down may cause illness (Kricher 1989; Bourdy et al. 2000). So how does a native tree[62] become the host of superstitions that are said to be only African traditions?

It is my contention that since folk knowledge was passed on orally, the descendents of slaves from the French West Indian islands and those born in Africa may have decided to rename the insufficiently understood Amerindian culture they had learnt in Trinidad as African. The phenotypically Negroid Black Caribs of Central America have preserved the culture of the Caribs of St. Vincent (Taylor 1949)[63]. A similar situation may exist in Trinidad since the Amerindians influenced the lifestyle of rural Trinidadians before they 'disappeared'. Amerindian contributions to Caribbean culture were not recognized by social scientists like Richard Adams (1959) who considered the natives to lie outside the process of Creolization. Adams and Niehoff and Niehoff (1960) may have assumed that the "extinction" of the Amerindians was paralleled by an erasure of their culture. Implicit in their work is the idea that no Amerindian[64] cultural patterns, whole or modified, could have endured to play a role in Creolization (Butt Colson and de Armellada 1983; Taylor 1949). The assumption that most Caribbean folk culture was African 'survivals', and 'retentions' is prevalent in the literature (Brathwaite 1971; Herskovits and Herskovits 1964 [1947]). Some of these so-called retentions are very similar to Amerindian practices described in Taylor (1950), Dennis (1988) and Duke (1970)[65]. M.G. Smith (1957) critiqued the theoretical claims of Herskovits and Herskovits while Mintz (1974) claims that social scientists attribute African origins to traditions because they are frustrated by the painstaking and inconclusive research required in order for origins to be traced. Given that I found considerably more Asian-origin than African-origin plants during my research (17 plants were of African origin and 41 were Asian) it is not possible to concur with the assertions of Niehoff and Niehoff (1960) that 'the Indians obtained a considerable amount of their beliefs from Negroes' [and that] the Indians depend heavily on the "bush" remedies which they have mostly borrowed from their Negroe neighbors' unless the plant borrowings that took place were those that originated in South America.

The mainland connection

Amerindian influence on local culture took place through the Spanish colonials and the 'peóns' of Venezuelan origin (Borde 1876; Brereton 1981). Trinidad was colonized and ignored by the Spanish until the island was surrendered to the British in 1797. During the Spanish period some Amerindians re-crossed the Gulf of Paria to the mainland, but those who stayed accepted the Spanish culture and Catholic faith and gradually became

---

[62] Cumucurapo - the Amerindian name for Port of Spain means "place of the Silk Cotton trees" (Besson, 2000).

[63] French missionaries recorded *karifuna* and *kalligonam* as the names of Dominican men and women. This may explain why the Black Caribs of St. Vincent, later deported to Belize, call themselves *Garifuna* (Hulme, 2000).

[64] Butt Colson and de Armellada (1983) base their arguments on ethnographic data derived from remote, mostly unacculturated Amerindian societies of the recent past and of today and historical evidence in 17th century literature on Carib peoples.

[65] 1. Boiling milk bush roots to make a tea which is given to the expectant mother to drink on **5 or 9** successive days 'it cools down the body.' they say for this medicine. The scissors used to cut the umbilical cord are put beneath the place the baby's head is to lie, and left there for **9** days when mother and child first emerge from the house. The new mother can assume full household duties after **9** days. When the baby and its mother emerge from the house **9** days after the birth, a ceremony is held to present the new member of the family to relatives and the family dead. (Herskovits and Herskovits, 1947)

2. A special bath is given eight or nine days after childbirth to the mother and another to the newborn infant. Plants used in the mother's bath are framboisin (*Ocimum micranthum*), coton noir (*Gossypium vitifolium*), rokou (*Bixa orellana*), verveine (*Stachytarpheta* species), semen contra (*Chenopodium ambrosioides*), sou marque (*Cassia bicapsularis*), pistache (*Arachis hypogaea*), and bouton blanc (*Egletes prostrate*) (Taylor, 1950; Hodge and Taylor, 1957). The second quotation refers to the Caribs in Dominica. The first quotation resembles the Amerindian practice of Couvade in which the underlying belief is that the souls of babies are weakly attached to their bodies and the practices of rest and dieting protect the baby's soul for the first nine days after birth (Butt Colson and de Armellada, 1983). However Herskovits and Herskovits (1947) refer to these practices as African survivals.

assimilated (Banks 1956). Spanish-Amerindian peoples, called 'cocoa panyols', were known as the poor but hospitable backbone of the cocoa economy, clearing the forest and cultivating the cocoa fields (Besson 2000).

One example of the Amerindian plant heritage was found in Tobago during research conducted in 1995. An individual remedy to induce oestrus included cedar bark (Cedrela odorata). The Tacanas in the Bolivian Amazon use a decoction of cedar bark for post partum haemorrhage (Bourdy et al., 2000). Amerindians do not operate from the dualisms that separate humans from spirits, animals, plants or things, mind and body, thinking and feeling or nature and culture (Lawrence, 1998; McCorkle and Green, 1998). They practised a universal belief in spirits of nature and deities were not worshiped (Besson, 2000). Medicine men served as curers and advisors due to their ability to contact spirits. Amerindian culture has personalistic explanations for sickness (Banks, 1956; Davis and Yost, 1983). Personalistic explanations of illness are explained by the active aggression of some agent, which might be human, non-human, or supernatural like souls, deities, demons, ancestors and sorcerers (Dressler, 1980; Davis and Yost, 1983). The sick person is a victim of aggression or punishment directed against him for reasons that concern only him (Butt Colson and de Armellada, 1983). Dressler (1980) wrongly subsumes all personalistic beliefs under the African-based tradition of Obeah. Wrongly because Warao [Amerindian] personalistic explanations dominate over those of natural causation and some of these explanations persist in the Caribbean (Wilbert, 1983a&b). There is an underlying aspect of some Amerindian culture claiming that all human relationships are potentially dangerous (Banks, 1956). It is claimed that this theme underlies their couvade[66] and other rituals and purifications and the Amerindian theory of sickness.

The Catholic missionaries of the Cisterciensan and Capuchin orders who set up missions along the east and south coasts of Trinidad are responsible for the Hispanicization of the Amerindians. The resulting Spanish-Amerindian culture has been documented in Moodie-Kublalsingh (1994). When the Amerindians intermarried with other groups, their language may have been lost but their cultural heritage was passed on through every day practices. In this chapter I illustrate the continuing existence of Amerindian culture in the ethnoveterinary uses of plants and insects by hunters. Trinidad hunters use various strategies in an attempt to make their dogs better hunters or catch certain game. There is literature establishing that native Trinidadians or Spanish-Amerindians participated in hunts with Creole hunters (Carr 1893). Farabee (1918) claims that dogs naturally become better hunters for certain animals. However Im Thurn (1883: 232) records that the Amerindians trained hunting dogs to hunt one sort of game. In Trinidad a combination of both occurs[67]. Amerindian use of hallucinogenic and other plants to improve hunting success is also recorded in Russo (1992: 202), Morton (1981) and Muñoz et al. (2000: 145).

Trinidad hunting practices are similar in many respects to the Amerindian traditions documented by Im Thurn (1883), Farabee (1918) and Roth (1915) and may reveal the kinship ties[68] between Trinidad Amerindians and the mainland tribes described by Figueredo and Glazier (1978) as the Guianas Tropical Forest Culture groups. Heinen and García-Castro (2000) claim that Waraoan groups in the Orinoco Delta have an oral tradition that the

---

[66] Couvade (Fr. couver, "to hatch"), widespread custom among native peoples, whereby the father, during or immediately after the birth of a child, complains of having labor pains, and is accorded the treatment usually shown to pregnant women. The social function of couvade is held to be the assertion by the father of his role in reproduction or of his legal rights to the child. The underlying belief is that the souls of babies are weakly attached to their bodies and the couvade and practices of rest and dieting protect the soul for the first nine days after birth (Taylor, 1950; Butt Colson and de Armellada, 1983).

[67] Boomert (2000) claims that as late as the 18th century Amerindians of Sabana Grande and Mayo specialised in training dogs to hunt peccaries and armadillos. Boomert also claims that throughout British colonial times short-legged hunting dogs named Warahoon (Guaraon) were traded between the Warao of the Orinoco delta and San Fernando.

[68] H. Dieter Heinen and Alvaro García-Castro (2000) claim the Carib (Kari'ña) of the mouth of the Guanipa and the "Island" Carib from Dominica were united linguistically by a common trade language, but only the former spoke a Carib language

people who originally lived there came over from Trinidad, providing further evidence of kinship ties[69].

Ethnoveterinary medicines used for hunting

As part of a larger study into ethnoveterinary medicine, research was conducted into medicinal plants used by hunters from 1997 to 1999 (Lans et al. 2001). A veterinarian-colleague was a long-standing member of a seven-member hunting group and facilitated participation in hunting activities in Guayaguayare, South Trinidad. The participant observation involved taking part in five hunts over the three years (going into the forest, observing the chase and capture, sharing a meal and sharing of take-home game). Unstructured interviews were also held with four individual hunters in North Trinidad (Paramin), two in Central Trinidad (Talparo) and four in Mayaro (South Trinidad). Paramin and Talparo retain Hispanic traditions either from the original Spanish colonists or from continuous small-scale immigration from Venezuela (Moodie-Kublalsingh 1994). The following information was collected from all respondents; the popular name, uses, part(s) used, mode of preparation and application. Plants were collected and identified at the Herbarium of the University of the West Indies.

The participant observation and interviews with other hunters was successful in recovering some of the undocumented knowledge of the stereotypical 'people without history'. Hunters claimed that their dogs either started hunting or hunted better after they had treated them in various ways with medicinal plants or other objects. The following game animals are most commonly hunted: agouti (*Dasyprocta agouti*), tatou (*Dasypus novemcinctus*), deer (*Mazama americana trinitatis*) lappe (*Agouti paca*) and wild hog/quenk (*Tayassu tajacu*). Hunting dogs are usually foxhounds, beagles, coonhounds and mixed breeds. These dogs are usually scent and not sight hounds. It was said that the mixed breeds (called 'common dogs') were quicker at catching game, "they hold the animal in 3 to 6 hours, now for now."

Hell (1996) developed a folk taxonomy of European hunters that distinguishes between red beasts (deer), black beasts (boar), and stinking beasts (fox). More hunting trips would be necessary to know how closely the Trinidad system fits this scale (see Figure . 98 below). In Trinidad the game animals are called beasts, and white meat (chicken) is classed at the bottom of the hierarchy, similarly to the European system (Hell 1996). Like the Amerindians studied by Im Thurn (1883: 228) Trinidadians rarely hunt alone. Collective hunting is deemed more socially acceptable than individual hunting as described by Hell (1996: 210) however the skill and landscape knowledge of the individual hunters who live off wild meat sales is acknowledged.

Women do not hunt. It was also claimed that women should not untie or tie hunting dogs or step over them during their menstrual cycle since that would "blight the dogs." However if a hunting dog was 'tied' by another hunter who was jealous that the dog was hunting better than his own, a woman was supposed to 'loose' it by bathing it in a river and making the dog pass between her legs. These mystical contagion[70] beliefs may be Amerindian in origin since Taylor (1950) and Rivière (1969: 41) claim that Dominican Caribs and the Trio respectively

---

[69] The *Warao* continued to come to San Fernando from the Orinoco delta until the 1940s on a pilgrimage to Naparima Hill - the home of their god Haburi. They collected quartz crystals for shaman's rattles at Naparima Hill and traded their own goods in the market, including for tobacco which could not be grown in the delta (Boomert, 2000).

[70] One hunter was bitten by a spider, and fell three times before he reached to the back of his house. When his wife called him he could not answer because before treating himself he had to: "Keep to yourself don't go by too much woman, if you see a pregnant woman you can't survive." He chewed three tref (*Aristolochia trilobata*) leaves found at the back of the house and recovered. Then he spoke to his wife. Mole (1924) records getting the same advice after he was bitten by a mapepire. He did see a pregnant woman and lived. Roth (1915: 304) documents the restrictions on pregnant women being nearby when poison for hunting was being prepared.

did not allow 'heaty' women (pregnant or menstruating) to eat hunted meat, handle dogs or guns since this would make the hunter's dogs 'spoiled' or slow and heavy.

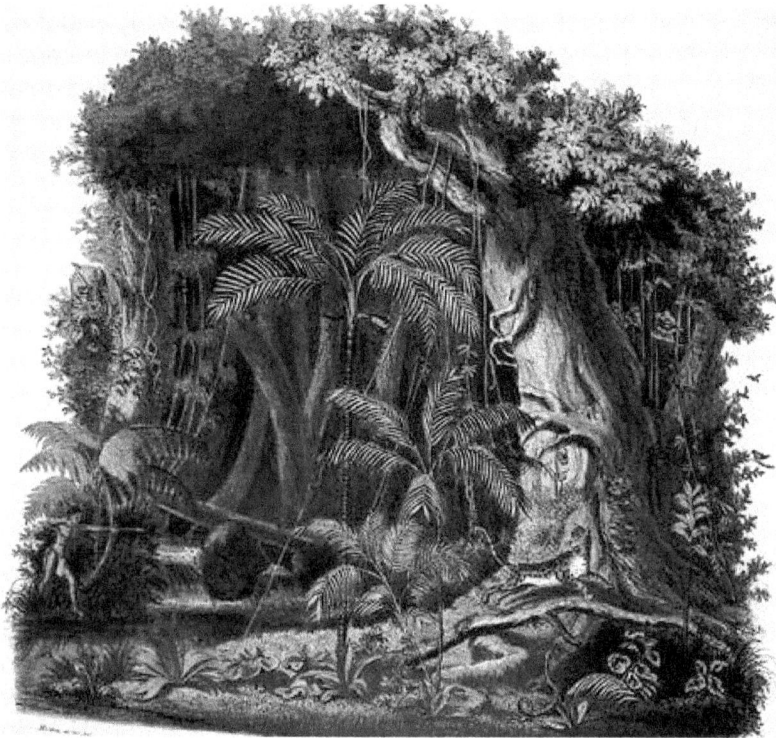

Figure 106. Amerindian hunting.
Source: Historia naturalis palmarum: opus tripartium / Carol. Frid. Phil. de Martius

Trinidad Scale

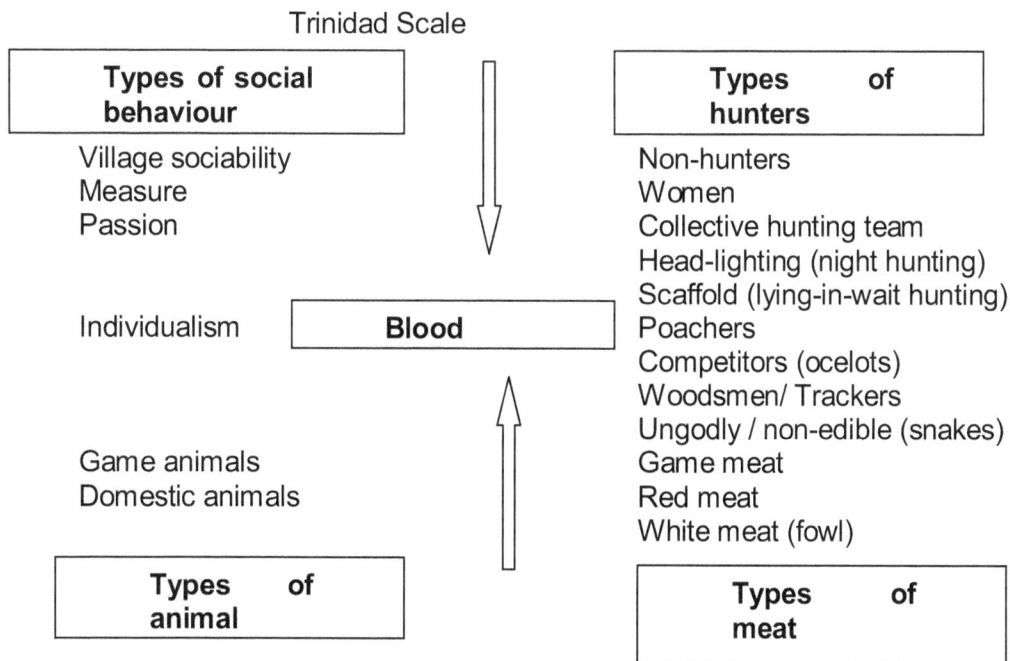

Types of social behaviour		**Types of hunters**
Village sociability		Non-hunters
Measure		Women
Passion		Collective hunting team
		Head-lighting (night hunting)
		Scaffold (lying-in-wait hunting)
Individualism	**Blood**	Poachers
		Competitors (ocelots)
		Woodsmen/ Trackers
		Ungodly / non-edible (snakes)
Game animals		Game meat
Domestic animals		Red meat
		White meat (fowl)
Types of animal		**Types of meat**

Figure 107. Trinidad taxonomy of hunting (adapted from Hell 1996: 214)

Im Thurn documents similar beliefs that pregnant women should not eat game, if they did spoiled guns or dogs could be blessed and put back to rights but this would affect the guilty woman. Women are also excluded from hunting in Europe since they do not have the 'black blood' said to be characteristic of the hunter and the game (Hell, 1996: 209). Hunters "compose" a snake bottle, often on Good Friday with plants collected on any Friday in Lent[71]. The tincture in the snake bottle is made from various plant parts and other ingredients, carried in a flask on hunting trips, and drunk when required. Snake bottles are composed of: caterpillars (*Battus polydamus*, Papilionidae) that eat the tref leaves (*Aristolochia trilobata*) are put into alcohol with mat root (*Aristolochia rugosa*), cat's claw (*Pithocellobium unguis-cati*), tobacco (*N. tabacum*), snake bush (*Barleria lupulina*) and obie seed (*Cola nitida*).

Medicinal plant baths are used frequently in the Amazon (Nunes 1996) and a similar situation exists among the hunters. Preparing dogs for hunting is called "steaming" and the plants employed are usually administered in baths and are considered to be mental and/or physical stimulants. The bush bath[72] for quenk-hunting dogs is prepared the day after the new moon. Dogs are put into the thick, foamy green liquid and "scrubbed from head to tail." Lappe and tatou hunters also bathe their dogs in the new moon using rotted leaves from the riverbed. Candle bush leaves (*Piper hispidum*) are used to make dogs "good" in the chase similarly to the Caribs of Dominica who considered *Piper* species to be charms (Hodge and Taylor 1957). One *Piper* species is used against spirits on Nicaragua's Atlantic coast (Barrett, 1994: 18). Mardi gras (*Renealmia alpinia*) berries and leaves used in plant baths are said to help dogs closely pursue the game. Mosetene Indians in Bolivia also use *Renealmia alpinia* to improve their dogs hunting ability. They mix the crushed plant with water and rub this preparation over the dog's body (Muñoz et al. 2000: 145). In Trinidad dry seeds of guinea pepper (*Aframomum melegueta*) are ground to a powder, and sprinkled on the dog's food. The use of guinea pepper (*Aframomum melegueta*) may be a syncretism of African and Amerindian practices since the Caribs of Dominica put seeds of '*poivre ginet*' into rum as a 'chauffe' to excite dogs. Hodge and Taylor (1957) identified '*poivre ginet*' as *Costus* species.

Steaming is also carried out with one type of insect (an unidentified solitary wasp that hunts spiders). Both the wasp and its spider prey are put into rum with guinea pepper (*Aframomum melegueta*) on a Friday. This solution is then given to the dog, or included in the bath water, as a stimulant. The use of the solitary wasp in the "steaming" process can also be linked to Amerindian traditions. The Waorani in the Ecuadorian Amazon believe that the characteristics of one entity or object may pass to another (Davis and Yost 1983: 281; Russo 1992: 196). This belief could explain the use of a wasp[73] that hunts successfully in baths or decoctions to turn dogs into better hunters. Amazonian Amerindians use most social wasps in hunting magic and rub wasp nests on the noses of hunting dogs to make them brave (Posey, 2002: 106). Additionally there are records of a specific ant[74] that was given to dogs by Guyanese Amerindians so that they would hunt with the same single-mindedness as the ants (Roth 1915). Amerindians also named their hunting dogs after ants and a wasp called "warribisi"[75] that caught prey. Plants are also placed in the dog's nose.

---

[71] Medicinal plants are also collected on Good Friday in Almería Spain (Martínez-Lirola et al., 1996: 43).

[72] Absorption routes of the active compounds are said to be the respiratory tract (volatile compounds carried by water vapour) and the skin (Nunes, 1996).

[73] Amazonian Amerindians also used *Melipona seminigra*, *Scaura longula*, *Oxytrigona* species and *Trigona amalthea* bee parts for hunting magic (Posey, 2002: 75).

[74] Posey documents that ants are considered by the Amazonian Amerindians to be like men because they walk and hunt on the ground. The special power of their stings is considered useful for hunting dogs and ants are used in concoctions to make dogs unafraid to keep their nose to the ground and to make them aggressive (Posey, 2002: 92).

[75] The northern Pemon are Carib-speaking Amerindians in the Guiana Highlands of the border areas of Venezuela, Brazil and Guyana. Pemon say the Wanawanari (an excavating sand wasp *Ammophila*) is a great shaman (Butt Colson and de Armellada, 1983).

158

Here it is expected that the plant will act as a nasal and chest decongestant and the dog will subsequently have a better sense of smell and improve its ability to follow a scent. One plant used in this way in Trinidad is bird pepper (*Capsicum frutescens*). Duke records that the Chocó Indians used *Capsicum frutescens* to give their hunting dogs more "energy" (Duke 1970: 356). The Chocó practice may be linked to the plant's ability to stimulate carbohydrate oxidation (Al-Qarawi and Adam 1999). In Trinidad ground kojo root (*Petiveria alliacea*) is used to bathe dogs so that they are more alert, while the Maya in Belize put *Petiveria alliacea* leaf on the dog's nose to improve its ability to follow a scent (Arnason et al. 1980: 359).

All of the above practices can be linked to those of the Guyanese Amerindians who conducted rituals in which ants and other insects were made to bite the nostrils of the hunting dog. Plant leaves and other plant parts including peppers were then rubbed into the wounds on the noses of the dogs. These practices were said to improve the power of scent in dogs since the nasal mucous membranes were cleaned, the nervous system of the dogs was irritated and thus responsive, the perceptions were sharpened, and the dog would keep its nose to the ground when hunting (Im Thurn 1883: 231; Roth 1915).

Im Thurn (1883: 230) and Roth (1915: 279) record how hunters from the Macusis, Arecunas and Ackawoi groups rubbed caterpillars on their chests or thighs in preparation rituals. The caterpillar hairs broke off easily and irritated the flesh causing a rash. There seemed to be a mental connection of success in acquisition of game with pain previously inflicted on the hunter and his dog (Im Thurn 1883: 231). There was also the belief that inflicting pain was a means of preparing the hunter and his dog to meet without flinching any pain or danger that could arise during the chase (Im Thurn 1883). This preparation was not ill-advised since the process of tracking deer was long and tedious and the pit viper 'mapepire z'annana' (*Lachesis muta muta*) often lives in the burrows of lappe and tatou (Farabee 1918; Mole 1924: 269).

Plants are also used for dogs that are "crossed." In this situation the hunters complain that the dog goes in the opposite direction from the game. The dog is faced upstream and bathed in a river with the water running east and rubbed with the crushed leaves of seven different plants found on the riverbed (sometimes the plants used have no other distinguishing characteristic). The dog is then turned to face downstream. Trinidad hunters bathe dogs for "cross" using the crushed leaves of sun bush (*Lepianthes peltata* syn. *Potomorphe peltata*). This practice is dissimilar to the practices of the Cuna and Chocó Indians and the Ese'eje tribe of Amerindians in Perú who use a cataplasm of the leaves for practical reasons such as various external ailments and to exterminate lice (Desmarchelier et al. 1996: 49; Duke 1970: 362, 1975: 291). The plant is used as a bath for intestinal pains by the Yanomani Indians of Brazil (Milliken and Albert 1997: 271). Plant tops of seed under leaf (*Phyllanthus urinaria*) are also used to bathe dogs for "cross." This is similar to the use of the plant by Caribs with other plants in a bath against bad luck (called 'piai') (Honychurch 1986). One respondent claimed that crossed dogs are really

"running spirits, evil things in the forest are humbugging them."

Bush baths were not universally seen as positive. Hunters with imported breeds claimed that only "hard-headed common dogs" were given bush baths, and that these baths especially those with bird pepper made the dogs look "miserable and hairless" and they "only last two seasons." As an alternative to bird pepper dogs were given mustard powder in rum. Other non-plant objects are also given to dogs. Deer liver and hooves are kept in a flask with puncheon rum and deer dogs are given a sniff before a deer hunt. The grated tail of tatou (*Dasypus novemcinctus*) is used similarly.

Cocoa panyols

The invisibility of the Amerindians is partly due to their practice of intermarrying and assimilating. The Amerindians influenced the original Spanish colonials and Spanish-Amerindian peoples were called 'cocoa panyols' (Besson 2000). Hispanicization of the Amerindians by Catholic missionaries was ongoing by 1787. An example of Hispanicization is the collection of medicinal plants on Good Friday, as is the practice in Almería, Spain (Martínez-Lirola et al. 1996). Talparo in central Trinidad retains some Spanish heritage. One Talparo respondent claimed that *Bixa orellana* root was to be cut on a Wednesday or Friday for dropsy, "this was a secret not Obeah, but for jaundice it could be cut at any time" (Lans 2001). Seasoning makers in Paramin (another area with strong Spanish heritage) spoke of a religious-based belief that "on Good Friday if someone dug up a clump of fowl foot grass (*Eleusine indica*) they would get a piece of coal below the roots." White/red physic nut (*Jatropha curcas / gossypifolia*, Euphorbiaceae), "if cut on Good Friday would produce the blood of Jesus" (Lans 2001).

The word *te* (tea) in Spanish refers to *Camellia sinensis*, but it is also used in Spain to refer to 70 different plant species. These are usually collected in the countryside, boiled dry or fresh, and drunk socially. Tes are used for stomach problems, and in as laxatives, antidiarrhoeics, and to reduce the blood pressure (Pardo de Santayana, 2005).The most important include *Chenopodium ambrosioides*, *Bidens aurea* and *Potentilla caulescens*.

Table 11 shows a fraction of the European contribution to local folk medicine including the Creole French and Spanish local names and the medicinal plant uses. This data was obtained from the field notes of Sylvia Moodie-Kublalsingh and was collected largely from 1977 - 1981. Moodie-Kublalsingh published some of this data in <u>The Cocoa Panyols of Trinidad</u>. Moodie (1982) describes special plants called 'turals[76]' that are a source of strength, good luck, and success in hunting and cock fighting and that are believed to protect people and their homes. These plants had to be rewarded with silver coins as a symbolic payment ('mounted') before removing some of the plant parts, or the respondents claimed that the entire plant or clump of plants would die. This payment was supposed to be placed in the hole from which the root was dug. These 'mounted' plants are planted on Good Friday or the first Friday in Lent, sprinkled with the blood of a dove or chicken and the roots are sprinkled with milk (Moodie 1982; Moodie-Kublalsingh 1994). Two of these turals were identified in Paramin during the research. Tref (*Aristolochia trilobata*) was one of the plants used by the hunters in their tinctures for snake bites. The only explanation given for the paying the plant was that it was not a "simple plant."

The European plant ruda (*Ruta graveolens*), was said to be a spiritual bush, and harvesters had to have clean hands to touch it, and could not be perspiring. The plant could not be told that it smelt funny or it would die. It had to be planted away from people since unclean people caused it to wither. "No evil meddles with it" respondents said of this plant. Hog tannia (*Xanthosoma brasiliense*, *Xanthosoma undipes*) was another plant that could not be planted too close to people since 'unclean' people would cause it to dry down and grow up somewhere else. Giving plants symbolic payments is an Amerindian belief according to Dennis (1988: 17). Miskito speaking people of eastern and southeastern Honduras consider that the plants have supernatural owners who require such payment and the payment is placed on the ground near the plant before it is picked and can be recovered later by the person who picked it (Dennis 1988). The belief in the supernatural ownership of plants was revealed by a Talparo informant who claimed that he used "no compelling" when hunting,

---

[76] Amazonian mestizos believe in magical plants that allow the healer to communicate directly with powerful beings (Jovel et al. 1996: 149). Roth (1915: 232) documented that *Caladium* plants could whistle to their owners and warn them of danger.

and his dogs used their "own mind" to hunt, implying that the plants hunters used compelled dogs to hunt.

Table 11. A selection of the European contribution to Trinidad folk medicine

Latin name	Family, uses	French Common name	Spanish Common name
Ambrosia cumanensis	Asteraceae. Herb teas for yellow fever	Altamis	Altamisa
Ambrosia cumanensis	Herb teas for constipation	Altamis	Altamisa
Ambrosia cumanensis	Herb tea for menorrhagia, postpartum depurants. Good for women if they are not seeing their health	Altamis	Altamisa
Ambrosia cumanensis	Root or herb infusions for colds, fever. During dry season 'it is hot".	Altamis	Altamisa
A.absinthium	Asteraceae		Ajenjo
C.ambrosioides	Chenopodiaceae	Simen contra	Pazote
Cyperus diffuses	Meliaceae	Corosi	Corosillo
Plantago major	Plantaginaceae		Llanten
Portulaca oleracea	Worms in children	Verdolaga	Verdolaga
Portulaca oleracea	Portulacaceae, Cooling	Verdolaga	Verdolaga
Portulaca oleracea	Portulacaceae, Herb tea	Verdolaga	Verdolaga
R. officinalis	Labiatae		Romero
Pimpinella anisum	Umbelliferae Good for bathing dogs and people, machuar la hoja, meterla en el agua		Hinojo
Pimpinella anisum	Leaves for making mauby		Hinojo
Pimpinella anisum	Leaf tea for settling stomach		Hinojo
	For women's disorders, leaf. Root par la barrija. La hoja cuando una mujer hace un muchachito y la sangre la para		Hoja de gato
Rumex crispus	Purify blood, thick leaf, roast then pound and squeeze, take for 9 days	Langue bef	Cuicuisa
Rumex crispus	For shortness of breath, make a tisane from the root with other roots	Langue bef	Cuicuisa
Sambucus intermedia insularis	Caprifoliaceae Asthma in combination with karap oil		Asaúco
Sambucus intermedia insularis	Flowers or leaves in infusions and decoctions for cough, flu, colds in chest, fever, consumption		Asaúco

Forgetting the Amerindian heritage

One of the few practices readily attributed to the Amerindian heritage is the use of roucou (*Bixa orellana*) in cooking to color meat. Gmelch and Gmelch (1996) have added the following contributions: fishing, crab catching, harvesting of sea turtles and the use of hammocks. There is a false consciousness in the Caribbean that gives little recognition to Amerindian customs (Drummond 1980). Burnett (2002) suggests how this false consciousness may have developed during colonialism when Europeans claimed the superiority of their own knowledge and culture and minimized Amerindian knowledge.

In the early years of slavery in Trinidad many of the slaves arrived in Trinidad during the French Revolution from the French West Indies, possessing a Creolized African-French-Caribbean culture and speaking Patois. The descendents of these slaves and those born in Africa may have decided to rename the Amerindian culture they had learnt as a reduced but

161

insufficiently understood native "cultural language" as African. When an herbalist reporting family folk practices claims that her source was her grandmother's mother who came from Africa, it does not mean that the knowledge itself was African. Similarly for the knowledge of the herbalist described as an old and skilled Orisha woman descended from slaves. Ditto for the slave medicine (based on native plants) meticulously described by Handler and Jacoby (1993). Brathwaite (1971) maintains that there is a tendency for Caribbean people to depend on the 'mother' countries for normative value-references rather than using residential traditions and the Amerindian heritage has been poorly documented. Drummond (1980) argues that Guyanese rename, redefine and reconstitute Amerindian practices as "English" and claims that there is a Creole insistence on defining behavior and belief according to persistent ethnic stereotypes.

The Amerindians themselves may have forgotten some of their own cultural beliefs. Im Thurn (1883) has recorded how the Guyanese Amerindians used 'beenas', as charms to entice any object or desire wanted. Beenas were used for hunting dogs, which were made to swallow specific pieces of roots and leaves for specific game animals. Roth (1915: 234) claimed that Guyanese Amerindians had forgotten that they used beenas because these plants were believed to possess associated spirits. Cultural explanations for plant use were not handed down so explanations are given using the Doctrine of Signatures[77]. It is difficult to say whether these explanations are culturally based[78] or created to fill a knowledge vacuum.

Trinidad hunters claimed that certain plants had characteristics with desirable qualities or had physical properties that resembled the desired game. These desirable qualities were transferred to the dog after the plant use in a bath. Im Thurn (1883) records that the beena for lappe had typical white markings similar to those of the lappe, while the beena for quenk had a leaf with a small secondary leaf under the surface that resembled either the scent gland of the quenk or its nostril tip. One Trinidad 'beena' is hog tannia. Trinidad hunters grind the root (or tannia) of hog tannia (*Xanthosoma brasiliense*, *Xanthosoma undipes*) and sprinkle this on the dog's food.

One explanation given is that the leaf of hog tannia has needles similar to the bristle-like hairs on the back and neck of the wild hog/quenk and that quenks also eat these tubers. A second explanation is that the hog tannia scratches the dog's throat so it has to keep moving. A third explanation may be that the Dominican Caribs used a *Xanthosoma species* called "chou poivre" which they rubbed on their bodies as a war charm (Plowman 1969: 118). There is a rational explanation for using a war charm when hunting wild hogs. They can be very aggressive, especially in a group of five or six[79].

One war story told of quenk hunting is documented in Carr (1893).
  '...it was found that the object of our chase had taken refuge within the hollow trunk of a gigantic balata tree...at the report of my shot and to our pleasant surprise, two more frightened members of the same band jumped right among us from the opening we had effected....After a short run, however, they were brought to bay by four of the dogs while the remaining five stood guarding the dead quank... Here were two full-grown quanks, foaming with rage...faced by the four dogs... The angered rovers of the woods put a stop to this truculent intrusion by frightfully mutilating with their tusks two of their annoyers...Exciting and not free from danger, as the foregoing might seem...there was... an encounter with the dreaded mapepire (Lachesis mutus) which had

---

[77] Davis and Yost (1983: 281) claim that the Waorani in Amazonian Ecuador have a similar logic to the Doctrine of Signatures. Certain plants that share a morphological similarity with a dangerous animal have the power to treat wounds caused by that animal.
[78] Nunes (1996) claims that Amazonian users of fragrant baths may not realize that they are ingesting a drug and therefore credit effects to magical or occult forces.
[79] One quenk hunter claimed he had been hunting from age nine to forty-eight and because of his use of bush baths had lost only two dogs to quenks.

162

inhabited or was asleep in the hollow of the balata tree in which the quanks had taken refuge...His snakeship had not been in the least disturbed until one of the most daring of the dogs that had, on our return to this, the scene of our first "kill", gone into the hollowed trunk rummaging in quest of further possible game, indecorously seized and dragged into the open this terrible animal...Before we could get near enough to kill this death-dealing brute, it had bitten four dogs, one dying almost immediately and another within fifteen minutes... the other two, one bitten on the neck and the other on the paw, were promptly attended to, and got well after a few days. The remedy used was a tincture I carried, prepared from roots, barks and seeds. The two sick patients, though conscious, were unable to walk and had to be carried home in guayares[80], an extemporised basket-like Indian palm-leaf and liane knapsack. (Carr 1893)

The above shows that the hunting practices and rituals used to capture specific game in Trinidad can be attributed to Amerindian knowledge and it is possible that this knowledge was first transmitted to the Spanish colonists in the 1700s. Due to the assimilation of the Amerindians and the Hispanic colonists more research is needed on the specifically Hispanic origin of some plant remedies. Rescue of the French and other European contribution will need what Gould (2000) described as exploration of unusual sources.

Conclusion

Voeks (1996) claims that the African slaves who became herbalists in the Caribbean played a limited role in introducing plant species from Africa but recognized some of the African species that did arrive opportunistically. There were also similar taxa in South America to medicinal plants in Africa. The non-experimental evaluation of the medicinal plants provided verifiable data on ethnoveterinary remedies used for hunting dogs. A 'reduced' body of knowledge (practising the rituals without knowing the underlying belief-system) was passed from the Amerindian hunters in the 1800s or before to their Creole co-hunters who then passed on this knowledge to family and friends.

Since the plants and practices are largely comparable to those of Amerindian groups in South America there is every reason to believe that Amerindian culture may lie at the base of Caribbean Creolization as suggested by Butt Colson and de Armellada (1983) and Johannes and Werner Wilbert (1983a; 1983b) who have done extensive work on Amerindian groups. The evidence of modification of this culture by African traditions could not be obtained from the literature. To paraphrase Balée (2000), the Rosetta Stone of Amerindian knowledge is not made of rock or found in archaeological digs, but in the living cultural practices of Caribbean peoples themselves.

---

[80] The guayare is another example of the Amerindian culture.

Table 11. Complete creole names of folk medicine in Trinidad

Latin name	Family, uses	French Common name	Spanish Common name
Andire inermis	Leguminosae	Angelin	
Begonia humilis	Begoniaceae Colds		
Mimosa pudica	Antidiarrhea. Mimosaceae Promote fertility in women. Use root with other bush for tisane. Take a tea for 9 days to take out 'cold' from system.		Adolmidero
Mimosa pudica	Bottles, 9 each time. After tisane take a purge and after that the woman should conceive. If woman does not conceive there is no hope		Adormidero
	Use with caraaili, cotton leaves and buchette		Adormidero
A. moschatus	Malvaceae. Put in rum for insect bites	Gombo mis	Aguajira, algalia
A. moschatus	Smoke seed in pipe for asthma		Aguajira, algalia
Abelmoschus moschatus	Grind seed and boil, make tea for pains, use for witchcraft.		Aguajira, algalia
Artemisia absinthium	Asteraceae		Ajenjo
Sesamum indicum	Pedaliaceae Make sweets		Ajonjoli
Ocimum micranthium	Labiatae, Drop a seed in eyes, after 2 hours impurities come out	Ti bom	Albahaca
Ocimum micranthium	For bathing corpses	Ti bom	Albahaca
Ocimum micranthium	Brew and put in milk for rheumatism	Ti bom	Albahaca
Gossypium barbadense	Malvaceae, worms in children and pups		Algodón
Vetiveria zizanoides	Graminae In making hats and bags	Vetivert	Almizquera
Vetiveria zizanoides	Wash root, put to dry. Boil root and make tea for fever, colds.	Vetivert	Almizquera
Ambrosia cumanensis	Asteraceae. Herb tea for menorrhagia, postpartum depurants. Good for women if they are not seeing their health. Tea for constipation, herb tea for yellow fever.	Altamis	Altamisa
Ambrosia cumanensis	Root or herb infusions for colds, fever.. Seen during dry season 'it is hot", not in rainy season	Altamis	Altamisa
Piper marginatum	Piperaceae Used in making mauby		Ánis
Potomorphe umbellate	Leaf good for bathing hunting dogs	Feuille soleil	Anîsillo
Annona muricata	Annonaceae		Anón
Bixa orellana	Boil root and make a tea for jaundice	Roucou	Anoto
Bixa orellana	Bixaceae. Food colouring, softening meat	Roucou	Anoto
Bixa orellana	Rum infusions of root for diabetes, flu, vd.	Roucou	Anoto
Impatiens balsomina			Arubamba
Ocimum gratissimum	Labiatae. Cough, colds		Arubamba
Sambucus intermedia insularis	Caprifoliaceae. Asthma in combination with karap oil		Asaúco
Sambucus intermedia insularis	Flowers or leaves in infusions and decoctions for cough, flu, colds in chest, fever, consumption.		Asaúco
Bambusa vulgaris	Gramineae Purgative, young sucker, pound it and add a little epsom salt after straining it.		Bambú
Bauhinia cumanensis,	Caesalpiniaceae Used in preparing tisane to clean blood, drink like a wine		Bejuco de cadena,
	For making whips		Bejuco de pesi
Gouania polygama	Rhamnaceae For rashes, skin problems. Se machuca las hojas y se hace un jabon. Se hace una expuma y se echa en la cabeza. For dandruff.	Liane savonette	Bejuco de rema, Hoho provå
Bauhinia excisa	Caesalpiniaceae Wine decoction for snake bites, scorpion stings, pain		Bejuco de tasajo

164

Table 11. Complete creole names of folk medicine in Trinidad (cont.)

Latin name	Family, uses	French Common name	Spanish Common name
Bauhinia excisa	Wine decoction for eczema, colds, heat, venereal disease		Bejuco de tasajo
Serjania diversifolia	Used in making tisane. Leaf with veins. Place in rum or wine. Drink for 'failing nature' , 3 times a day. Seven pieces of dry vine, and 7 pieces of black incense and 7 pieces of root of langue boeuf (lengue de vaca)		Bejuco moreno
Heliconia bihai	Heliconiaceae Making mats, ink.		Bijao
Heliconia bihai	Young leaf for wrapping pastilles, burns.		Bijao
Cassia occidentalis	Caesalpiniaceae Scorpion sting used with Cecropia peltata	Z'herbe puante	Brusca
Cassia occidentalis	Used with root decoctions and infusions for womb inflammation, abortifacients, purgative, postpartum depurants.	Z'herbe puante	Brusca
Cassia occidentalis	Seed decoction for palpitation, colds. Congestive heart failure	Z'herbe puante	Brusca
Urena sinuata	Malvaceae	Cousin maho	Cadillo de caballo
Desmodium incanum	Papilionaceae. Fever, vomiting, bad stomach	Patte chien	Cadillo de maní
Urena lobata	Malvaceae. Colds		Cadillo de perro
Urena lobata	Place leaf on affected area for dog bites. As the leaf becomes drier the victim improves, but the dog which bit him languishes by degrees		Cadillo de perro
Coffee arabica	Rubiaceae. Root for snake bites		Café
Croton flavens	Euphorbiaceae. Cold, root for snake bite.		Calcanapé
			Caldón
Ageratum conyzoides	Labiatae. Herb teas for heat, flu, cough, pneumonia. Root decoction for diabetes.	Z'herbe à femme	Calero macho, Calero hembra
Ageratum conyzoides	Herb teas for women's disorders and root decoctions postpartum clotting		Calero macho, Calero hembra
Musa paradisiaca var sapientum	Musaceae Leaves and bark for diarrhea. Dry leaf for pain in waist.		Cambure de moco
Paspalum conjugatum	Poaceae Fever, colds, pleurisy		Cambute
Croton conduplicatus	Euphorbiaceae Pass 3 leaves over the fire, squeeze the juice into the ear when ears are blocked or when they have wind		Cancanapire
Leonotis nepetifolia	Lamiaceae Colds, cough, pheumonia	Chandilier	Candelero
Renealmia alpinia	Zingiberaceae For bathing dogs		Canopia
Renealmia alpinia	Bush bath for humans, making ink.		Canopia
Renealmia alpinia	Pound leaves and put in a piece of cloth, apply to piles, and swollen feet.		Canopia
Hibiscus rosa-sinensis	Flowers for stomach problems, colds.		Cardón
Annona muricata	Annonaceae Leaves for cooling, heat, lack of sleep	Cowosol	Catuche
Eleutherine bulbosa	Iridaceae For dysentery		Cebolleta morá
Eleutherine bulbosa	Poultice made of grated cebolleta mixed with fine bachac earth (flor de tierra de bachaco) and lamp oil		Cebolleta morá
Eupatorium odoratum	Compositae. Bath for colds, mix with ramoncillo, citronera, verbena, pawpaw etc to make loch for cold, headache	Fleuri noel	Cigarrón
Cymbopogon citratus	Gramineae. Grass and rhizome teas for colds, flu, fever, pneumonia and malarial fever		Citronera
Eclipta alba	Asteraceae. Boil in milk for marasmus		Congolala

Table 11. Complete creole names of folk medicine in Trinidad (cont.)

Latin name	Family, uses	French Common name	Spanish Common name
Eclipta alba	Boil very strong for asthma		Congolala
Peperomia rotundifolia	Piperaceae. Make tea with 2 or 3 leaves with pinch of salt	Mowon	Coralillo
Cyperus diffuses	Meliaceae Make a tea with root for stomach pains, mix with salt for fever	Corosi	Corosillo
Xiphidium caeruleum	Haemodoraceae		Corrimiento
Rumex crispus	Purify blood, thick leaf, roast then pound and squeeze, take for 9 days	Langue bef	Cuicuisa
Rumex crispus	For shortness of breath, make a tisane from the root with other roots	Langue bef	Cuicuisa
Eryngium foetidum	Umbelliferae. Extract juice from leaves and drink for colds and abdominal pains	Chadron bénée	Culantro
Eryngium foetidum	Use leaves for seasoning	Chadron bénée	Culantro
Momordica charantia	Cucurbitaceae. Antidiabetic	Mesichen	Cundeamor
Momordica charantia	Fruit good for fever, malaria, venereal disease. Juice for rashes.	Mesichen	Cundeamor
Polypodium latum			Curapasmo
Scoparia dulcis	Scrophulariaceae. For maljo (bad eye), put plant in child's hand, give some plant juice to drink mixed with infant boy's urine	Balier doux	Escobilla
Scoparia dulcis	Extract juice with salt or olive oil and give for gastroenteritis	Balier doux	Escobilla
Luffa operculata	Cucurbitaceae. Leaf tea antidote for snake bite, scorpion sting, sinusitis.	Torchon	Esponjilla
Luffa operculata	Leaf tea as purgative use with care	Torchon	Esponjilla
Gurania spinulosa	Curcurbitaceae. Leaf tea as purgative		Estrolog
Tagestes patula	Compositae Tea of plant or flower for toothache. Loch of leaf or flower for flu	Souci	Flor de muerto
Tagestes patula	Used for bathing dead people	Souci	Flor de muerto
Capraria biflora	Scrophulariaceae. Purifies blood, take after drinking castor oil	Du thé pays	Fregosa
Xylopia grandiflora	Asthma, seeds with nutmeg con un grano de ajo y concha de naranja		Fruta de burro
Sataria pouretiana	Use root for haemorrhage in women		Gamelote
Fleurya aestuans	Urticacea. Stoppage of water	Zoti rouge, zoti blanc	Guanitoto
Fleurya aestuans	Bich with aloes to "dress" children Stoppage of water. Colic in horses	Zoti rouge, zoti blanc	Guanitoto
Cecropia peltata	Moraceae. 3 pieces of root for any kind of sting. Dry leaf for pressure.	Bois canôt	Guarumo
Cecropia peltata	Used for dancing cocoa	Bois canôt	Guarumo
Guazuma ulmifolia	Sterculiaceae. Pound bark and use it for dancing the cocoa		Guásimo
Guazuma ulmifolia	Sterculiaceae. Band waist with shiny skin and add puncheon rum as it gets dry		Guásimo
Myrospermum frutescens	Papilionaceae. Cold, pneumonia, rheumatism		Guatamare
		Marasma	Guineo criollo
			Hierba de carpiento
Eleusine indica	Poaceae. Grass or root decoctions for cystitis, heat pay plant to help. Take part of it for drinking, bath, etc.		Hierba de chival
Eleusine indica	Grass or root decoctions for pneumonia		Hierba de chival
Peperomia pellucida	Piperaceae. For thrush make an infusion and wash, apply honey after. Cooling.		Hierba de sapo
Solanum americanum	Cooling. Ward off evil. Juice applied on body with escobilla.	Agouma	Hierba mora, Yerba mora

Table 11. Complete creole names of folk medicine in Trinidad (cont.)

Latin name	Family, uses	French Common name	Spanish Common name
			Hierba salwaje
Ricinus communis	Euphorbiaceae. Purgative after aloes has been taken.		Higuereta
Ricinus communis	Ward off evil eye, la hoja dolol. Extract oil for seed par la parreja		Higuereta
Didymopanax morototoni	Araliaceae. Wood for making matches		Higuereton
Pimpinella anisum	Umbelliferae. Good for bathing dogs and people, machuar la hoja, meterla en el agua		Hinojo
Pimpinella anisum	Leaves to make mauby, settling stomach		Hinojo
	For women's disorders, leaf. Root par la barrija. La hoja cuando una mujer hace un muchachito y la sangre la para		Hoja de gato
Neurolaena lobata	Compositae.1 tbs. of leaf juice in brandy (vermouth) leave in dew at night, take every other day		Hoja de lanza
Neurolaena lobata	Leaf tea for fever, colds, malaria, bites.		Hoja de lanza
Neurolaena lobata	Leaf tea for women's disorders		Hoja de lanza
Kalanchoe pinnata	Crassulaceae. Boil water, drink tea for skin diseases, sores, eczema	Feuille pavo, Caractère des hommes	Hoja de libertad
Kalanchoe pinnata	Apply leaf to sores for swollen feet	Feuille pavo, Caractère des hommes	Hoja de libertad
Manilkara zapota	Sapotaceae. Stoppage of water		Hoja de níspero
Hura crepitans	Euphorbiaceae. Wood used for making coffins, matches		Jabillo, jarillo
Jasminum officinale	Leaf tea for calming nerves		Jazmin
Trixis radialis	Compositae. Scorpion bite		Juan de la calle
Trixis radialis	Plant with money for good luck		Juan de la calle
Trixis radialis	Bathing dogs and people for good luck		Juan de la calle
Trixis radialis	Use 3 leaves with white musk powder and pigeon pea leaf for colds		Juan de la calle
	Gall from Lappe put over fire and boil for pain. Use for diabetes.		La hiel de la lapa
Pimenta racemosa	Myrtaceae	Laurier	Laurel
Polypodium phyllitides	Polypodiaceae. Colds, coughs, take a small part of the leaf and with sirio flowers and mowon, make a loch		Lengua de sierpe
	Dysentery, sprain finger and ankle		Lengua de vaca
Plantago major	Plantaginaceae. Extract juice and apply drops to eyes		Llanten
Portulaca pilosa	Portulacaceae. Herb tea for worms		Lombricero
	To ward off the evil eye from cultivated land		Maldiohera
Petiveria alliacea	Put root in brandy or urine and sap joints for rheumatism	Mapurite	Mapurite
Petiveria alliacea	Put in rum, put on cloth for headaches, scorpion bite,	Mapurite	Mapurite
Petiveria alliacea	Root for colds. With rum for gas.	Mapurite	Mapurite
Gomphrena globosa			Margarita
Hyptis suaveolens	Labiatae, Leaf teas and baths for colds	Matrang	Matransa
Anacardium occidentale	Anacardiaceae. Use leaves, fruit and bark for diarrhea		Merey
Myristica fragrans	Myristicaceae. Use grated nutmeg to avoid cold, for pneumonia, salla, gastric problems, fleta par pasmo con vela	Muscade	Nuez moscada

Table 11. Complete creole names of folk medicine in Trinidad (cont.)

Latin name	Family, uses	French Common name	Spanish Common name
Myristica fragrans	Blandita y son par gas. Dolol de diente. Con son fuelte en el hoyo, worm in gum eating you, put remedy. When you do(n't) have toothache, that is when the worm have de head up	Muscade	Nuez moscada
Myristica fragrans	Cold, cuando quiere evitar un resfriado se mete un mêh mõhká en la boca	Muscade	Nuez moscada
Coleus aromaticus	Labiatae. Earache: cocinar 3 hojas de o.f., 1 cucharadita de aceite de pescao (opresción de frió) of aciete de coco fresco (de calor). Stroke: 1 puño de orégano molido. 1 cucharada de aceite de carapa colds (frio). 1 puño de orégano con sal y azúcar se toma 5, 7 0r 9 noches hasta que se colte	Thym	Orégano francés, Orégano chiquito, orégano grande
Pogostemon cablin	Labiatae	Pachouli	Pachulí
	Leaf decoction for neuralgia, put warm in mouth		Pata de paloma, correrimento
Cissampelos pareira	Menispermaceae. Leaf and roots good for liver, spleen complaints, swollen face, cancer		Patacon
Chenopodium ambrosioides	Chenopodiaceae. Boil stalks for worms, use with lepozen	Simen contra	Pazote
Mucuna pruriens	For worms		Pica pica, surin
Piper nigrum	Piperaceae. Use with other bush for stroke		Pimienta (hoja de)
Afromomum melegueta	Zingiberaceae. Good for gas		Pimienta de guinea
Afromomum melegueta	Give seed to 'warm up' hunting dogs		Pimienta de guinea
Jatropha curcas	Euphorbiaceae. Ward off evil if planted in 4 corners of yard. Leaf for pains, headaches.	Medicien beni/ blanc	Piñón
Jatropha curcas	Use stem to make a garrote or a cross to keep off soucouyant bruja	Medicien beni/ blanc	Piñón
Jatropha curcas	Boil leaves till they are soft, add cooking oil and salt apply to sores. Cooking oil prevents leaf from adhering to sores	Medicien beni/ blanc	Piñón
Amaranthus spinosus	Amaranthaceae		Pira
	Asclepidaceae		Platanilla
Manilkara bidentata	Sapotaceae. Milk or gum for making whips, make a ball to play cricket	Balata	Pulgo macho
Justicia secunda	Acanthaceae. Bathe child with St. John's bush for marasmus	Shanshanmuns hin	Quiebra quiebra
Heliotropium indicum	Boraginaceae. Wash and boil leaves, apply liquid to eyes	Verveine lacher rate	Rabo de alacrán
Aristolochia rugosa	Aristolochiaceae. Root tea for snakebites, scorpion stings, indigestion	Rey de parel	Raiz de mato
Rauwolfia ligustrina	Apocynaceae. Snake bites, scorpion bites		Raiz de pareira
	Put in water with 1 or 2 grains of corn. Number depends on number of teeth to be cut, give child water to drink		Rama
Lantana camara	Verbenaceae, Colds, chest colds		Ramoncillo
Cordyline terminalis			Rayo
Dorstenia contrajerva	Moraceae. Colds, bellyaches, use root make a tea		Resfriado
Dorstenia contrajerva	Dolor de barrija, use root make a tea		Resfriado

Table 11. Complete creole names of folk medicine in Trinidad (cont.)

Latin name	Family, uses	French Common name	Spanish Common name
Rosmarinus officinalis	Labiatae. Bad eye, boil in afternoon and put in dew, then wash face with decoction. Burn leaves and rub down with it. Burn with bless palm and santawai the child.		Romero
	Colds. Some rudas are trees		Rura extranjera
Aloe barbadensis	Liliaceae, Blows, falls, sores, marasma.		Sábila
Aloe barbadensis	To regulate menstrual cycle, bich, almorrana. Mix gel with milk or egg or garlic and give to drink for jaundice		Sábila
Aloe barbadensis	Mix gel with rum and give to drink for pneumonia		Sábila
Pluchea symphytifolia	Compositae. Pass leaves over fire, get veins flat with soft candle, put on forehead with headaches		Salvia
Pluchea symphytifolia	3 cogollitos se cocina par frio, colds		Salvia
Pluchea odorata	Compositae		Salvia
Lippia alba	Verbenaceae, Boil 3 tops and drink for colds and stomach problems.	Santa maria	Santa maría
	Grate seed and boil and drink for ring worm and decomposition. Boil skins for pain.		Secua
Gomphrena globosa	Amaranthaceae, Venereal disease	Marguerite blanc	Siempreviva
Alternanthera ficoridea	Amaranthaceae		Suelda con suelda
Commelina diffusa	Commelinaceae	Z'herbe grasse	Suelda con suelda
Acnistus arborescens	Solanaceae. Apply leaf with soft candle for headache. Take 5 leaves, 0.5 cup water, squeeze juice in water and warm with soft candle 'vela blandits. For cold in eye.'		Tabaco guarey
Ochroma pyramidale	Bombacaceae. Use flowers to make mattresses		Tacarigua
Cassia alata	Take whole pod and senna leaves for purgative to prevent senna from griping, put in wine to clean blood		Tarantán
Dracontium asperum	Araceae. Tuber is used in preparation for snake bite		Tigrilla
Physalis pubescens	Solanaceae	Topatop	Topotopo
Jatropha gossypifolia	Euphorbiaceae		Tuba tuba
Nopalea cochenillifera	Cactaceae. Inflammation in feet, roast over ashes and peel, sprinkle fine salt on it, place on inflamed area		Tuna
Nopalea cochenillifera	Irritation in chest, drink decoction		Tuna
Uncaria tormentosa	Rubiaceae		Uña de gowilán
Mactadgena uncata	Cough		Uña de morciélago
Stachytarpheta jamaicensis	Verbenaceae. Juice with salt, par pechuwela asthma, calming nerves.		Verbena
Stachytarpheta jamaicensis	Juice with salt for haemorrhage, fresco, cooling, increase milk in nursing mothers.		Verbena
Portulaca oleracea	Portulacaceae, Cooling, worms in children, herb tea.	Verdolaga	Verdolaga
Hyptis atrorubens	Labiatae. To prevent vomiting make tea, soak in hops bread, put against chest. Soak in urine, put against chest to prevent vomiting		Yerba buena

Table 11. Complete creole names of folk medicine in Trinidad (cont.)

Latin name	Family, uses	French Common name	Spanish Common name
Cariospermum microcarpum	Sapindaceae		Yerba de bicho
Justicia pectoralis			Yerba de carpintero
Euphorbia hirta	Euphorbiaceae		Yerba de malomé
			Yerba de polla
Justicia secunda	Acanthaceae. Bush bath to prevent vomiting, mix with mint. Pound with salt, good for lash, bicho		Yerba de San Juan
Manihot esculenta	Euphorbiaceae. Para un golpe el almidón bien seco la catebilla. Se toma la catebilla que derrite la sangre	Yuca agria	Yuca agria
Entada polystachya	Minosaceae. Boil leaf and touch head of your cock, the opponent's cock gets 'edged', cooling, eyes.	Yuquilla	Yuquilla

The search for original continents

The origin of the ethnoveterinary knowledge indicates why things are done in certain ways, and if there are any theories behind the practice. Table 12 traces the possible origin of some of the medicinal plants. Difficulties arise because of the remigration of some Indian indentured labourers, the repatriation of some freed African slaves and the migration of Caribbean peoples throughout South America. References used are Joseph (1837), Williams and Williams (1969), Morton (1981) INRA-CARDI (1991) and Pacific Island Ecosystems at Risk (www.hear.org/pier/scinames.htm. Native in the geographical origin column means Latin America and the Caribbean.

Table 12. Possible origin of the ethnoveterinary medicinal plants

0	Scientific name	Common name	Geographical Origin
1.	Abelmoschus esculentus	Okro	Africa
2.	Abelmoschus moschatus	Gumbo musque	S.E. Asia
3.	Abrus precatorius	Jumbie bead	Native
4.	Achyranthes indica	Man better man	Asia
5.	Acnistus arborescens	Wild tobacco	Native
6.	Acrocomia aculeata	Gru gru boeuf	Native
7.	Aframomum melegueta	Guinea pepper	Africa
8.	Ageratum conyzoides	Z'herbe á femme	Native
9.	Allium sativum	Garlic	Europe
10.	Aloe vera	Aloe	Africa
11.	Ambrosia cumanenesis	Altamis	Native
12.	Anacardium occidentale	Cashew	Native
13.	Annona muricata	Soursop	Native
14.	Antigonon leptopus	Coralita	Native
15.	Apium graveolens	Celery	Europe
16.	Areca catechu	Betel nut	Malaysia

Table 12. Possible origin of the ethnoveterinary medicinal plants (cont.)

17.	*Aristolochia rugosa*	Mat root, racin mat	Native
18.	*Aristolochia tribolata*	Tref	Native
19.	*Artemisia absinthium*	Wormwood	Europe
20.	*Artocarpus altilis*	Breadfruit	Pacific
21.	*Asclepias curassavica*	Red top	Native
22.	*Azadirachta indica*	Neem	Asia
23.	*Bambusa vulgaris*	Bamboo	Asia
24.	*Barleria lupulina*	Snake bush	Mauritius
25.	*Bauhinia cumanensis*	Monkey step	Native
26.	*Begonia humilis*	Lozeille	Native
27.	*Bidens pilosa*	Needle grass	Native
28.	*Bixa orellana*	Roukou	Native
29.	*Bontia daphnoides*	Olive bush	Native
30.	*Brownea latifolia*	Cooper hoop	Native
31.	*Cajanus cajan*	Pigeon pea	Africa, India
32.	*Calotropis gigantea*	Madar	Asia
33.	*Cannabis sativa*	Ganja	Asia
34.	*Capraria biflora*	Du thè pays	Native
35.	*Capsicum frutescens/annum*	Pepper	Native
36.	*Carica papaya*	Papaya	Native
37.	*Catharanthus roseus*	Periwinkle	Native
38.	*Cecropia peltata*	Bois canôt	Native
39.	*Cedrela odorata*	Cedar	Native
40.	*Centropogon cornutus*	Crepe coq	Native
41.	*Chamaesyce hirta*	Mal nommée	Native
42.	*Chenopodium ambrosioides*	Worm grass	Native
43.	*Chromolaena odorata*	Christmas bush	Native
44.	*Chrysobalanus icaco*	Ipecak	Native
45.	*Cissus verticillata*	Blister bush	Native
46.	*Citharexylum spinosum*	Bois côtelette	Native
47.	*Citrus aurantifolia*	Lime	Asia
48.	*Citrus aurantium*	Sour orange	Asia
49.	*Citrus limonia*	Lemon	Asia
50.	*Citrus nobilis*	Portugal	Asia
51.	*Citrus paradisi*	Grapefruit	Native
52.	*Citrus sinensis*	Orange	Asia
53.	*Cocos nucifera*	Coconut	Pacific
54.	*Coffee arabica*	Coffee	Africa
55.	*Cola nitida*	Obie seed	Native
56.	*Coleus aromaticus*	Spanish thyme	Asia, Africa
57.	*Commelina* species	Water grass	Native
58.	*Cordia curassavica*	Black sage	Native
59.	*Costus scaber*	Wild cane	Native
60.	*Crescentia cujete*	Calabash	Native
61.	*Crotalaria retusa*	Shack shack	Pantropical
62.	*Croton gossypifolius*	Blood bush	Native
63.	*Curcuma domestica*	Turmeric	Asia

Table 12. Possible origin of the ethnoveterinary medicinal plants (cont.)

64.	*Cuscuta americana*	Love vine	Native
65.	*Cymbopogon citratus*	Fever grass	India
66.	*Cynodon dactylon*	Dube	Pantropical
67.	*Cyperus rotundus*	Nut grass	Eurasia
68.	*Datura stramonium*	Datur	India
69.	*Dendropanax arboreus*	Fei jein	Native
70.	*Desmodium canum*	Sweet heart bush	Native
71.	*Dorstenia contrayerva*	Refriyau	Native
72.	*Eclipta prostrata*	Congo lala	Native
73.	*Eleusine indica**	Dead man's grass	India
74.	*Eleutherine bulbosa*	Dragon blood	Native
75.	*Entada polystachya*	Mayoc chapelle	Native
76.	*Eryngium foetidum*	Chadron bénée	Native
77.	*Erythrina pallida*	Immortelle	Native
78.	*Eupatorium macrophyllum*	Z'herbe chatte	Native
79.	*Eupatorium triplinerve*	Japanne	Native
80.	*Fleurya aestuans*	Stinging nettle	Pantropical
81.	*Flemingia strobilifera*	Kidney bush	Asia, Malaysia
82.	*Gomphrena globosa*	Bachelor button	India
83.	*Gossypium species*	Cotton bush	Native
84.	*Hibiscus rosa-sinensis*	Hibiscus	Asia
85.	*Hibiscus sabdariffa*	Sorrel	Asia
86.	*Hippobroma longiflora*	Ipecac	Native
87.	*Hyptis sauveolens*	Matrank	Native
88.	*Jatropha curcas*	Physic nut	Native
89.	*Jatropha gossypifolia*	Physic nut	Native
90.	*Justica pectoralis*	Carpenter grass	Native
91.	*Justica secunda*	St. John's bush	Native
92.	*Kalanchoe pinnata*	Wonder / world	Asia
93.	*Lantana camara*	Kayakeet	Native
94.	*Laportea aestuans*	Red stinging nettle	Asia, Paciific
95.	*Lawsonia inermis*	Mehndi	N. Africa, Asia
96.	*Leonotis nepetaefolia*	Shandileer	Africa
97.	*Lepianthes peltata*	Lani bois, sun bush	Native
98.	*Lippia alba*	Santa Maria	Naitve
99.	*Mammea americana*	Mammy apple	Native
100.	*Mangifera indica*	Mango	Asia
101.	*Manilkara zapota*	Sapodilla	Native
102.	*Microtea debilis*	Alantukai	Native
103.	*Mimosa pudica*	Ti marie	Native
104.	*Momordica charantia*	Caraaili	Asia
105.	*Monstera dubia*	Sei jein	Native
106.	*Morinda citrifolia*	Noni	Asia, Australia
107.	*Morus alba*	Pawi bush	China
108.	*Mucana pruriens*	Cowitch	Pantropical
109.	*Musa species*	Plantain	Asia
110.	*Myristica fragrans*	Nutmeg	Moluccas
111.	*Nasturtium officinale*	Water cress	Europe

Table 12. Possible origin of the ethnoveterinary medicinal plants (cont.)

112.	Neurolaena lobata	Z'herbe á pique	Native
113.	Nicotiana tabacum	Tobacco	Native
114.	Nopalea cochenillifera	Rachette	Native
115.	Clusia rosea?	Matapal	Native
116.	Not yet identified	Turpentine bush	-------
117.	Ocimum campechianum	Ti bom	Native
118.	Ocimum gratissimum	Fon bazin	Pantropical
119.	Ocimum sanctum	Tulsi	Asia
120.	Oryza sativa	Rice	Asia
121.	Ottonia ovata	Pot bush	Native
122.	Panicum maximum*	Wiz/ Guinea grass	Africa
123.	Parinari campestris	Bois bandé	Native
124.	Parthenium hysterophorus	White head broom	Native
125.	Paspalum virgatum	Razor grass	Native
126.	Passiflora foetida	Marie gourgeois	Native
127.	Passiflora quadrangularis	Barbadine	Native
128.	Passiflora suberosa	No name known	Native
129.	Pelargonium zonale	Geranium	South Africa
130.	Peperomia pellucida	Shining bush	Native, Africa
131.	Persea americana	Avocado	Mexico
132.	Petiveria alliacea	Kojo root	Native
133.	Peperomia rotundifolia	Giron fleur	Africa, Native
134.	Phyllanthus niruri	Seed under leaf	Native
135.	Phyllanthus urinaria	Red Seed under leaf	Native
136.	Pilea microphylla	Du thé bethelmay	Native
137.	Pimenta racemosa	Bayleaf	Native
138.	Piper hispidum	Candle bush	Native
139.	Piper marginatum	Agouti bush	Native
140.	Pithocellobium unguis-cati	Cat's claw	Native
141.	Pityrogramma calomelanos	Egyptian secret	Native
142.	Plantago major	Planten	Native
143.	Pluchea symphytifolia	Guèrir toute	Native
144.	Pogostemon heyneanus	Pachouli	Asia
145.	Portulaca oleracea	Pussley	Eurasia
146.	Pouteria sapota	Mammy sapote	Native
147.	Psidium guajava	Guava	Native
148.	Pueraria phaseoloides	Kudzu	Asia, Pacific
149.	Punica granatum	Pomegranate	Eurasia
150.	Renealmia alpinia	Wild balisier	Native
151.	Richeria grandis	Bois bandé	Native
152.	Ricinus communis	Castor oil leaf	Africa
153.	Rosmarinus officinalis	Rosemary	Europe
154.	Roupala montana	Bois bandé	Native
155.	Ruellia tuberosa	Minny root	Native
156.	Ruta graveolens	Ruda	Europe
157.	Saccharum officinarum	Sugar cane	Asia
158.	Sambucus simpsonii*	Syrio [Sabugueiro]	Native
159.	Sansevieria guineensis	Langue bouef, lash	S. Africa

Table 12. Possible origin of the ethnoveterinary medicinal plants (cont.)

160.	Scoparia dulcis	Sweet broom	Native
161.	Senna alata	Senna	Native
162.	Senna occidentalis	Wild coffee	Native
163.	Sida acuta	Garaba broom	Pantropical
164.	Siparuna guianensis	Dead man's bush	Native
165.	Solanum americanum	Agouma, gouma	Native
166.	Solanum melongena	Melongene	India
167.	Solanum species	Devil pepper	-------
168.	Spiranthes acaulis	Lappe bush	Native
169.	Spondias mombin	Hogplum	Native
170.	Stachytarpheta cayennensis	Rat tail vervine	Native
171.	Stachytarpheta jamaicensis	Vervine	Native
172.	Syngonium podophyllum	Matapal-kit	Native
173.	Tagetes patula	Marigold	Mexico
174.	Tamarindus indica	Tamarind	E. Africa
175.	Theobroma cacao	Cocoa	Native
176.	Tournefortia hirsutissima	Chigger bush	Native
177.	Triumfetta lapula	No name known	Native
178.	Unknown	Eyebright	------
179.	Urena lobata	Cousin Mahoe	Asia
180.	Urena sinuata	Patte chien	Asia
181.	Vernonia scorpioides	Ruckshun	Pantropical
182.	Vetiveria zizanioides	Vetivert	India
183.	Vitex trifolia	No name known	S.E. Asia
184.	Wedelia trilobata	Venven Caribe	Old tropics
185.	Xanthosoma brasiliense	Hog tannia	Native
186.	Xanthosoma undipes	Hog tannia	Native
187.	Xiphidium caeruleum	Walk fast	Native
188.	Zea mays	Corn	Native
189.	Zingiber officinale	Ginger	Asia

Conclusion

Caribbean folk medicine is based on a marriage-á-cinq of European folk medicine; scientific medicine; African-based practices; Amerindianmedicine and Indian-based medicine. It is a product of inter-group borrowing based on cultural traditions.

This chapter has examined some of the cultural traditions and the socio-historical 'baggage' of the Caribbean. There are people in the Caribbean who prefer to live in the present and try to skip parts of their history, especially the five centuries of colonisation (Douglas, 1995; Price and Price, 1997). The irony of Creolization is that it is the same destructive double consciousness of the colonized subject that paradoxically generates the creation of rich creolized cultural forms (Barnes, 1998). African and Indian identities built on half-forgotten collective memories are being strategically used by political and cultural interest-seekers for their own political, social or economic agendas (Ryan, 1999).

Part of this phenomenon can be explained in terms of self-perceived subalterns now claiming an equal space in the 'rainbow society'. Brathwaite (1971) claims that the original white élite's political weakness[81] and their dependence on Europe for normative value-references created a pattern of behaviour which has since continued with the equally weak Afro-Saxons. Currently non-residential traditions are being sought not only in Britain, the colonial mother country, but also in North America, Africa and India.

During indenture East Indian families and immigrants from the same villages or regions were sent to the same estates (Weller, 1968). This has always been said to have allowed for a greater retention of Asian cultures and traditions than the practice of slavery did for African traditions. The issue to be debated is whether all African survivals are indeed so or whether Amerindian culture provides the base of creolization. If the African survivals were indeed limited then the tendency for Afro Creoles to imitate their white masters imitation of Europe as claimed by Brathwaite (1971) is only partly a rejection of their own culture. In the early years of slavery in Trinidad many of the slaves were born in Martinique and Guadeloupe and arrived in Trinidad already possessing a creolized African-French-Caribbean culture that included Patois as the main language. The descendents of these slaves and those born in Africa may have decided to reject or rename the Amerindian culture they had learnt as a reduced but insufficently understood native 'cultural language'. Those who accuse others of erasure of their heritage have to correct the historical record with care (Haslip-Viera et al., 1997).

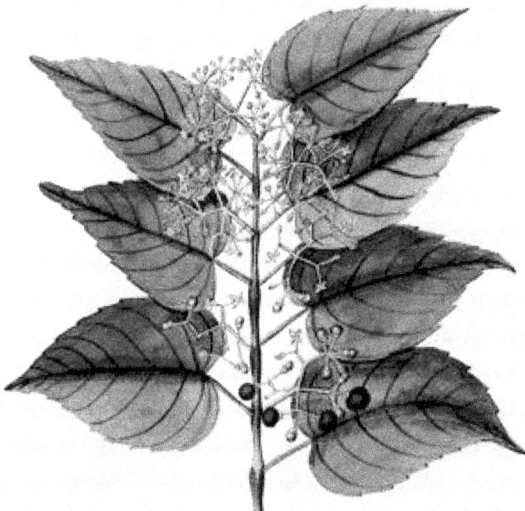

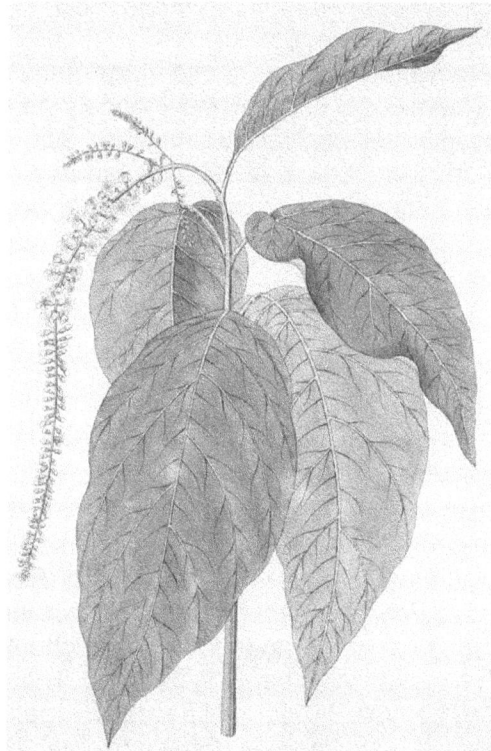

Figure 108. Cissus sicyoides
Figure 109. Citharexylum spinosum

---

[81] Local whites in Trinidad had their own internal tensions based on their different European origins (Wood, 1968).

Conclusions

"to enumerate all the fantastic recommended therapy based on witchcraft, hearsay and superstition and to describe all the authentic efforts to refute it is impossible in one article" (McCollough and Gennaro, 1970 cited by Martz, 1992)

12. Conclusions

Livestock producers are generally low resource farmers who if given an opportunity can continue to make a contribution to the development of the islands. The current economic environment of globalisation and trade liberalisation is removing traditional markets and reducing the competitiveness of the domestic production sector. Sustainable production systems and economic viability for small farmers means low cost, technically appropriate management, minimising of most types of risks, and increased independence from imported inputs (Evans, 1992). Ethnoveterinary practices are already one component of sustainable production. The objective of this book was to document ethnoveterinarymedicinal knowledge in Trinidad and Tobago and to explore whether ethnoveterinarymedicinal knowledge could usefully complement formal veterinary and medicinal knowledge; and if so, how? The non-experimental validation used for each plant gave indications that several of the plants had chemical compounds that justified their ethnomedicinal use. Ethnoveterinary remedies based on these uses may be cheaper than Western drugs.

Ethnomedicine and ethnoveterinary medicines are complementary rather than separate fields. The majority of the ethnoveterinary practices had parallel uses in ethnomedicine in the Caribbean, other tropical countries and sometimes in Europe. Culture and religion also play a role in the choice of ethnoveterinaryplants. Creolized technology development by Caribbean immigrants involved matching available knowledge from their different origins to available plants that were or were not botanically related to previously known plants for emergent health needs. Creolization in folk medicine is similar but different to Creolization in languages. A coherent body of Creolized Caribbean folk knowledge was created that was structured and ordered (but reduced in terms of content and explanations) and passed on to subsequent generations as such.

Those plants that were not being used similarly in other places are tentatively judged to be 'indigenous' to Trinidad and Tobago. These ethnomedicinal plants are *Antigonon leptopus*, *Justicia secunda*, *Microtea debilis*, *Eupatorium macrophyllum*, *Centropogon cornutus*, *Bontia daphnoides*, *Brownea latifolia*, *Xiphidium caeruleum*, *Icaco chrysobalanus*, *Sansevieria guineensis*, *Richeria grandis*, *Roupala montana*, *Eupatorium triplinerve, Persea americana* and *Hippobroma longifolia*. Indigenous to Trinidad implies that the Amerindian knowledge found throughout South and Central America is excluded. It is difficult to judge whether Trinidad and Tobago folk medicine has influenced that in other countries as well as being influenced. For example Morton (1981) considers that periwinkle (*Catharanthus roseus*) is native to the West Indies, but it was first described from Madagascar. A wider view might be required which recognises folk medicine in the Caribbean basin as one entity. During and after colonialism East Indians and Creoles went to South America especially to Venezuela (Weller, 1968). The Caribbean basin countries included in TRAMIL studies are Colombia, Costa Rica, Guatemala (Livingston, Antilleans on the Atlantic coast), Panama (Antilleans in Colon), Honduras (Garífunas on the Atlantic coast), and Nicaragua (Creole and Garífuna on the Atlantic coast) (Girón *et al.*, 1991; Barrett, 1994; Coe and Anderson, 1996a) (see Map 1). 'Bush doctors' are found in Miskito communities in Eastern Nicaragua (Dennis, 1988). Medicinal plants of the Caribbean basin would include *Mimosa pudica*, *Tagetes patula*, *Eryngium foetidum*, *Piper hispidum*, *Cissus*

176

sicyoides, *Pityrogramma calomelanos*, *Persea americana*, *Neurolaena lobata*, *Wedelia trilobata*, *Peperomia pellucida*, *Scoparia dulcis* and *Chamaesyce hypericifolia*.

A wider view of 'indigenous knowledge' is also necessary based on the experience of other researchers. Of 216 introduced plant species used by populations in northern South America (Brazil, Colombia, Ecuador and Peru) 80% were of European, Mediterranean or Asian origin, 9% were of African origin and 8% were from the New World (Bennett and Prance, 2000). Voeks (1996) found that 36% of the taxa used in the Altlantic forests of Bahia, Brazil for which origins could be established came from Africa, Asia and Europe. Voeks concurs with Davis and Yost (1983) on the plant pharmacopoeia in South America: it is cultivated, exotic and opportunistic and based on home gardens, roadsides and secondary forest rather than on indigenous species from the primary forests that were alien to the new settlers. Davis and Yost (1983) found that some isolated Amerindian tribes had smaller pharmacopoeias than the acculturated tribes and speculated that these latter benefited from the chaos of contact and the accelerated experimentation that was necessary to combat the diseases encountered in post-contact times. However other explanations for this finding exist: male ethnobotanists may not have recorded women's knowledge for various reasons or their research focus may have been on shamanic medicine and hallucinogens (Milliken and Albert, 1996). The non-experimental validation of the ethnoveterinary medicines was undertaken in recognition of the fact that western science has become the main means of determining the validity of knowledge. Biomedicine like other dominant world-views maintains its stability and resilience by dismissing alternatives as illogical or unscientific (Banuri, 1990). Marglin (1990a) talks about the failure of those who cannot imagine the creation of a space for the dynamic transformation of indigenous culture without validation in western terms. Rather than an imaginative failure, this research attempts to reduce the cultural confrontation between science and tradition by showing scientists in western scientific terms that ethnoveterinary medicine can provide an economic alternative to some western technology. This is a pragmatic approach given the recognition that most sciences, including medicine do not critically reflect on their own underlying philosophical assumptions (Nandy and Visvanathan, 1990). Biomedical paradigm-defenders will have the choice of ignoring the research, dismissing it because of various flaws (i.e. no lodging of voucher specimens) or assimilating the new information (Dolby, 1979).

An action/collaborative approach was taken to document the ethnoveterinary medicinal plants used by hunters, pet and livestock owners. The result was a non-random, culturally-informed account of pharmacologically active plants, some of which may warrant further phytochemical and/or pharmacological analysis (Etkin, 1993). Information was captured on medicinal plants used for pigs, poultry including game cocks, ruminants, horses, pet dogs, hunting dogs, ruminant reproductive health and ethnomedicine currently not related to ethnoveterinary medicine. Future clinical trials or research projects will establish in scientific terms whether the Creole legacy of folk medicine is of positive value for human and animal health.

The school essay method was chosen as a method that would be quick, clean, cheap and alter the researcher's role as an interviewer. This last is important since ethnoveterinary knowledge is cultural knowledge that is shared in networks of relationships. The time limits of the first phase did not allow for the identification and development of relationships with key informants. The essays thus provided much needed 'entrance'. The method also provided more respondents in Trinidad than the veterinarians and AHA/Extension officers. As part of the collaborative approach used in the first research phase, the school principals' request for questionnaires was agreed to. However student essays proved better than the questionnaires. Questionnaires may have seemed too inflexible and too political for students and for informal oral knowledge like folk medicine. Some schools can be considered to have given their students more choice to collaborate with the research or not. This may account for the high non-response in some schools, and may also explain why one student felt obliged to invent information because he could not identify a respondent. The School essay method brought folk medicine into the education system for one brief moment.

This research has disproved the view of Sutton and Orr (1991) who say that the essay method should not be extended beyond its capabilities, and that it is unlikely to yield useful quantitative data. The student responses give a list of plants, their uses and sometimes exactly how they are to be prepared. Thirty diseases, twenty-five plants and eight non-plants were described in the responses. Some responses also indicated whether the moon phase was applicable to picking the plant or treating the animal. The school essay method was an effective means of identifying respondents. The difference in the responses from the schools was very apparent. Carapichaima Junior Secondary and its very supportive principal produced the best results. The principals who actively supported this research with their students rather than merely giving permission impacted on the information quality of the essays. Other criteria like geographic location in choosing schools played a lesser role.

The workshops provided the basis for preparing practical booklets on poultry and ruminants for farmers to use, and for discussing the information gathered with the informants. The booklets of ethnoveterinary practices provided to participants in the workshops, if used, could provide a form of corrective action at a local inclusive level (Rappaport, 1993). This corrective action would be based on local knowledge guided by local people and should thus be more culturally sensitive, nuanced and less disruptive than a program imposed by remote, central regulators. Action based on local knowledge also strengthens rather than undermines local institutions, strengthens the correcting capacities that local systems have and could restore adaptiveness to an agricultural system deformed by maladaptions (Rappaport, 1993).

Validation of ethno [veterinary] knowledge is important because it cannot be assumed that all of the practices are effective. Workshops like that of IIRR (1994) are forms of group validation. The experiments of Dr. Brown of the Poultry Surveillance Unit (PSU) and Carlton Snipe are also validation processes. Validity for ethnoveterinary knowledge based on most farmers' criteria would mean practices that fit their farm performances. Empiricism (informal clinical trials, observations and experiments) was seen in the informal clinical trials that are conducted on commercial poultry. Expert 1 conducted his own experiments; with wonder of the world (*Kalanchoe pinnata*), on combating debeaking stress and on vaccination stress. He also tested to see if caraaili (*Momordica charantia*) reduced mortality from Aspergillosis and found that garlic reduced a flock's respiratory reaction to the Newcastle Disease Virus vaccine. He also encouraged his 18 contract farmers to use those plants which proved effective. Lubchenco (1998) suggests a new social contract for science in which science is seen as both part of the problem and a source of solutions. In this research an attempt was made to use a type of science that produces 'socially robust knowledge'. Socially robust knowledge has three aspects: it is valid inside and outside the laboratory; its validity is achieved through involving an extended group of experts, including 'lay' experts; and thirdly this participatory-generated knowledge is likely to be less contested in the future (Funtowicz and Ravetz, 1993; Gibbons, 1999). Research would become a co-learning activity that develops mutual accountability (Jiggins and Gibbon, 1997). Co-learning develops ways of understanding the world that re-enter society and affect action in society (Jiggins and Gibbon, 1997). Co-learning was seen in the case of the PSU.

The PSU operated on the basis that farmers need help in searching out and selecting information that is relevant to them (Nitsch, 1991). This implies continuous learning about the farming situation by advisors like the PSU who then assess and suggest alternatives (like medicinal plants) to farmers to coordinate their complex farming systems (Nitsch, 1991). The Caribbean does not have a strong livestock extension service so the PSU is perhaps an example of one of the new types of support structure that the Caribbean states can provide for livestock-based extension. Shiva (1993) assessed that 'local knowledge systems throughout the world have been conquered through the politics of disappearance'. Feminist researchers have shown the power that can be defined over women, and their subjugated [traditional] knowledges through researchers defining objective knowledge as superior to personal experience (Holland and Ramazanoglu, 1994). Non-scientific knowledge often disappears with its holders because it is considered in the short term to have no economic importance, and it seems that no one is in charge of the long term, for according to Allport (1990), [some] 'social science never solves any problems, it just gets tired of them'.

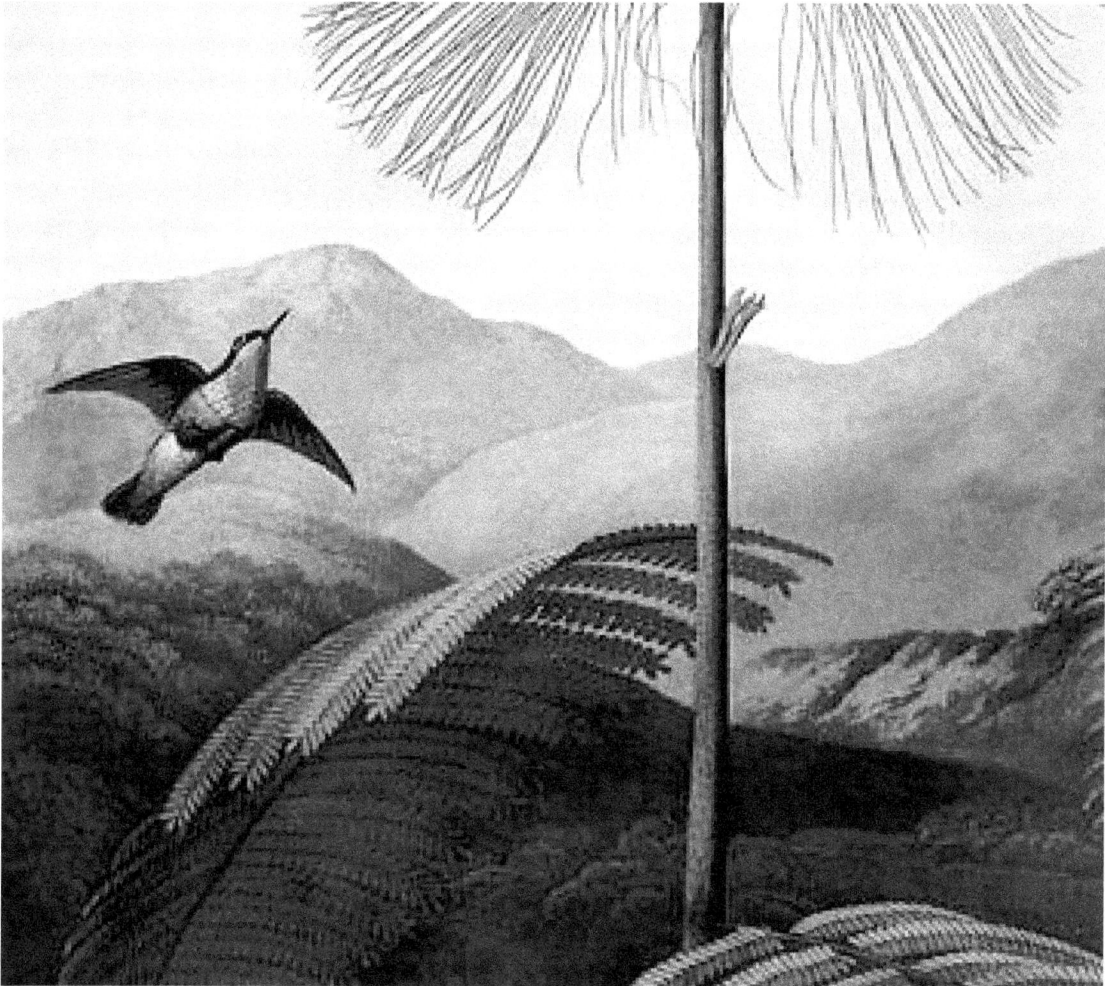

Figure 110. Cairi - land of the hummingbird
Source: New illustration of the sexual system of Carolus von Linnaeus: and the temple of Flora, or garden of nature.

References

Abdel-Kader, M.S., Bahler, B.D., Malone, S., Werkhoven, M.C.M., van Troon, F., David, Wisse, J.H., Bursuker, I., Neddermann, K.M., Mamber, S.W., Kingston, D.G. 1998. DNA-damaging steroidal alkaloids from *Eclipta alba* from the Suriname rainforest. Journal of Natural Products 61 (10), 1202 - 1208.

Abdel-Sattar, E., Mossa, J.S., el-Askary, H.I. 2000. Hirsutinolides from *Vernonia cinerascens*. Pharmazie 55 (2), 144-5.

Abdon AP, Leal-Cardoso JH, Coelho-de-Souza AN, Morais SM, Santos CF: Antinociceptive effects of the essential oil of *Croton nepetaefolius* on mice. Braz J Med Biol Res. 2002, 35(10):1215-9.

Abo KA, Ogunleye VO, Ashidi JS. 1999. Antimicrobial potential of *Spondias mombin*, *Croton zambesicus* and *Zygotritonia crocea*. Phytother Res. 13(6):494-7.

Achola, K.J., Munenge, R.W. 1998. Bronchodilating and uterine activities of *Ageratum conyzoides* extract. Pharmaceutical Biology 36 (2), 93 - 96.

Acosta SL, Muro LV, Sacerio AL, Pena AR, Okwei SN: Analgesic properties of *Capraria biflora* leaves aqueous extract. Fitoterapia 2003, 74 (7-8): 686-8.

Adams, Richard. 1959. On the relation between plantation and "Creole cultures." In Plantation Systems of the New World. Social Science Monographs, VII. Vera Rubin, ed. pp. 73 - 79. Washington: Pan American Union.

Adeboye, J., Fajonyomi, M., Makinde, J., Taiwo, O. 1999. A preliminary study on the hypotensive activity of *Persea americana* leaf extracts in anaesthetized normotensive rats. Fitoterapia 70 (1), 15 - 20.

Adesiyun, A.A. and Krishnan, C. 1995. Occurrence of *Yersinia enterocolitica* 0:3, *Listeria monocytogenes* 0:4 and thermophilic *Campylobacter* spp. in slaughter pigs and carcasses in Trinidad. Food Microbiology (London) 12 (2), 99-107.

Adesiyun, A.A., Cazabon, E.P. 1996. Seroprevalence of brucellosis, Q-fever and toxoplasmosis in slaughter livestock in Trinidad. Revue d'Elevage et de Medicine Veterinaire des Pays Tropicaux 49 (1), 28 - 30.

Adeyemi OO, Okpo SO, Ogunti OO. 2002. Analgesic and anti-inflammatory effects of the aqueous extract of leaves of *Persea americana* Mill (Lauraceae). Fitoterapia 73 (5): 375-80.

Afifi, F.U., Abu-Irmaileh, B. 2000. Herbal medicine in Jordan with special emphasis on less commonly used medicinal herbs. Journal of Ethnopharmacology 72 (1-2), 101 - 110.

Afzal, M., Ali. M., Hassan. R.A.H., Sweedan, N., Dhami, M.S.I. 1991. Identification of some prostanoids in *Aloe vera* extracts. Planta Medica 57, 38-40.

Agar, M., MacDonald, J. 1995. Focus groups and ethnography. Human Organization 54 (1), 78 - 86.

Agbonon, A., Aklikokou, K., Kwashie, E.G., Gbeassor, M. 2004. Anti-cholinergic effect of *Pluchea ovalis* (pers.) Dc. (asteraceae) root extract on isolated Wistar rat tracheae. Ann Pharm Fr. 62 (5): 354-8. [Article in French]

Ahmad, F., Holdsworth, D. 1994. Medicinal plants of Sabah, Malaysia, Part II. The Muruts. International Journal of Pharmacognosy 32 (4), 378 - 383.

Ahmad, I., Beg, A.Z. 2001. Antimicrobial and phytochemical studies on 45 Indian medicinal plants against multi-drug resistant human pathogens. Journal of Ethnopharmacology 74 (2), 113 - 123.

Ahmad, M., Akhtar, M.F., Miyase, T., Ueno, A., Rashid, S., Usmanghani, K. 1993. Studies on the medicinal herb *Ruellia patula*. International Journal of Pharmacognosy 31 (2), 121 - 129.

Ahmad, S., Khan, A. 1991. Nematicidal action of *Antigonon leptopus* against *Meloidogyne incognita* race 1. Current Nematology 2(1), 3-4.

Ahmed, A.A., Abou-Douh, A.M., Mohammed, A., Hassan, M.E., Karchesy, J. 1999. A new chromene glucoside from *Ageratum conyzoides*. Planta Medica 65 (2), 171 - 172.

Ahmed, S. 1999. 'She'll wake up one of these days and find she's turned into a nigger': passing through hybridity. Theory, Culture and Society 16 (2), 87 - 106.

Aho, W.R., Minott, K. 1977. Creole and doctor medicine: folk beliefs, practices, and orientations to modern medicine in a rural and an industrial suburban setting in Trinidad and Tobago, the West Indies. Social Science and Medicine 11 (5), 349 - 355.

Ajao, A.O., Shonukan, O., Femi-Onadeko, B. 1985. Antibacterial effect of aqueous and alcohol extracts of *Spondias mombin* and *Alchornea cordifolia* - two local antimicrobial remedies. International Journal of Crude Drug Research 23 (2), 67 - 72.

Akhtar, M., Alam, M.M 1989. Evaluation of nematicidal potential in some medicinal plants. International Nematology Network Newsletter 6 (1), 8 - 10.

Akindahunsi AA, Olaleye MT: Toxicological investigation of aqueous-methanolic extract of the calyces of *Hibiscus sabdariffa* L. J Ethnopharmacol. 2003, 89(1):161-4.

Akinpelu DA. 2000. Antimicrobial activity of *Bryophyllum pinnatum* leaves. Fitoterapia. 71(2):193-4.

Akinsinde, K.A., Olukoya, D.K. 1995. Vibriocidal activities of some local herbs. J. Diarrhoeal Dis. Res. 13 (2), 127-9.

Alarcon de la Lastra, C., Martin, M.J., La Casa, C., Motilva, V. 1994. Antiulcerogenicity of the flavonoid fraction from *Bidens aurea*: comparison with ranitidine and omeprazole. Journal of Ethnopharmacology 42 (3),161-8.

Alarcon-Aguilara, F.J., Roman-Ramos, R., Perez-Gutierrez, S., Aguilar-Contreras, A., Contreras-Weber, C.C., Flores-Saenz, J.L. 1998. Study of the anti-hyperglycemic effect of plants used as antidiabetics. Journal of Ethnopharmacology 61(2), 101-10.

Alatas, S.F. 1993. On the indigenization of academic discourse. Alternatives 18, 307 - 338.

Alcazar, M.D., Garcia, C., Rivera, D., Obon, C. 1990. Lesser-known herbal remedies as sold in the market at Murcia and Cartegena (Spain). Journal of Ethnopharmacology 28 (2), 243 - 247.

Al-Hader, A.A., Hasan, Z.A., Aqel, M.B. 1994. Hyperglycemic and insulin release inhibitory effects of *Rosmarinus officinalis*. Journal of Ethnopharmacology 43 (3), 217 - 221.

Al-Hindawi, M.K., Al-Deen, I.H., Nabi, M.H., Ismail, M.A. 1989. Anti-inflammatory activity of some Iraqi plants using intact rats. Journal of Ethnopharmacology 26 (2), 163-8.

Ali BH, Mousa HM, El-Mougy S. 2003. The effect of a water extract and anthocyanins of *Hibiscus sabdariffa* L on paracetamol-induced hepatoxicity in rats. Phytother Res. 17(1):56-9.

Ali, Abdul, M., Mackeen, M.M., El-Sharkawy, S., Hamid, J., Ismail, N., Ahmad, F., Lajis, N. 1996. Antiviral and cytotoxic activities of some plants used in Malaysian indigenous medicine. Pertanika Journal of Tropical Agricultural Science 19 (2/3), 129 - 136.

Ali, M.B., Salih, W.M., Mohamed, A.H., Homeida, A.M. 1991. Investigation of the antispasmodic potential of *Hibiscus sabdariffa* calyces. Journal of Ethnopharmacology 31 (2), 249 - 257.

Ali, Z. 1995. Neonatal meningitis: a 3-year retrospective study at the Mount Hope Women's Hospital, Trinidad, West Indies. Journal of Tropical Pediatrics 41 (2), 109-11.

Ali-Shtayeh, M.S., Yaniv, Z., Mahajna, J. 2000. Ethnobotanical survey in the Palestine area: a classification of the healing potential of medicinal plants. Journal of Ethnopharmacology 73 (1-2), 221 - 232.

Allen, P.C., Lydon, J., Danforth, H.D.1997. Effects of components of *Artemisia annua* on coccidia infections in chickens. Poultry Science 76 (8), 1156-63.

Alleyne, S., Cruickshank, J.K. 1990. The use of informal medication - particularly bush teas - in Jamaican patients with diabetes mellitus. Cajanus 23 (1), 57 - 67.

Alleyne, S.I., Morrison, E.Y., St. A., Richard, R.R. 1979. Some social factors related to control of diabetes mellitus in adult Jamaican patients. Diabetes Care 2, 401 - 408.

Allport, G. cited by Banuri, T. 1990. Development and the politics of knowledge. In: Marglin, F.A. and Marglin, S.A. (eds) Dominating Knowledge; Development, Culture, and Resistance. Pp. 29 - 72.

Almeida, A.P., Da Silva, S.A., Souza, M.L., Lima, L.M., Rossi-Bergmann, B., de Moraes, V.L., Costa, S.S. 2000. Isolation and chemical analysis of a fatty acid fraction of *Kalanchoe pinnata* with a potent lymphocyte suppressive activity. Planta Medica 66 (2), 134-7.

Almeida, F.C.G., Lemonica, I.P. 2000. The toxic effects of *Coleus barbatus* B. on the different periods of pregnancy in rats. Journal of Ethnopharmacology 73 (1-2), 53 - 60.

Al-Qarawi, A.A., Adam, S.E.I. 1999. Effects of red chilli (*Capsicum frutescens* L.) on rats. Vet. Human Toxicol. 41 (5), 293 - 295.

al-Sereiti, M.R., Abu-Amer, K.M., Sen, P. 1999. Pharmacology of rosemary (*Rosmarinus officinalis* Linn.) and its therapeutic potentials. Indian J Exp Biol. 37(2):124-30.

Alvarado-Panameno, J.F., Lopez Caceres, F.E., Escolan Jovel, N.A. 1994. Evaluation of aqueous and ethanol extracts of mammey seed (*Mammea americana*) for tick control in bovines. (In Spanish). Facultad de Ciencias Agronomicas, San Salvador, 130 pp.

Álvarez Arias, B.T. 2000. Ichthyotoxic plants used in Spain. Journal of Ethnopharmacology 73 (3), 505 - 512.

Alvarez, A., Pomar, F., Sevilla, M.A., Montero, M.J. 1999. Gastric antisecretory and antiulcer activities of an ethanolic extract of *Bidens pilosa* L. var. radiata Schult. Bip. Journal of Ethnopharmacology 67 (3), 333-340.

Alvarez, L., Marquina, S., Villarreal, M.L., Alonso, D., Aranda, E., Delgado, G. 1996. Bioactive polyacetylenes from *Bidens pilosa*. Planta Medica 62 (4), 355-7.

Alves de Paulo, C., Teruszkin Balassiano, I., Henriques Sliva, N., Oliveira Castilho, R., Coelho Kaplan, M., Currie Cabral, M., da Costa Carvalho, M. 2000. *Chrysobalanus icaco* L. extract for antiangiogenic potential observation. International Journal of Molecular Medicine 5 (6), 667 - 669.

Ammon, H.P.T., Safayhi, H., Mack, T., Sabieraj, J. 1993. Mechanism of antiinflammatory actions of curcumine and boswellic acids. Journal of Ethnopharmacology 38 (1), 113 - 119.

Anderson, J.E., Cleland, J.G. 1984. The world fertility survey and contraceptive prevalence surveys: a comparison of substantive results. Studies in Family Planning 15, p. 7. In: Riddle, J.M. 1991. Oral contraceptives and early-term abortifacients during Classical Antiquity and the Middle Ages. Past and Present 132, 3 - 32.

Angell, M., Kassirer, J.P. 1998. Alternative medicine - the risks of untested and unregulated remedies. Editorial. The New England Journal of Medicine 339, 839 - 841.

Anis, M., Iqbal, M. 1994. Medicinal plantlore of Aligarh, India. International Journal of Pharmacognosy 32 (1), 59 - 64.

Ankli, A., Sticher, O., Heinrich, M. 1999. Medical ethnobotany of the Yucatec Maya: healers' consensus as a quantitative criterion. Economic Botany 53 (2), 144 - 160.

Anon, 1999. Caution: Traditional knowledge: principles of merit need to be spelt out in distinguishing valuable knowledge from myth. Nature 401 (6754), 623.

Anonymous, 1988. Trinidad Guardian, 19 April 1988. Article by a medical doctor. Headline: Nature a mixture of good and evil.

Anthony, M. 1999. King George V Park best for Emancipation. Letter to the Editor. Express July 22, 1999.

Anto, R.S., Kuttan, G., Dinesh Babu, K.V., Rajasekharan, K.N., Kuttan, R. 1998. Anti-inflammatory activity of natural and synthetic curcuminoids. Pharm. Pharmacol. Commun. 4, 103 - 106.

Apisariyakul, A., Vanittanakom, N., Buddhasukh, D. 1995. Antifungal activity of turmeric oil extracted from *Curcuma longa* (Zingiberaceae). Journal of Ethnopharmacology 49 (3), 163 - 169.

Appleby, John. 1996. English settlement in the Lesser Antilles during War and Peace, 1603 – 1660. In Robert Paquette and Stanley Engerman (eds.), The Lesser Antilles in the Age of European Expansion. University Press of Florida. Pp 86 – 104.

Archana, R., Namasivayam, A. 2000. Effect of *Ocimum sanctum* on noise induced changes in neutrophil functions. Journal of Ethnopharmacology 73 (1-2), 81 - 85.

Arenas, P., Azorero, R.M. 1977. Plants of common use in Paraguayan folk medicine for regulating fertility. Economic Botany 31, 298 - 301.

Argyris, C., Schon, D.A. 1974. Theory in Practice: Increasing professional effectiveness. Jossey-Bass Inc., San Francisco.

Arnason, T., Uck, F., Lambert, J., Hebda, R. 1980. Maya medicinal plants of San Jose Succotz, Belize. Journal of Ethnopharmacology 2 (4), 345 - 364.

Arnold, A. James. 1994. The erotics of colonialism in contemporary French West Indian literary culture. New West Indian Guide / Nieuwe West-Indische Gids 68 (1-2), 5 - 22.

Arnold, W.N. 1988. Vincent van Gogh and the thujone connection. Journal of the American Medical Association 260 (20), 3042-4.

Asano, S., Mizutani, M., Hayashi, T., Morita, N., Takeguchi, N. 1990. Reversible inhibitions of gastric H+,K(+)-ATPase by scopadulcic acid B and diacetyl scopadol. New biochemical tools of H+,K(+)-ATPase. Journal of Biological Chemistry 265 (36), 22167-73.

Asprey, G.F. and Thornton, P. 1953 -1955. Medicinal Plants of Jamaica, Parts 1 - 4. West Indian Journal 2 (4), 233-252; 3 (1), 17 - 41; 4(2), 69-82; 4(3), 145 - 168.

Atawodi, S., Mende, P., Pfundstein, B., Preussmann, R., Spiegelhalder, B. 1995. Nitrosatable amines and nitrosamide formation in natural stimulants: *Cola acuminata*, *C. nitida* and *Garcinia cola*. Food and Chemical Toxicology 33 (8), 625 - 630.

Atta, A.H., Alkofahi, A. 1998. Anti-nociceptive and anti-inflammatory effects of some Jordanian medicinal plant extracts. Journal of Ethnopharmacology 60 (2), 117 - 124.

Autumn, S. 1996. Anthropologists, development and situated truth. Human Organization 54 (4), 480 - 487.

Auvin-Guette, C., Baraguey, C., Blond, A., Pousset, J-L., Bodo, B. 1997. Cyclogossine B, a cyclic octapeptide from *Jatropha gossypifolia*. Journal of Natural Products 60 (11), 1155 - 1157.

Ayala Flores, F. 1984. Notes on some medicinal and poisonous plants of Amazonian Peru. Advances in Economic Botany 1, 1 - 8.

Ayers S, Sneden AT. Caudatosides A-F: new iridoid glucosides from *Citharexylum caudatum*. J Nat Prod. 2002 65(11):1621-6.

Ayoka, A.O., Akomolafe, R.O., Iwalewa, E.O., Akanmu, M.A., Ukponmwan, O.E. 2006. Sedative, antiepileptic and antipsychotic effects of *Spondias mombin* L. (Anacardiaceae) in mice and rats. J Ethnopharmacol. 103(2):166-75.

Aziba, P.I., Adedeji, A., Ekor, M., Adeyemi, O. 2001. Analgesic activity of *Peperomia pellucida* aerial parts in mice. Fitoterapia 72 (1), 57-58.

Aziba, P.I., Bass, D., Elegbe, Y. 1999. Pharmacological investigation of *Ocimum gratissimum* in rodents. Phytotherapy Research 13(5), 427-9.

Baber, Z. 1992. Sociology of scientific knowledge. Review essay. Theory and Society 21 (1), 105 - 199.

Baer, H.A. 1993. How critical can Clinical Anthropology be? Medical Anthropology 15, 299 - 317.

Baer, H.A. 1996. Bringing political ecology into Critical Medical Anthropology: A challenge to biocultural approaches. Medical Anthropology 17, 129 - 141.

Baer, H.A. 1997. Introduction to symposium: on-going studies in Critical Medical Anthropology. Social Science and Medicine 44 (10), 1563.

Bailey, C.J., Day, C., Turner, S.L., Leatherdale, B.A. 1985. Cerasee, a traditional treatment for diabetes. Studies in normal and streptozotocin diabetic mice. Diabetes Research 2 (2), 81 - 84.

Balée, William. 2000. Antiquity of traditional ethnobiological knowledge in Amazonia: The Tupí-Guaraní family and time. Ethnohistory 47 (2): 399 - 422.

Balick, M.J., Mendelsohn, R. 1992. Assessing the economic value of traditional medicines from tropical rain forests. In: Farnsworth, N.R. 1993. Ethnopharmacology and future drug development: the North American experience. Journal of Ethnopharmacology 38 (2-3), 145-152.

Balutansky, K.M. 1997. Appreciating C.L.R. James, a model of modernity and creolization. Review essay. Latin American Research Review 32 (2), 233 -243.

Bamba, D., Bessière, J-M., Marion, C., Pélissier, Y., Fourasté, I. 1993. Essential oil of *Eupatorium odoratum*. Planta Medica 59 (2), 184 - 185.

Banks, E.P. 1956. A Carib village in Dominica. Social and Economic Studies 5 (1), 74 - 86.

Banuri, T. 1990. Development and the politics of knowledge: A critical intepretation of the social role of modernization theories in the development of the Third World. In: Marglin, F.A. and Marglin, S.A. (eds) Dominating Knowledge; Development, Culture, and Resistance. Pp. 29 - 72.

Barata, L., Mors, W.B., Kirson, I., Lavie, D. 1970. A new withanolide from *Acnistus arborescens* Schlecht. (Solanaceae) from the State of Guanabara, Brazil. Acad. Brasil. Cienc. An. 42 (suppl.), 401 - 407.

Barbour EK, Al Sharif M, Sagherian VK, Habre AN, Talhouk RS, Talhouk SN: Screening of selected indigenous plants of Lebanon for antimicrobial activity. *J Ethnopharmacol.* 2004 93(1):1-7.

Bardouille, V., Mootoo, B.S., Hirotsu, K., Clardy, J. 1978. Sesquiterpenes from *Pityrogramma calomelanos* [Pteridophyta]. Phytochemistry 17 (2), 275 - 277.

Barnes, Barry, Edge, David 1996. (Eds.). Science in context: readings in the sociology of science. The Open University Press.

Barnes, F.R. 1998. Book review. Signs 23 (2), 513 - 516.

Barreto GS: Effect of butanolic fraction of *Desmodium adscendens* on the anococcygeus of the rat. Braz J Biol. 2002, 62(2):223-30.

Barrett, B. 1994. Medicinal plants of Nicaragua's Atlantic coast. Economic Botany 48 (1), 8 - 20.

Barrett, B. 1997. Identity, ideology and inequality: methodologies in medical anthropology, Guatemala 1950 - 1995. Social Science and Medicine 44 (5), 597 - 587.

Barsh, R. 1997. The epistemology of traditional healing systems. Human Organisation 56 (1), 28 - 37.

Bawden, R. 2000. The Importance of Praxis in Changing Forestry Practice (prelim. title). Invited Keynote Address for 'Changing Learning and education in Forestry: A Workshop in Educational Reform', held at Sa Pa, Vietnam, April 16 - 19, 2000.

Bayley, I. 1949. The bush teas of Barbados. Journal of the Barbados Museum Historical Society 16 (3), 103 - 109.

Begum, S., Raza, S.M., Siddiqui, B.S., Siddiqui, S. 1995. Triterpenoids from the aerial parts of *Lantana camara*. Journal of Natural Products 58 (10), 1570 - 1574.

Bello, M., Gomez, A., Amor, D., Perez-Amador, M.C., Bratoeff, E.A. 1991. Chemical study of the latex of *Euphorbia tanquahuete* Sesse et. Moc. (Euphorbiaceae) Phyton (Buenes Aires) 52 (1), 69-71.

Beltrame FL, Ferreira AG, Cortez DA. 2002. Coumarin glycoside from *Cissus sicyoides*. Nat Prod Lett. 16 (4): 213-6.

Bennett, B.C., Prance, G.T. 2000. Introduced plants in the indigenous pharmacopoeia of northern South America. Economic Botany 54 (1), 90 - 102.

Bennett, S. 1986. Sheep rearing at Circle B Ranch Ltd. Caribbean Agricultural Research and Development Institute (CARDI). Small Ruminant and Rabbit Health production Workshop. April 28 - 29, Mount Hope, Tobago.

Bentley, M.E., Pelto, G.H., Straus, W.L., Schumann, D. A., Adegbola, C.A., de la Pena, E., Oni, G.A., Brown, K.H., Huffman, S.L. 1988. Rapid ethnographic assessment: applications in a diarrhea management program. Social Science and Medicine 27 (1), 107 - 116.

Berchieri JA, Alessi AC, Paulillo AC, Moraes FR and Rocha UF. 1984. Trials of the anthelmintic activity of *Chenopodium ambrosioides* (L) against nematodes of chickens. 9 Encontro de Pesquisas Veterinarias, 8 – 9 Novembro de 1984, Resumos 52. (in Portuguese).

Berlin, B., Berlin, E.A. 1994. Anthropological issues in medical ethnobotany. Ciba Foundation Symposium 185, 246 - 259.

Bernart, M.W., Cardellina, J., Balaschak, M., Alexander, M., Shoemaker, R., Boyd, M. 1996. Cytotoxic falcarinol oxylipins from *Dendropanax arboreus*. Journal of Natural Products 59 (8), 748 - 753.

Besson, Gerard. 2000. The 'Land of Beginnings'. A historical digest, Newsday Newspaper Sunday August 27, 2000.

Besson, Jean. 1993. Reputation and respectability reconsidered: a new perspective on Afro-Caribbean peasant women. In: Janet Momsen 1993. (Ed.). Women and change in the Caribbean: a Pan-Caribbean perspective. James Curreye Ltd. Ian Randle Publishers. Pp. 15 - 37.

Best R, Lewis DA, Nasser N. 1984. The anti-ulcerogenic activity of the unripe plantain banana (*Musa* species). Br J Pharmacol. 82(1):107-16.

Betancur-Galvis, L., Saez, J., Granados, H., Salazar, A., Ossa, J. 1999. Antitumor and antiviral activity of Colombian medicinal plant extracts. Mem Inst Oswaldo Cruz. 94 (4): 531-5.

Bhamarapravati S, Pendland SL, Mahady GB, 2003. Extracts of spice and food plants from Thai traditional medicine inhibit the growth of the human carcinogen *Helicobacter pylori*. In Vivo 17(6): 541-4.

Bhargava, A.K., Lal, J., Vanamayya, P.R., Kumar, P.N. 1989. Experimental evaluation of a few indigenous drugs as promotors of wound healing. Indian Journal of Animal Sciences 59 (1), 66 - 68.

Bhaskaran S and Kshama D. 1999. Anti-implantation and anti-oestrogenic activity of a herbal preparation. *Indian Journal of Pharmacology* 31: 319 - 320.

Bhaskaran, S., Kshama, D. 1999. Anti-implantation and anti-oestrogenic activity of a herbal preparation. Indian Journal of Pharmacology 31 (4), 319 - 320.

Bhat, R. B., Etejere, E.O., Oladipo, V.T. 1990. Ethnobotanical studies from central Nigeria. Economic Botany 44 (3), 382 - 390.

Bhattarai, N. 1994. Folk herbal remedies for gynaecological complaints in Central Nepal. International Journal of Pharmacognosy 32 (1), 13 - 26.

Bianchi C, Ceriotti G. 1975. Chemical and pharmacological investigations of constituents of *Eleutherine bulbosa* (Miller) Urb. (Iridaceae). J. Pharm. Sci. 64 (8),1305-8.

Binutu, O.A., Lajubutu, B.A. 1994. Antimicrobial potentials of some plant species of the Bignoniaceae family. African Journal of Medicine and Medical Sciences 23 (3), 269 - 273.

Bishnodat, Persaud. 1988. Agricultural Administration and Extension 29, 35-51.

Bittar M, de Souza MM, Yunes RA, Lento R, Delle Monache F, Cechinel Filho V: Antinociceptive activity of I3,II8-binaringenin, a biflavonoid present in plants of the Guttiferae. Planta Med. 2000, 66(1):84-6.

Blanco, E., Macia, M.J., Morales. R. 1999. Medicinal and veterinary plants of El Caurel (Galicia, northwest Spain). Journal of Ethnopharmacology 65 (2), 113-24.

Block, L.C., Santos, A.R., de Souza, M.M., Scheidt, C., Yunes, R.A., Santos, M.A., Monache, F.D., Cechinel Filho, V. 1998b. Chemical and pharmacological examination of antinociceptive constituents of *Wedelia paludosa*. Journal of Ethnopharmacology 61 (1), 85 - 89.

Block, L.C., Scheidt, C., Quintao, N.L., Santos, A.R., Cechinel-Filho, V. 1998a. Phytochemical and pharmacological analysis of different parts of *Wedelia paludosa* DC. (Compositae). Pharmazie 53 (10), 716 - 718.

Blunden, G., Patel, A.V., Armstrong, N.J., Gorham, J. 2001. Betaine distribution in the Malvaceae. Phytochemistry 58 (3): 451-4.

Blunt, W., Raphael, S. 1994. The Illustrated Herbal. Thomas and Hudson Inc., New York. 190 pp.

Bohlmann, F., Ziesche, J., King, R.M., Robinson, H. 1981. Eudesmanolides and diterpenes from *Wedelia trilobata* and an *ent*-kaurenic acid derivative from *Aspilia parvifolia*. Phytochemistry 20 (4), 751 - 756.

184

Bojo, A., Garcia, E., Quibyan, T., Poosidio, G. 1997. Isolation and characterization of the major antibacterial compounds of the plant *Peperomia pellucida* (1.) HBK, Family Piperaceae. Philippine Journal of Biotechnology 6 (1), 62 - 63.

Boomert, Arie. 2000. Trinidad, Tobago and the Lower Orinoco Interaction Sphere: An archaeological/ethnohistorical study. Alkmaar: Cairi Publications.

Boomert, A. 2006. Between the mainland and the islands: The Amerindian cultural geography of Trinidad. Paper to be presented at the symposium 'Caribbean Archaeological Research at the Peabody Museum of Natural History, Yale University: In Memory of Irving Rouse', Seventy-first Annual Meeting of the Society for American Archaeology, San Juan, Puerto Rico, April 2006

Bonet, M.A., Blanché, C., Xirau Vallès, J. 1992. Ethnobotanical study in the River Tenes valley (Catalonia, Iberian Peninsula). Journal of Ethnopharmacology 37 (3), 205 - 212.

Bonet, M.A., Parada, M., Selga, A., Xirau Vallès, J. 1999. Studies on pharmaceutical ethnobotany in the regions of L'Ált Emporada and Les Guilleries (Catalonia, Iberian Peninsula). Journal of Ethnopharmacology 68 (1 - 3), 145 - 168.

Bontis, N., Choo, C.W. 2002 (Eds.). The strategic management of intellectual capital and organisational knowledge: a collection of readings. Oxford University Press, New York.

Borde, P.G.L. 1876. The history of the island of Trinidad under the Spanish Government. Part 1. 1498-1622. Discovery, Conquest and Colonisation. Paris Masionneuve et C. Libraires-Editeurs, 25, Quai Voltaire, 15. Republished in 1982 by Paria Publishing Co. Ltd, Trinidad, W.I.

Borges-del-Castillo, J., Manresa-Ferrero, M., Rodríguez-Luis, F., Vázquez-Bueno, P., Gupta, M.P., Joseph-Nathan, P. 1982. Panama flora. II. New sesquiterpene lactones from *Neurolaena lobata*. Journal of Natural Products 45 (6), 762 - 765.

Borkosky, S, Alvarez Valdés, D., Bardón, A., Díaz, J., Herz, W. 1996. Sesquiterpene lactones and other constituents of *Eirmocephala megaphylla* and *Cyrtocymura cincta*. Phytochem 42 (6), 1637 - 1639.

Borthakur, S.K. 1997. Plants in the folklore and folk life of the Karbis (Mikirs) of Assam. In: Jain, S.K. (Ed.) 1997. Contribution to Indian Ethnobotany, 3rd Edition. Scientific Publishers, India, pp. 169 - 178.

Bos, R., Hendriks, H., van Os, F.H. 1983. The composition of the essential oil in the leaves of *Coleus aromaticus* Bentham and their importance as a component of the species antiaphthosae. Ph. Ned. Ed. V. Pharm. Weekbl. Sci. 5 (4), 129-30.

Botelho FV, Eneas LR, Cesar GC, Bizzotto CS, Tavares E, Oliveira FA, Gloria MB, Silvestre MP, Arantes RM, Alvarez-Leite JI: Effects of eggplant (*Solanum melongena*) on the atherogenesis and oxidative stress in LDL receptor knock out mice (LDLR(-/-)). Food Chem Toxicol. 2004, 42(8):1259-67.

Botta B, Gacs-Baitz E, Vinciguerra V, Delle Monache G: Three isoflavanones with cannabinoid-like moieties from *Desmodium canum*. Phytochemistry 2003, 64(2):599-602.

Bourdy, G., DeWalt, S.J., Chávez de Michel, L.R., Roca, A., Deharo, E., Muñoz, V., Balderrama, L., Quenevo, C., Gimenez, A. 2000. Medicinal plants uses of the Tacana, an Amazonian Bolivian ethnic group. Journal of Ethnopharmacology 70 (2), 87 - 109.

Bourdy, G., Walter, A. 1992. Maternity and medicinal plants in Vanuatu. 1. The cycle of reproduction. Journal of Ethnopharmacology 37 (1), 179 - 196.

Bourne, R.K., Egbe, P.C. 1979. A preliminary study of the sedative effects of *Annona muricata* (Soursop). West Indian Medical Journal. 28, 106-110. University of the West Indies, Jamaica.

Bradshaw, G.A., Borchers. J.G. 2000. Uncertainty as information: Narrowing the science-policy gap. Conservation Ecology 4 (1), 7. [online] URL:http://www.consecol.org/vol4/iss/art7.

Braga LC, Shupp JW, Cummings C, Jett M, Takahashi JA, Carmo LS, Chartone-Souza E, Nascimento AM: Pomegranate extract inhibits *Staphylococcus aureus* growth and subsequent enterotoxin production. *J Ethnopharmacol.* 2005, 96(1-2):335-9.

Brandäo, M.G., Krettli, A.U., Soares, L.S., Nery, C.G., Marinuzzi, H.C. 1997. Antimalarial activity of extracts and fractions from *Bidens pilosa* and other *Bidens* species (Asteraceae) correlated with the presence of acetylene and flavonoid compounds. Journal of Ethnopharmacology 57(2), 131-8.

Brandäo, M.G.L., Grandi, T.S.M., Rocha, E.M.M., Sawyer, D.R., Krettli, A.U. 1992. Survey of medicinal plants used as antimalarials in the Amazon. Journal of Ethnopharmacology 36 (2), 175 - 182.

Brandäo, M.G.L., Nery, C.G.C., Mamão, M.A.S., Krettli, A.U. 1998. Two methoxylated flavone glycosides from *Bidens pilosa*. Phytochemistry 48 (2), 397 - 399.

Brander, G.C., Pugh, D.M., Bywater, R.J., Jenkins, W.I. 1993. Veterinary applied pharmacology and therapeutics. Balliere Tindall, London, 624 pp.

Bras, G., Jelliffe, D.B., Stuart, K.L. 1954. Arch. Path., 57, 285.

Brathwaite, E. 1971.The Development of Creole Society in Jamaica 1770-1820, Clarendon Press, Oxford, 374 pp.

Brereton, B. 1981. A history of modern Trinidad 1783 - 1962. Kingston, Jamaica: Heineman.

Brereton, B. 1995. Text, testimony and gender: an examination of some texts by women on the English-speaking Caribbean from the 1770s to the 1920s. In: V. Shepherd, B. Brereton, B. Bailey 1995. (Eds.). Engendering History:Caribbean women in historical perspective. Ian Randle Pub, Jamaica. pp. 63- 93.

Broadway, W.E. 1893. The natural order of the Compositae - Part II. Journal of the Trinidad Field Naturalists' Club 1, 208 -216.

Brodwin, P. 1998. The cultural politics of biomedicine in the Caribbean. Review article. New West Indian Guide / Nieuwe West-Indische Gids 72 (1-2), 101 - 109.

Brown, P. and E.J. Mikkelson 1990 (Eds.). No Safe Place. Toxic Waste, Leukemia and Community Action. University of California Press, California

Browner, C.H. 1985. Plants used for reproductive health in Oaxaca, Mexico. Econ Bot 39 (4), 482 - 504.

Browner, C.H., Ortiz de Montellano, B.R., Rubel, A.J. 1988. A methodology for cross-cultural ethnomedical research. Current Anthropology 29 (5), 681 - 702.

Bruni, A., Ballero, M., Poli, F. 1997. Quantitative ethnopharmacological study of the Campidano Valley and Urzulei district, Sardinia, Italy. Journal of Ethnopharmacology 57 (2), 97 - 124.

Brzezinska-Siebodzinska, E., Miller, J.K., Quigley, J.D.,III, Moore, J.R., Madsen, F.C. 1994. Antioxidant status of dairy cows supplemented prepartum with vitamin E and selenium. Journal of Dairy Science 77, 3087 - 3095.

Buchler, I.R. 1964. Caymanian folk medicine: a problem in applied anthropology. Human Organisation 23 (1), 48 - 49.

Burke, B., Nair, M. 1986. Phenylpropene, benzoic acid and flavonoid derivatives from fruits of Jamaican *Piper* species. Phytochemistry 25 (6), 1427 - 1430.

Burnett, D. Graham. 2002. "It Is Impossible to Make a Step without the Indians": Nineteenth-Century Geographical Exploration and the Amerindians of British Guiana. Ethnohistory 49 (1) 3-40.

Burton, M. L., Schoepfle, G.M., Miller, M.L. 1986. Natural resource anthropology. Human Organization 45 (3), 261 - 269.

Burton, R. 1993. Ki moun nou ye? The idea of difference in contemporary French West Indian thought. New West Indian Guide 67 (1-2), 5 - 32.

Busch, L., Lacy, W.B. 1983. Science, Agriculture and the Politics of Research. Westview Special Studies in Agriculture, Science and Policy.

Butt Colson A.B., de Armellada, C. 1983. An Amerindian derivation for Latin American creole illnesses and their treatment. Social Science and Medicine 17 (17), 1229-48.

Caballero-George, C., Vanderheyden, P., Solis, P., Pieters, L., Shabat, A., Gupta, M., Vauquelin, G., Vlietinck, A. 2001. Biological screening of selected medicinal Panamanian plants by radioligand-binding techniques. Phytomedicine 8 (1), 59 - 70.

Cáceres, A., Alvarez, A.V., Ovando, A.E., Samayoa, B.E. 1991. Plants used in Guatemala for the treatment of respiratory diseases. 1. Screening of 68 plants against gram-positive bacteria. J Ethnopharmacol. 31(2):193-208.

Cáceres, A., Cano, O., Samayoa, B., Aguilar, L. 1990. Plants used in Guatemala for the treatment of gastrointestinal disorders. 1. Screening of 84 plants against enterobacteria. Journal of Ethnopharmacology 30 (1), 55 - 73.

Cáceres, A., Figueroa, L., Taracena, A.M., Samayoa, B. 1993. Plants used in Guatemala for the treatment of respiratory diseases. 2: Evaluation of activity of 16 plants against gram-positive bacteria. Journal of Ethnopharmacology 39 (1), 77 - 82.

Cáceres, A., Figueroa, L., Taracena, A.M., Samayoa, B. 1993c. Plants used in Guatemala for the treatment of respiratory diseases. 2: Evaluation of activity of 16 plants against gram-positive bacteria. Journal of Ethnopharmacology 39 (1), 77 - 82.

Cáceres, A., Fletes, L., Aguilar, L., Ramirez, O., Figueroa, L., Taracena, A.M., Samayoa, B. 1993b. Plants used in Guatemala for the treatment of gastrointestinal disorders. 3. Confirmation of activity against enterobacteria of 16 plants. Journal of Ethnopharmacology 38 (1), 31 - 38.

Cáceres, A., Jauregui, E., Herrera, D., Logemann, H. 1991b. Plants used in Guatemala for the treatment of dermatomucosal infections. 1. Screening of 38 plant extracts for anticandidal activity. Journal of Ethnopharmacology 33 (3), 277 - 283.

Cáceres, A., Lopez, B., Giron, M., Logemann, H. 1991a. Plants used in Guatemala for the treatment of dermatophytic infections. 1. Screening for antimycotic activity of 44 plant extracts. Journal of Ethnopharmacology 31 (3), 263 - 276.

Cáceres, A., López, B., González, S., Berger, I., Tada, I., Maki, J. 1998. Plants used in Guatemala for the treatment of protozoal infections. 1. Screening of activity to bacteria, fungi and American trypanosomes of 13 native plants. Journal of Ethnopharmacology 62 (3), 195 - 202.

Cáceres, A., Torres, M.F., Ortiz, S., Cano, F., Jauregui, E. 1993a. Plants used in Guatemala for the treatment of gastrointestinal disorders. IV. Vibriocidal activity of five American plants used to treat infections. Journal of Ethnopharmacology 39 (1), 73 - 75.

Calixto, J.B., Santos, A.R.S., Cechinel Filho, V.C., Yunes, R.A. 1998. A review of the plants of the genus *Phyllanthus*: their chemistry, pharmacology, and therapeutic potential. Medicinal Research Reviews 18 (4), 225 - 258.

Callon, M. 1987. Society in the making: the study of technology as a tool for sociological analysis. In: Bijker, W.E, Hughes, T.P. and Pinch, T.J. 1987 (Eds.). The social construction of technological systems. New directions in the sociology and history of technology. Cambridge, MIT Press. Pp. 83 - 103.

Callon, Michel. 1991. Techno-economic networks and irreversibility. In: John Law 1991 (Ed.) A sociology of monsters: essays on power, technology and domination. Sociological Review Monograph 38, Routledge & Kegan Paul, London. Pp. 132 - 164.

Cambie, R.C. 1997. Anti-fertility plants of the Pacific. CSIRO Publishing, Australia.

Campbell TW, Bartley EE, Bechtle RM, Dayton AD. 1976. Coffee grounds. I. Effects of coffee grounds on ration digestibility and diuresis in cattle, on in vitro rumen fermentation, and on rat growth. J Dairy Sci. 59(8):1452-60.

Camporese A, Balick MJ, Arvigo R, Esposito RG, Morsellino N, De Simone F, Tubaro A: Screening of anti-bacterial activity of medicinal plants from Belize (Central America). *J Ethnopharmacol.* 2003, 87(1):103-7.

Caparros-Lefebvre, D., Elbaz, A. 1999. Possible relation of atypical parkinsonism in the French West Indies with consumption of tropical plants: A case-control study. Lancet 354 (9175), 281- 6.

Carbajal, D., Casaco, A., Arruzazabala, L., Gonzalez, R., Tolon, Z. 1989. Pharmacological study of *Cymbopogon citratus* leaves. Journal of Ethnopharmacology 25 (1), 103-7.

Carlini, E.A. 2003. Plants and the central nervous system. Pharmacology, Bichemistry and Behaviour 75: 501 – 512.

Carlini, E.A., Contar, J. de D.P., Silva-Filho, A.R., da Silveira-Filho, N.G., Frochtengarten, M.L., Bueno, O.F. 1986. Pharmacology of lemongrass (*Cymbopogon citratus* Stapf). I. Effects of teas prepared from the leaves on laboratory animals. Journal of Ethnopharmacology 17(1), 37-64.

Carr, Albert. 1893. A quank "hunt." Club Papers. Journal of the Trinidad Field Naturalist Club, 1, 269 - 277.

Carstens, E, Anderson, K A, Simons, C T, Carstens, M I, Jinks, S L: Analgesia induced by chronic nicotine infusion in rats: differences by gender and pain test. *Psychopharmacologia* 2001, 157 (1): 40-45.

Cazabon, E.P.I., Berment, M.P., and Supersad, N. 1978. *Salmonella* infection in market swine in Trinidad and Tobago. Bulletin of the Pan American Health Organisation 12 (10), 51-54.

Cernea, M.M. 1995. Social organization and development anthropology. Malinowski Award Lecture. Human Organization 54 (3), 340 - 352.

Chadband, Connell Henry Branson. 1987. Trinidad Express Newspaper Advertisement. August 9th, 1987.

Chan, K., Islam, M.W., Kamil., M., Radhakrishnan, R., Zakaria, M.N.M., Habibullah, M., Attas, A. 2000. The analgesic and anti-inflammatory effects of *Portulaca oleracea* L. subsp. sativa (Haw.) Celak. Journal of Ethnopharmacology 73 (3), 445 - 451.

Chang FR, Liaw CC, Lin CY, Chou CJ, Chiu HF, Wu YC., 2003. New adjacent Bis-tetrahydrofuran Annonaceous acetogenins from *Annona muricata*. Planta Medica. 69 (3): 241-6.

Chang SL, Chang CL, Chiang YM, Hsieh RH, Tzeng CR, Wu TK, Sytwu HK, Shyur LF, Yang WC: Polyacetylenic compounds and butanol fraction from *Bidens pilosa* can modulate the differentiation of helper T cells and prevent autoimmune diabetes in non-obese diabetic mice. Planta Med. 2004, 70(11):1045-51.

Chang, F.R., Yang, P.Y., Lin, J.Y., Lee, K.H,, Wu, Y.C. 1998. Bioactive kaurane diterpenoids from *Annona glabra*. Journal of Natural Products 61(4), 437-9.

Charles, V., Charles, S.X. 1992. The use and efficacy of *Azadirachta indica* ADR ('Neem') and *Curcuma longa* ('Turmeric') in scabies. A pilot study. Tropical and Geographical Medicine 44 (1-2), 178 - 181.

Chassagne, M., Barnouin, J. 1992. Circulating $PgF_{2\alpha}$ and nutritional parameters at parturition in dairy cows with and without retained placenta: Relation to prepartum diet. Theriogenology 38, 407 - 418.

Chen, C., Huang, Y., Ou, J., Lin, C., Pan, T. 1993. Three new prenylflavones from *Artocarpus altilis*. Journal of Natural Products 56 (9), 1594 - 1597.

Chen, L. 1991. Polyphenols from leaves of *Euphorbia hirta* L. Chung Kuo Chung Yao Tsa Chih. 16 (1), 38-9, 64 [Article in Chinese].

Chen, L., Mohr, S.N., Yang, C.S. 1996. Decrease of plasma and urinary oxidative metabolites of acetaminophen after consumption of watercress by human volunteers. Clin. Pharmacol. Ther. 60 (6), 651-60.

Chen, Z-P., Cai, Y., Phillipson, J. David. 1994. Studies on the anti-tumour, anti-bacterial, and wound-healing properties of Dragon's Blood. Planta Medica 60 (6), 541 - 545.

Cherian T. 2000. Effect of papaya latex extract on gravid and non-gravid rat uterine preparations *in vitro*. *Journal of Ethnopharmacology* 70: 205-212.

Chih, H.W., Lin, C.C., Tang, K.S. 1995. Anti-inflammatory activity of Taiwan folk medicine "ham-hong-chho" in rats. American Journal of Chinese Medicine 23 (3-4), 273-8.

Chin, H.W., Lin, C.C., Tang, K.S. 1996. The hepatoprotective effects of Taiwan folk medicine ham-hong-chho in rats. American Journal of Chinese Medicine 24 (3-4), 231-40.

Chinnah, A.D., Baig, M.A., Tizard, I.R., Kemp, M.C. 1992. Antigen dependent adjuvant activity of a polydispersed β-(1-4)-linked acetylated mannan (acemannan). Vaccine 10 (8), 551 - 557.

Chinnock, R.J., Ghisalberti, E.L., Jeffries, P.R. 1987. (-)-Epingaione from *Bontia daphnoides*. Phytochemistry 26 (4), 1202 - 1203.

Chippaux JP, Rakotonirina VS, Rakotonirina A, Dzikouk G. 1997. Drug or plant substances which antagonize venoms or potentiate antivenins. Bull Soc Pathol Exot. 90(4):282-5. Article in French.

Chiossone, V. 1938. Flora Medica del Estado Lara. Coop. De Artes Graficas, Caracas. In: Morton, J.F. 1975. Current folk remedies of northern Venezuela. Quarterly Journal of Crude Drug Research 13, 97 - 121.

Chirol, N., Jay, M. 1995. Acylated anthocyanins from flowers of *Begonia*. Phytochemistry 40 (1), 275 - 277.

Chistokhodova N, Nguyen C, Calvino T, Kachirskaia I, Cunningham G, Howard Miles D: Antithrombin activity of medicinal plants from central Florida. J Ethnopharmacol. 2002, 81(2):277-80.

Chithra, P., Sajithlal, G.B., Chanrakasan, G. 1998. Influence of *Aloe vera* on the glycosaminoglycans in the matrix of healing dermal wounds in rats. Journal of Ethnopharmacology 59 (3), 179 - 186.

Choudhury, M.N., Bhattacharyya, B., Ahmed, S. 1993. Incidence, biochemical and histopathological profiles of retained placenta in cattle and buffalo. Environment and Ecology 11, 34 - 37.

Christoplos, Ian, Nitsch, Ulric. 1996. Pluralism and the Extension Agent: Changing Concepts and Approaches in Rural Extension. Publications on Agriculture: No. 1. Sweden: Swedish University of Agricultural Sciences, Department for Natural Resources and the Environment.

Cichewicz, R.H., Thorpe, P.A. 1996. The antimicrobial properties of chile peppers (*Capsicum* species) and their uses in Mayan medicine. Journal of Ethnopharmacology 52 (2), 61 - 70.

Clavin, M.L., Gorzalczany, S., Mino, J., Kadarian, C., Martino, V., Ferraro, G., Acevedo, C. 2000. Antinociceptive effect of some Argentine medicinal species of *Eupatorium*. Phytotherapy Research 14 (4),275-7

Coates, N.J., Gilpin, M.L., Gwynn, M.N., Lewis, D.E., Milner, P.H., Spear, S.R., Tyler, J.W. 1994. SB-202742, a novel beta-lactamase inhibitor isolated from *Spondias mombin*. Journal of Natural Products 57 (5), 654 - 657.

Code, Lorraine. 1993. Taking Subjectivity into Account. In: Linda Alcoff, and Elizabeth Potter (Eds.) Feminist Epistemologies, Routledge, New York and London, Pp. 15 - 48.

Coe, F.G., Anderson, G.J. 1996a. Screening of medicinal plants used by the Garífuna of Eastern Nicaragua for bioactive compunds. Journal of Ethnopharmacology 53 (1), 29 - 50.

Coe, F.G., Anderson, G.J. 1996b. Ethnobotany of the Garífuna of eastern Nicaragua. Economic Botany 50 (1), 71 - 107.

Collins, D.O., Gallimore, W.A., Reynolds, W.F., Williams, L.A., Reese, P.B. 2000. New skeletal sesquiterpenoids, caprariolides A-D, from *Capraria biflora* and their insecticidal activity. Journal of Natural Products 63 (11), 1515-1518.

Collins, H.M. 1981. The place of the core-set in modern science: social contingency with methodological propriety in science. Cited in Pinch, T.J., Bijker, W.E. 1987. The social construction of facts and artifacts: or how sociology of science and the sociology of technology might benefit each other. Pp. 17-50.

Comerford, S.C. 1996. Medicinal plants of two Mayan healers from San Andrés, Petén, Guatemala. Economic Botany 50 (3), 327 - 336.

Consolini AE, Ragone MI, Migliori GN, Conforti P, Volonte MG. 2006. Cardiotonic and sedative effects of *Cecropia pachystachya* Mart. (ambay) on isolated rat hearts and conscious mice. J Ethnopharmacol. Jan 12; [Epub ahead of print]

Conway, G.A., Slocumb, J.C. 1979. Plants used as abortifacients and emmenagogues by Spanish New Mexicans. Journal of Ethnopharmacology 1(3), 241-61.

Corthout, J., Pieters, L., Claeys, M., Geerts, S., Berghe, D., van den, Vlietinck, A. 1994. Antibacterial and molluscicidal phenolic acids from *Spondias mombin* L. Planta Medica 60 (5), 460 - 463.

Corthout, J., Pieters, L., Claeys, M.,Vlietinck, A.J. 1990b. Isolation and characterisation of geraniin and galloyl-geraniin from *Spondias mombin*. Planta Medica 56 (6), 584 - 585. [Poster].

Corthout, J., Pieters, L., Janssens, J., Vlietinck, A.J. 1990a. The long-chain phenolic acids of *Spondias mombin*. Planta Medica 56 (6), 584. [Poster]

Cos P, Hermans N, De Bruyne T, Apers S, Sindambiwe JB, Vanden Berghe D, Pieters L, Vlietinck AJ: Further evaluation of Rwandan medicinal plant extracts for their antimicrobial and antiviral activities. J Ethnopharmacol. 2002, 79(2):155-63.

Costa, S.S., Jossang, A., Bodo, B., Souza, M.L., Moraes, V.L. 1994. Patuletin acetylrhamnosides from *Kalanchoe brasiliensis* as inhibitors of human lymphocyte proliferative activity. Journal of Natural Products 57 (11), 1503-10.

Cox, H. 1997. Professional responsibility to the communities in which they work and live. Human Organization 56 (4), 490 - 492.

Cozier, J.D., Robertson, L. 1994. Memories of the turf: the history of horse racing in Trinidad and Tobago. Caribbean Information Systems and Services Ltd. Trinidad and Tobago, 191 pps.

Cragg, G.M., Newman, D.J., Sue Yang, S. 1998. Bioprospecting for drugs. Letter to the editor. Nature 393, 301.

Craig, K., Lans, C. 1993. Lamb tasting session: Tobago. Caribbean Agricultural Research and Development Institute (CARDI), Trinidad and Tobago.

Craveiro, A., Alencar, J., Matos, F., Andrade, C., Machado, M. 1981. Essential oils from Brazilian Verbenaceae. Genus *Lippia*. Journal of Natural Products 44 (5), 598 - 601.

Crockett, C.O., Guede-Guina, F., Pugh, D., Vangah-Manda, M., Robinson, T.J., Olubadewo, J.O., Ochillo, R.F. 1992. *Cassia alata* and the preclinical search for therapeutic agents for the treatment of opportunistic infections in AIDS patients. Cell. Mol. Biol. 38 (5), 505-11. Erratum in: Cell. Mol. Biol. 1992 Sep;38(615).

Croom, E.M. Jr. 1983. Documenting and evaluating herbal remedies. Economic Botany 37 (1),13 - 27.

CSO, 1997. Central Statistical Office, Vol. 13, No. 243, November 1997. Quarterly survey of pig farmers. Office of the Prime Minister, Republic of Trinidad and Tobago.

CSO, 2002. Central Statistical Office. Quarterly pig production survey. Ministry of Planning and Development. Government of the Republic of Trinidad and Tobago cso.gov.tt/statistics/pdf/Tables11-12_2002.pdf

Cummings E, Hundal HS, Wackerhage H, Hope M, Belle M, Adeghate E, Singh J. *Momordica charantia* fruit juice stimulates glucose and amino acid uptakes in L6 myotubes. Mol Cell Biochem. 2004, 261(1-2):99-104.

Dafallah, A.A., al-Mustafa, Z. 1996. Investigation of the anti-inflammatory activity of *Acacia nilotica* and *Hibiscus sabdariffa*. American Journal of Chinese Medicine 24 (3-4), 263-9.

Dalen, J. 1998. Editorial. "Conventional" and "unconventional" medicine: Can they be integrated? Arch. Intern. Med. 158 (20), 2179 - 2181.

Damodaran, S., Venkataraman, S. 1994. A study on the therapeutic efficacy of *Cassia alata* Linn. leaf extract against *Pityriasis versicolor*. Journal of Ethnopharmacology 42 (1),19-23.

D'Armas, H.T., Mootoo, B.S., Reynolds, W.F. 2000. An unusual sesquiterpene derivative from the Caribbean gorgonian *Pseudopterogorgia rigida*. Journal of Natural Products 63 (11), 1593-5.

Das B, Tandon V, Saha N: Effects of phytochemicals of *Flemingia vestita* (Fabaceae) on glucose 6-phosphate dehydrogenase and enzymes of gluconeogenesis in a cestode (*Raillietina echinobothrida*). Comp Biochem Physiol C Toxicol Pharmacol. 2004, 139(1-3):141-6.

Das, B., Rao, S. Padma, Srinivas, K.V.N.S., Das, R. 1996. Jatrodien, a lignan from stems of *Jatropha gossypifolia*. Phytochemistry 41 (3), 985 - 987.

Das, B., Venkataiah, B., Kashinatham, A. 1999. (+)-Syringaresinol from *Parthenium hysterophorus*. Fitoterapia 70 (1), 101 - 102.

Dasgupta T, Banerjee S, Yadava PK, Rao AR: Chemopreventive potential of *Azadirachta indica* (Neem) leaf extract in murine carcinogenesis model systems. *J Ethnopharmacol.* 2004, 92(1):23-36.

da-Silva, M.H.L., Zoghbi, M.G.B., Andrade, E.H.A., Maia, J.G.S., da Silva, M.H.L. 1999. The essential oil of *Peperomia pellucida* Kunth and *P. circinnata* Link var. *circinnata*. Flavour and Fragrance Journal 14 (5), 312 - 314.

da-Silva, V.A., de Freitas, J.C., Mattos, A.P., Paiva-Gouvea, W., Presgrave, O.A., Fingola, F.F. 1991. Neurobehavioral study of the effect of beta-myrcene on rodents. Braz. J. Med. Biol. Res. 24 (8), 827-31.

Datta, S., Sinha, S., Bhattacharyya, P. 1999. Effect of a herbal protein, CI-1, isolated from *Cajanus indicus* on immune response of control and stressed mice. Journal of Ethnopharmacology 67 (1), 259 - 267.

Datubo-Brown D.D., Blight, A. 1990. Inhibition of human fibroblast growth *in vitro* by a snake oil. Br. J. Plast. Surg. 43 (2), 183-6.

Davis, E., Yost, J. 1983. The ethnomedicine of the Waorani of Amazonian Ecuador. Journal of Ethnopharmacology 9 (2-3), 273 - 297.

Davis, R.H., Donato, J.J., Hartman, G.M., Haas, R.C. 1994. Anti-inflammatory and wound healing activity of a growth substance in *Aloe vera*. Journal of the American Podiatric Medical Association 84 (2), 77 - 81.

Davis, W.G. and Persaud, T.N.V. 1970. Recent studies on the active principles of Jamaican medicinal plants. West Indian Medical Journal 19,101.

de Fatima Arrigoni-Blank M, Dmitrieva EG, Franzotti EM, Antoniolli AR, Andrade MR, Marchioro M: Anti-inflammatory and analgesic activity of *Peperomia pellucida* HBK (Piperaceae). J Ethnopharmacol. 2004, 91(2-3):215-8.

de Mello FB, Jacobus D, de Carvalho KC, de Mello JR, 2003. Effects of *Lantana camara* (Verbenaceae) on rat fertility. Vet Hum Toxicol. 45 (1): 20-3.

de Moura RM, Pereira PS, Januario AH, Franca Sde C, Dias DA: Antimicrobial screening and quantitative determination of benzoic acid derivative of *Gomphrena celosioides* by TLC-densitometry. Chem Pharm Bull (Tokyo). 2004, 52(11):1342-4.

de-Barros Viana, G.S., do Vale, T.G., Silva, C.M., de Abreu Matos, F.J. 2000. Anticonvulsant activity of essential oils and active principles from chemotypes of *Lippia alba* (Mill.) N.E. Brown. Biol. Pharm. Bull. 23 (11), 1314-7.

de-Guzman, C.C. 1999. Hydroponic culture of pansit-pansitan (*Peperomia pellucida*). PCARRD highlights '98: Summary of the Proceedings of the 1998 Regional Research and Development Symposia. Philippine Council for Agriculture, Forestry and Natural Resources Research and Development, Los Banos, Philippines. Pp. 45.

Deichmann, Ute, Müller-Hill, Benno. 1998. The Fraud of Abderhalden's Enzymes. Nature 393 (6681), 109 - 111.

de-Lima, T.C., Morato, G.S., Takahashi, R.N. 1991. Evaluation of antinociceptive effect of *Petiveria alliacea* (Guine) in animals. Memorias do Instituto Oswaldo Cruz, 86 Suppl 2, 153-158.

Dennis, P.A. 1988. Herbal medicine among the Miskito of Eastern Nicaragua. Economic Botany 42 (1), 16 - 28.

Deokule, S. 1991. Phytochemical studies on roots of *Mucuna pruriens* (Linn.) DC. Biovigyanam 17 (2), 111 - 114.

De-Oliveira AC, Silva IB, Manhaes-Rocha DA, Paumgartten FJ. 2003. Induction of liver monooxygenases by annatto and bixin in female rats. Braz J Med Biol Res. 36(1):113-8.

Descola, P. 1996. Constructing natures: symbolic ecology and social practice. In: Descola, P., Pálsson, G. 1996. (Eds). Nature and society: anthropological perspectives. Routledge, London, pp. 82 - 102.

Desmarchelier, C., Barros, S., Repetto, M., Latorre, L.R., Kato, M., Coussio, J., Ciccia, G. 1997a. 4-Nerolidylcatechol from *Pothomorphe* spp. scavenges peroxyl radicals and inhibits Fe (II)-dependent DNA damage. Planta Medica 63 (6), 561 - 563.

Desmarchelier, C., Gurni, A., Ciccia, G., Giulietti, A.M. 1996. Ritual and medicinal plants of the Ese'ejas of the Amazonian rainforest (Madre de Dios, Perú). Journal of Ethnopharmacology 52 (1), 45 - 51.

Desmarchelier, C., Mongelli, E., Coussio, J., Ciccia, G. 1997b. Inhibition of lipid peroxidation and iron (II)-dependent DNA damage by extracts of *Pothomorphe peltata* (L). Miq. Braz. J. Med. Biol. Res. 30 (1), 85-91.

Desmarchelier, C., Slowing, K., Ciccia, G. 2000. Anti-inflammatory activity of *Pothomorphe peltata* leaf methanol extract. Short Report. Fitoterapia 71 (5), 556-558.

Deshpande, R.S., Dhoble, R.L., Sawale, A.G. 1999. Clinical evaluation of newly developed herbal drug in treatment of post-partum anoestrus in buffaloes. Journal of Maharashtra Agricultural Universities 24 (2), 195 - 196.

de-Verteuil, L. A. A. 1884. Trinidad: Its geography, natural resources, administration, present condition and prospects. London, Paris, New York: Cassell & Co., Ltd.

de-Verteuil, L.A.A. 1889. Native medicinal plants. Agricultural Record of Trinidad. 1, 17 - 24.

de-Vries J.X., Tauscher, B., Wurzel, G. 1988. Constituents of *Justicia pectoralis* Jacq. 2. Gas chromatography/mass spectrometry of simple coumarins, 3-phenylpropionic acids and their hydroxy and methoxy derivatives. Biomed. Environ. Mass Spectrom. 15 (8), 413-7.

Dhawan, K., Dhawan, S., Sharma, A. 2004. Passiflora: A review update. J Ethnopharmacol. 94(1):1-23.

Diaz-Carballo D, Seeber S, Strumberg D, Hilger RA. 2003. Novel antitumoral compound isolated from *Clusia rosea*. Int J Clin Pharmacol Ther. 41(12):622-3.

Dickson, D. 1999. ICSU seeks to classify 'traditional knowledge'. News. Nature 401 (6754), 631.

Didier, J.M., Bundy, D.A.P., McKenzie, H.I. 1988. Traditional treatment and community control of gastrointestinal helminthiasis in St. Lucia, West Indies. Transactions of the Royal Society of Tropical Medicine and Hygiene 82 (2), 303 - 304.

Diehl MS, Atindehou KK, Tere H, Betschart B. 2004. Prospect for anthelminthic plants in the Ivory Coast using ethnobotanical criteria. *J Ethnopharmacol*. 95(2-3):277-84.

Dimo, T., Rakotonirina, S., Kamgang, R., Tan, P., Kamanyi, A., Bopelet, M. 1998. Effects of leaf aqueous extract of *Bidens pilosa* (Asteraceae) on KCL- and norepinephrine-induced contractions of rat aorta. Journal of Ethnopharmacology 60 (2), 179 - 182.

Dindial, P. 1991. Livestock production in Trinidad and Tobago: An overview. In: FAO (1991), Report of the round table on small farmers' livestock development in the Caribbean. Port of Spain, Trinidad and Tobago, 24 - 26 July, 1991. FAO Regional Office for Latin America and the Caribbean, Santiago, Chile.

Dissanayake, W. 1992. Knowledge culture and power: some theoretical issues related to the agricultural knowledge and information system framework. Knowledge and Policy 5 (1), 65 - 76.

Djibo, A., Bouzou, S.B. 2000. Acute intoxication with "sobi-lobi" (Datura). Four cases in Niger. Bull. Soc. Pathol. Exot. 93 (4), 294 - 297.

Dolby, R.G.A. 1979. Reflections on deviant science. In: Wallis, R. 1979 (Ed.). On The Margins of Science: The Social Construction of Rejected Knowledge. Sociological Review Monograph 27. University of Keele, Keele, Staffordshire, UK. Pp. 9-47.

Dong-lei Y, Xue-dong Y, Jian G, Li-zhen X and Shi-lin Y. 2000. Studies on chemical constituents of *Erythrina arborescens* Roxb. *Zhongguo Zhongyao Zazhi* 25: 353 - 355. (in Chinese).

Douglas, M. 1995. Forgotten knowledge. In: Marilyn Strathern (Ed.) 1995. Shifting contexts: Transformations in anthropological knowledge. Routledge, London and New York, pp.13 - 29.

Dressler, W. 1980. Ethnomedicinal beliefs and patient adherence to a treatment regimen: a St. Lucian example. Human Organization 39 (1), 88 - 91.

Drummond, Lee 1977. On being Carib. In Carib-speaking indians: Culture, society and language. Anthropological papers of the University of Arizona no. 28. Ellen Basso, ed. pp. 76 - 88. Tuscon: The University of Arizona Press.

Drummond, Lee. 1980. The cultural continuum: A theory of intersystems. Man 15: 352 – 374.

Dubey, N.K., Kishore, N. 1987. Fungitoxicity of some higher plants and synergistic activity of their essential oils. Tropical Science 27 (1), 23 - 27.

Duke, J. A. 2000. Phytochemical and Ethnobotanical Databases. USDA-ARS-NGRL, Beltsville Agricultural Research Center, Beltsville, Maryland, USA.

Duke, J.A. 1970. Ethnobotanical observations on the Chocó Indians. Economic Botany 24 (3), 343 - 366.

Duke, J.A. 1975. Ethnobotanical observations on the Cuna Indians. Economic Botany 29 (3), 278 - 293.

Duke, J.A. 1989. Handbook of medicinal herbs. CRC Press, Boca Raton, Florida, 677 pp.

Duke, J.A. 1992. Handbook of phytochemical constituents of GRAS herbs and other economic plants. Boca Raton, Florida. CRC Press.

Duke, J.A., duCellier, J., Beckstrom-Sternberg. 1998. Western Herbal Medicine: Traditional Materia Medica in: Allen M. Schoen and Susan Wynn (Eds.). Complementary and Alternative Veterinary Medicine. Mosby, Inc: Missouri, pp. 299 - 336.

Duker-Eshun G, Jaroszewski JW, Asomaning WA, Oppong-Boachie F, Brogger Christensen S. 2004. Antiplasmodial constituents of Cajanus cajan. Phytother Res. 18 (2):128-30.

Dunstan, C.A., Noreen, Y., Serrano, G., Cox, P., Perera, P., Bohlin, L. 1997. Evaluation of some Samoan and Peruvian medicinal plants by prostaglandin biosynthesis and rat ear oedema assays. Journal of Ethnopharmacology 57 (1), 35 - 56.

Eigner, D., Scholz, D. 1999. *Ferula asa-foetida* and *Curcuma longa* in traditional medical treatment and diet in Nepal. Review article. Journal of Ethnopharmacology 67 (1), 1 - 6.

Elam, M. 1999. Living dangerously with Bruno Latour in a hybrid world. Theory, Culture and Society 16 (4), 1 - 24.

Eldridge, J. 1975. Bush medicine in the Exumas and Long Island, Bahamas: A field study. Economic Botany 29, 307-332.

Elisabetsky, E, Posey, D.A. 1989. Use of contraceptive and related plants by the Kayapo Indians (Brazil). Journal of Ethnopharmacology 26 (3), 299 - 316.

Elisabetsky, E., de Moraes, J.A.R. 1990. Ethnopharmacology: a technological development strategy. In: Ethnobiology: implications and applications. Proceedings of the First International Congress of Ethnobiology (2), 111 -118. Museu Paraense Emílio Goeldi, Belém, Brazil.

Elisabetsky, E., Wannmacher, L. 1993. The status of ethnopharmacology in Brazil. Journal of Ethnopharmacology 38 (2-3), 137 - 143.

Ellen, R. 1996a. Anthropological approaches to understanding the ethnobotanical knowledge of rainforest populations. In: D.S. Edwards, W.S. Booth and S.C. Choy (Eds.), Tropical rainforest research: current issues. Kluwer: Dordrecht, pp. 457 - 465.

Ellen, R. 1996b. The cognitive geometry of nature. In: Descola, P., Pálsson, G. 1996. (Eds.). Nature and society: Anthropological perspectives. Routledge, London.

Emele, F.E., Agbonlahor, D.E., Ahanotu, C. 1998. *Euphorbia hirta* leaves and *Musa sapientum* fruits in culture media for fungi. Mycoses 41 (11-12), 529-33.

Emeruwa, A. 1982. Antibacterial substance from *Carica papaya* fruit extract. Journal of Natural Products 45 (2), 123 - 127.

Engerman, Stanley, 1996. Europe, the Lesser Antilles, and European expansion, 1600 – 1800. In Paquette, Robert and Engerman, Stanley (eds.), The Lesser Antilles in the Age of European Expansion. University Press of Florida. Pp. 147 – 164.

Eno, A.E., Owo, O.I., Itam, E.H., Konya, R.S. 2000. Blood pressure depression by the fruit juice of *Carica papaya* in renal and DOCA-induced hypertension in the rat. Phytotherapy Research 14 (4), 235-9.

Escobar, A. 1999. After nature: steps to an antiessentialist political ecology. Current Anthropology 40 (1), 1 - 30.

ESSA, 2005. Food and Agriculture Indicators. Trinidad and Tobago. FAO, Rome, Italy. www.fao.org/es/ess/compendium_2005/pdf/ESS_TRI.pdf

Etkin, N.L. 1988. Ethnopharmacology: biobehavioral approached in the Anthropological study of indigenous medicines. Annual Review of Anthropology 17, 23 - 42.

Etkin, N.L. 1993. Anthropological methods in Ethnopharmacology. Journal of Ethnopharmacology 38 (2 - 3), 93 -104.

Evans, E. 1992. The economics of small ruminant production systems of resource-poor farmers in selected Caribbean countries. A paper presented at the CARDI/CIDA regional small ruminant workshop. September 15 - 17, 1992. CARDI, Barbados.

Evans, E., Ganteaume - Farrell, J. 1993. Economic liberalization and its likely impact on cost of production and returns in the livestock sector. Proc. Workshop on the survival of the livestock industry; marketing strategies for sheep, goats and cattle. CARDI, Trinidad and Tobago.

Ewen, E.D. 1896. Notes on the economic uses of the Compositae. Journal of the Trinidad Field Naturalists' Club 2, 204 -210; 225-231.

Fabry, W., Okemo, P., Ansorg, R. 1996. Fungistatic and fungicidal activity of east African medicinal plants. Mycoses 39 (1-2), 67-70.

Facey, P.C., Pascoe, K.O., Porter, R.B., Jones, A.D. 1999. Investigation of plants used in Jamaican folk medicine for anti-bacterial activity. Journal of Pharmacy and Pharmacology 51, 1455 - 1460.

FAO, 1997. Medicinal plants for forest conservation and health care. Non-wood Forest Products Series, No. 11. Global Initiative for Traditional Systems (GIFTS) of Health. Rome, Italy.

Farabee, William Curtis. 1918. The Central Arawaks. Anthropological Publications Vol. IX. The University Museum, Pennsylvania: University of Pennsylvania.

Farage, Nadine. 2003. Rebellious memories: The Wapishana in the Rupununi uprising, Guyana, 1969. In: Neil L. Whitehead (ed.) Histories and historicities in Amazonia. University of Nebraska Press, Lincoln and London. Pp. 107 – 120.

Farine, J-P., Legal, L., Moreteau, B., Le Quere, J-L. 1996. Volatile components of ripe fruits of *Morinda citrifolia* and their effects on *Drosophila*. Phytochemistry 41 (2), 433 - 438.

Farnsworth, N. R. 1993. Ethnopharmacology and future drug development: The North American experience. Journal of Ethnopharmacology 38 (2-3), 145 - 152.

Fatehi M, Farifteh F, Fatehi-Hassanabad Z. Antispasmodic and hypotensive effects of *Ferula asafoetida* gum extract. *J Ethnopharmacol*. 2004 91(2-3):321-4.

Felzenszwalb, I., Valsa, J.O., Araujo, A.C., Alcantara-Gomes, R. 1987. Absence of mutagenicity of *Potomorphe umbellata* and *Potomorphe peltata* in the salmonella/mammalian-microsome mutagenicity assay. Braz. J. Med. Biol. Res. 20 (3-4), 403-5.

Feng, P. C., Haynes, L. J., Magnus, K. E., Plimmer, J. R. 1964. Further pharmacological screening of some West Indian medicinal plants. Journal of Pharmacy and Pharmacology 16, 115.

Feresin, G., Tapia, A., Bustos, D. 2000. Antibacterial activity of some medicinal plants from San Juan, Argentina. Fitoterapia 71 (4), 429 - 432.

Feresin GE, Tapia A, Sortino M, Zacchino S, de Arias AR, Inchausti A, Yaluff G, Rodriguez J, Theoduloz C, Schmeda-Hirschmann G. 2003. Bioactive alkyl phenols and embelin from *Oxalis erythrorhiza*. Journal of Ethnopharmacology 88 (2-3): 241-7.

Ferguson, K.E. 1997. Book review. Signs 22 (4), 1037 - 1040.

Fernandes J, Castilho RO, da Costa MR, Wagner-Souza K, Coelho Kaplan MA, Gattass CR: Pentacyclic triterpenes from Chrysobalanaceae species: Cytotoxicity on multidrug resistant and sensitive leukemia cell lines. Cancer Lett. 2003, 190(2):165-9.

Fernando, M.R., Thabrew, M.I., Karunanayake, E.H. 1990. Hypoglycaemic activity of some medicinal plants in Sri Lanka. Gen. Pharmacol. 21 (5), 779 - 782.

Ferradás, C. 1998. Comment. In: Sillitoe, P. 1998. The development of indigenous knowledge. Current Anthropology 39 (2), 223 - 252.

Ferraz, M.B., Pereira, R.B., Coelho Andrade, L.E., Atra, E. 1991. The effectiveness of tipi in the treatment of hip and knee osteoarthritis--a preliminary report. Memorias do Instituto Oswaldo Cruz, 86 Suppl 2, 241-243.

Ferreira-Machado SC, Rodrigues MP, Nunes AP, Dantas FJ, De Mattos JC, Silva CR, Moura EG, Bezerra RJ, Caldeira-de-Araujo A: Genotoxic potentiality of aqueous extract prepared from *Chrysobalanus icaco* L. leaves. Toxicol Lett. 2004, 151(3):481-7.

Feyerabend, P. 1975. Against Method: Outline of an Anarchistic Theory of Knowledge. New Left Books, London.

Ficarra, R., Ficarra, P., Tommasini, S., Calabro, M.L., Ragusa, S., Barbera, R., Rapisarda, A. 1995. Leaf extracts of some *Cordia* species: Analgesic and anti-inflammatory activities as well as their chromatographic analysis. Farmaco 50 (4), 245-56.

Fielding, D. 2000. Ethnoveterinary medicine in the tropics - key issues and the way forward? Internet publication.

Figueredo, Alfredo, and Glazier, Stephen. 1978. A revised aboriginal ethnohistory of Trinidad. Seventh International Congress for the study of Pre-Columbian cultures of the Lesser Antilles (pp 259 - 262). Caracas: Centre de recherches Caraibes (Montreal 1978).

Filipov, A. 1994. Medicinal plants of the Pilagá of central Chaco. Journal of Ethnopharmacology 44 (3), 181 - 193.

First Citizens Bank, 2004. Sustaining our agriculture sector in an era of free trade. First Citizens Bank Newsletter October 2004. Vol 7 No 4.

Fleischer TC, Ameade EP, Mensah ML, Sawer IK. 2003. Antimicrobial activity of the leaves and seeds of *Bixa orellana*. Fitoterapia 74(1-2):136-8.

Flemming, Rebecca. 2000. Medicine and the making of Roman women: Gender, nature, and authority from Celsus to Galen Oxford; New York: Oxford University Press.

Flora, Cornelia B. 1992. Reconstructing Agriculture: The Case for Local Knowledge. Rural Sociology 57, 92 - 97.

Foster, G.M. 1953. Relationships between Spanish and Spanish-American folk medicine. Journal of American Folklore 66, 201- 217.

Foucault, M. 1971. The order of discourse. In: Scoones, I., and Thompson, J. (Eds.) 1994. Beyond Farmer First: Rural People's Knowledge, Agricultural Research and Extension Practice. Intermediate Technology Publications, London.

Foucault, M. 1979. Discipline and punish: The birth of the prison. Harmondsworth, Penguin.

Foucault, M. 1980. Power/Knowledge: Selected Interviews and Other Writings 1972-77. Translated by C.Gordon, Brighton, Sussex: Harvester Press.

Francis, M.J.O. 1972. Biosynthesis of sesquiterpenes in *Pogostemon cablin* leaf discs. Planta Medica 22 (2), 201 - 204.

François, G., Passreiter, C.M., Woerdenbag, H.J., van Looveren, M. 1996. Antiplasmodial activities and cytotoxic effects of aqueous extracts and sesquiterpene lactones from *Neurolaena lobata*. Planta Medica 62 (2), 126 - 129.

Franklin, S. 1995. Science as culture, cultures as science. Ann. Rev. Anthropol. 24, 163 - 184.

Franssen, F., Smeijsters, L., Berger, I., Medinilla Aldana, B. 1997. *In vivo* and *in vitro* antiplasmodial activities of some plants traditionally used in Guatemala against malaria. Antimicrobial Agents and Chemotherapy 41 (7), 1500 - 1503.

Franzotti, E.M., Santos, C.V.F., Rodrigues, H.M.S.L., Mourão, R.H.V., Andrade, M.R., Antoniolli, A.R. 2000. Anti-inflammatory, analgesic activity and acute toxicity of *Sida cordifolia* L. (Malva-branca). Journal of Ethnopharmacology 72 (1-2), 273 - 278.

Frei, B., Baltisberger, M., Sticher, O., Heinrich, M. 1998. Medicinal ethnobotany of the Zapotecs of the Isthmus-Sierra (Oaxaca, Mexico): Documentation and assessment of indigenous uses. Journal of Ethnopharmacology 62 (1), 149 - 165.

Freire, M. de F.I, Abreu, H. dos. S., Cruz, L.C.H. da, Freire, R.B. 1996. Inhibition of fungal growth by extracts of *Vernonia scorpioides* (Lam.) Pers. Revista de Microbiologia 27 (1), 1-6.

Freire, S.M., Torres, L.M., Roque, N.F., Souccar, C., Lapa, A.J. 1991. Analgesic activity of a triterpene isolated from *Scoparia dulcis* L. (Vassourinha). Memorias do Instituto Oswaldo Cruz 86 Suppl 2, 149 - 151.

Friedman, J. 1999. The hybridization of roots and the abhorence of the bush. In: M. Featherstone and S. Lash 1999. (Ed.). Spaces of culture:city, nation, world. Sage Publications Ltd. Pp 230 - 256.

Frutuoso, V.S., Gurjao, M.R., Cordeiro, R.S., Martins, M.A. 1994. Analgesic and anti-ulcerogenic effects of a polar extract from leaves of *Vernonia condensata*. Planta Medica 60 (1), 21-5.

Funtowicz, S.O., Ravetz, J.R. 1993. Science for the post-normal age. Futures 25, (7), 739-755.

Galvez, J., Zarzuelo, A., Crespo, M.E., Lorente, M.D., Ocete, M.A., Jiménez, J. 1993. Antidiarrhoeic activity of *Euphorbia hirta* extract and isolation of an active flavonoid constituent. Planta Medica 59 (4), 333-6.

Ganai, G., Jha, G. 1991. Immunosuppression due to chronic *Lantana camara* L. toxicity in sheep. Indian Journal of Experimental Biology 29 (8), 762 - 766.

Garcia, M.D., Fernandez, M.A., Alvarez, A., Saenz, M.T. 2004. Antinociceptive and anti-inflammatory effect of the aqueous extract from leaves of *Pimenta racemosa* var. ozua (Mirtaceae). Journal of Ethnopharmacology 91(1): 69-73.

Garcia, C.C., Talarico, L., Almeida, N., Colombres, S., Duschatzky, C., Damonte, E.B. 2003. Virucidal activity of essential oils from aromatic plants of San Luis, Argentina. Phytother Res. 17(9):1073-5.

García, M.D., Quílez, A.M., Sáenz, M.T., Martínez-Domínguez, M.E., de la Puerta, R. 2000. Anti-inflammatory activity of *Agave intermixta* Trel. and *Cissus sicyoides* L., species used in the Caribbean traditional medicine. Journal of Ethnopharmacology 71(3), 395-400.

García, M.D., Saenz, M.T., Gomez, M.A., Fernandez, M.A. 1999a. Topical antiinflammatory activity of phytosterols isolated from *Eryngium foetidum* on chronic and acute inflammation models. Phytotherapy Research 13 (1), 78 - 80.

García, M.D., Saenz, M.T., Puerta, R., Quilez, A., Fernandez, M.A. 1999b. Antibacterial activity of *Agave intermixta* and *Cissus sicyoides*. Fitoterapia 70 (1), 71 - 73.

Garcia, X., Cartas-Heredia, L., Lorenzana-Jimenez, M., Gijon, E. 1997. Vasoconstrictor effect of *Cissus sicyoides* on guinea-pig aortic rings. Gen Pharmacol 29 (3), 457-62.

Geissberger, P., Sequin, U. 1991. Constituents of *Bidens pilosa* L.: Do the components found so far explain the use of this plant in traditional medicine? Acta Trop 48 (4), 251-61.

Ghisalberti, E.L. 2000. Lantana camara L. (Verbenaceae). Fitoterapia 71 (5): 467-86.

Ghosal, S., Singh, S., Bhattacharya, S. 1971. Alkaloids of *Mucuna pruriens* chemistry and pharmacology. Planta Medica 19 (3), 280 - 284.

Giarelli, G. 1996. Broadening the debate: The Tharaka participatory action research project. Indigenous Knowledge and Development Monitor 4 (2), 19 - 22.

Gibbons, M. 1999. Science's new social contract with society. Nature 402, Suppl. C81-C84.

Gilbert, L. 1998. Dispensing doctors and prescribing pharmacists: A South African perspective. Social Science and Medicine 46 (1), 83 - 95.

Gilkes, A.C. 1999. Wisdom for Solomon. Letter to the Editor, Sunday Express November 7th 1999.

Girón, L.M., Aguilar, G.A., Cáceres, A., Gerardo, L. 1988. Anticandidal activity of plants used for the treatment of vaginitis in Guatemala and clinical trial of a *Solanum nigrescens* preparation. Journal of Ethnopharmacology 22 (3), 307 - 313.

Girón, L.M., Freire, V., Alonzo, A., Cáceres, A. 1991. Ethnobotanical survey of the medicinal flora used by the Caribs of Guatemala. Journal of Ethnopharmacology 34 (2-3), 173 - 187.

Glucksmann, M. 1994. The work of knowledge and the knowledge of work. In: Maynard, M. and Purvis, J. (Eds.) 1994. Researching Women's Lives from a Feminist Perspective. Taylor and Francis, London.

Gmelch, George and Sharon Gmelch. 1996. Barbados's Amerindian past. Antrhopology Today 12 (1): 11 - 15.

Goda, Y., Hoshino, K., Akiyama, H., Ishikawa, T., Abe, Y., Nakamura, T., Otsuka, H., Takeda, Y., Tanimura, A., Toyoda, M. 1999. Constituents in watercress: inhibitors of histamine release from RBL-2H3 cells induced by antigen stimulation. Biol. Pharm. Bull. 22 (12), 1319-26.

Goff, J.P., Horst, R.L. 1997. Physiological changes at parturition and their relationship to metabolic disorders. J. Dairy Science 80 (7), 1260 - 8.

Goldsby, G., Burke, B. 1987. Sesquiterpene lactones and a sesquiterpene diol from Jamaican *Ambrosia peruviana*. Phytochemistry 26 (4), 1059 - 1063.

González, A.G., Bazzocchi, I.L., Moujir, L., Ravelo, A.G., Correa, M.D., Gupta, M.P. 1995. Xanthine oxidase inhibitory activity of some Panamanian plants from Celastraceae and Lamiaceae. Journal of Ethnopharmacology 46 (1), 25 - 29.

González-Tejero, M.R., Molero-Mesa, J., Casares-Porcel, M., Martínez-Lirola, M.J. 1995. New contributions to the ethnopharmacology of Spain. Journal of Ethnopharmacology 45 (3), 157 - 165.

Good, M. 1995. Cultural studies of biomedicine: an agenda for research. Social Science and Medicine 41 (4), 461 - 473.

Goodenough, W.H. 1996. Navigation in the Western Carolines: A traditional science. In: Laura Nader 1996. (Ed.) Naked Science: Anthropological inquiry into boundaries, power, and knowledge. Routledge, New York and London. Pp 29 - 42.

Gooding, E.G.B. 1940. Facts and beliefs about Barbadian plants. Journal of the Barbados Museum Historical Society 7 (4), 170 - 174.

Goodwin, J.S., Tangum, M.R. 1998. Battling quackery: attitudes about micronutrient supplements in American academic medicine. Arch. Intern. Med. 158 (20), 2187 - 2191.

Gordon, E.A., Guppy, L.J., Nelson, M. 2000. The antihypertensive effects of the Jamaican Cho-Cho (*Sechium edule*). West Indian Medical Journal 49 (1), 27 - 31.

Gore MA, Akolekar D: Evaluation of banana leaf dressing for partial thickness burn wounds. Burns 2003, 29(5):487-92.

Gorinstein S, Caspi A, Libman I, Katrich E, Lerner HT, Trakhtenberg S. 2004. Fresh israeli jaffa sweetie juice consumption improves lipid metabolism and increases antioxidant capacity in hypercholesterolemic patients suffering from coronary artery disease: studies in vitro and in humans and positive changes in albumin and fibrinogen fractions. J Agric Food Chem. 52(16):5215-22.

Gould, Stephen Jay. 2000. The creation myths of Cooperstown. Pp 520 – 531. In: Oates, Joyce Carol (ed.), Atwan, Robert (co-editor), 2000. The best American essays of the century. Boston, [MA]: Houghton Mifflin Company.

Gracioso, J.S., Hiruma-Lima, C.A., Souza Brito, A.R. 2000. Antiulcerogenic effect of a hydroalcoholic extract and its organic fractions of *Neurolaena lobata* R.BR. Phytomedicine 7 (4), 283 - 289.

Gracioso, J.S., Paulo, M.Q., Hiruma-Lima, C.A., Souza Brito, A.R. 1998. Antinociceptive effect in mice of a hydroalcoholic extract of *Neurolaena lobata* R.Br. and its organic fractions. Journal of Pharmacy and Pharmacology 50 (12), 1425 - 1429.

Gray, M., Jones, D.P. 2004. The effect of different formulations of equivalent active ingredients on the performance of two topical wound treatment products. Ostomy Wound Manage. 50 (3): 34-8, 40, 42-4.

Green, E.C. 1998. Etiology in human and animal ethnomedicine. Agriculture and Human Values 15 (2), 127 - 131.

Greenspan Gallo, L., Allee, L.L., Gibson, D.M. 1996. Insecticidal effectiveness of *Mammea americana* (Guttiferae) extracts on larvae of *Diabrotica virgifera virgifera* (Coleoptera: Chrysomelidea) and *Trichoplusia Ni* (Lepidoptera: Noctuidae). Economic Botany 50 (2), 236 - 242.

Grmek, Mirko, D. (ed.). 1998. Western medical thought from antiquity to the Middle Ages. Coordinated by Bernardino Fantini; translated by Antony Shugaar. Cambridge, Mass: Harvard University Press.

Grosvenor, P.W., Gothard, P.K., McWilliam, N.C., Suprionon, A., Gray, D.O. 1995. Medicinal plants from Riau Province, Sumatra, Indonesia. Part 1: Uses. Journal of Ethnopharmacology 45, 75 - 95.

Grover JK, Yadav S, Vats V. 2002. Medicinal plants of India with anti-diabetic potential. J Ethnopharmacol. 81(1):81-100.

Grover, J.K., Yadav, S.P. 2004. Pharmacological actions and potential uses of *Momordica charantia*: A review. J Ethnopharmacol. 93(1):123-32.

Guan, L., Quan, L.H., Xu, L.Z., Cong, P.Z. 1994. Chemical constituents of *Pogostemon cablin* (Blanco) Benth. Zhongguo Zhong Yao Za Zhi 19(6):355-6, 383 [Article in Chinese].

Guarrera, P.M. 1999. Traditional antihelmintic, antiparasitic and repellent uses of plants in Central Italy. Journal of Ethnopharmacology 68 (1-3), 183 - 192.

Guerrero MF, Puebla P, Carron R, Martin ML, Arteaga L, Roman LS. 2002. Assessment of the antihypertensive and vasodilator effects of ethanolic extracts of some Colombian medicinal plants. J Ethnopharmacol. 80(1):37-42.

Guèye, E. F. 1999. Ethnoveterinary medicine against poultry diseases in African villages. World's Poultry Science Journal, 55, 187 - 198.

Guilliford, M.C., Mahabir, D. 1997. Use of medicinal plants for diabetes in Trinidad [abstract]. Paper presented at the 42nd Annual Scientific Meeting of the Commonwealth Caribbean Medical Research Council, St. Maarten, April 16 - 19, 1997. West Indian Medical Journal 46 (Suppl. 2), 47.

Guilliford, M.C., Mahabir, D. 1998. Social inequalities in morbidity from diabetes mellitus in public primary care clinics in Trinidad and Tobago. Social Science and Medicinie 46 (1), 145 - 149.

Guimaraes, P.R., Galvao, A.M., Batista, C.M., Azevedo, G.S., Oliveira, R.D., Lamounier, R.P., Freire, N., Barros, A.M., Sakurai, E., Oliveira, J.P., Vieira, E.C., Alvarez-Leite, J.I. 2000. Eggplant (*Solanum melongena*) infusion has a modest and transitory effect on hypercholesterolemic subjects. Braz. J. Med. Biol. Res. 33 (9),1027-36.

Gupta M, Mazumder UK, Chaudhuri I, Chaudhuri RK, Bose P, Bhattacharya S, Manikandan L, Patra S. 2002. Antimicrobial activity of *Eupatorium ayapana*. *Fitoterapia* 73(2):168-70.

Gupta, A. 1990. Peasant knowledge -who has rights to use it? ILEIA Newsletter, March 1990 pg 24.

Gupta, M. P., Mireya, D., Correa, A., Solís, P. N., Jones, A., Galdames, C., Guionneau-Sinclair, F. 1993. Medicinal plant inventory of Kuna Indians: Part 1. Journal of Ethnopharmacology 40 (2), 77-109.

Gupta, M., Mazumder, U.K., Chakrabarti, S., Bhattacharya, S., Rath, N., Bhowal, S.R. 1997. Anti-epileptic and anti-cancer activity of some indigenous plants. Indian Journal of Physiology and Allied Sciences 51 (2), 53 - 56.

Gurib-Fakim, A., Sewraj, M., Gueho, J., Dulloo, E. 1993. Medicalethnobotany of some weeds of Mauritius and Rodrigues. Journal of Ethnopharmacology 39 (3), 175-85.

Gurib-Fakim, A., Sewraj, M.D., Gueho, J. Dullo, E. 1996. Medicinal plants of Rodrigues. International Journal of Pharmacognosy 34 (1), 2 - 14.

Guyer, J., Richards, P. 1996. The invention of biodiversity: social perspectives on the management of biological variety in Africa. Africa 66 (1), 1 - 13.

Gwehenberger, B., Rist, L., Huch, R., von Mandach, U. 2004. Effect of *Bryophyllum pinnatum* versus fenoterol on uterine contractility. *Eur J Obstet Gynecol Reprod Biol*. 113 (2):164-71.

Habtemariam, S. 1998. Extract of corn silk (stigma of *Zea mays*) inhibits the tumour necrosis factor-α- and bacterial lipopolysaccharide-induced cell adhesion and ICAM-1 expression. Planta Medica 64 (4), 314 - 318.

Habtemariam, S., Harvey, A.L., Waterman, P.G. 1993. The muscle relaxant properties of *Portulaca oleracea* are associated with high concentrations of potassium ions. Journal of Ethnopharmacology 40 (3), 195 - 2000.

Hammerton, J. 1989. Medicinal weeds. Caribbean Agricultural Research and Development Institute (CARDI), Trinidad and Tobago.

Handler, J.S., Jacoby, J. 1993. Slave medicine and plant use in Barbados. Journal of the Barbados Museum and Historical Society 41, 74 - 98.

Hansawasdi C, Kawabata J, Kasai T. 2000. Alpha-amylase inhibitors from roselle (*Hibiscus sabdariffa* Linn.) tea. Biosci. Biotechnol. Biochem. 64 (5), 1041-3.

Hansel, R., Leuschke, A., Bohlmann, F. 1980. A new isobutylamide from *Ottonia ovata* [the aerial parts of]. Planta Medica 40 (2), 161 - 163.

Harborne, J.B. 1975. Flavonoid bisulphates and their co-occurrences with ellagic acid in the Bixaceae, Frankeniaceae and related families. Phytochemistry 14 (5-6), 1331 - 1337.

Harris, R. 1991. Local Herbs Used in the Chinese Way (Tonics). Book 1. The Traditional Chinese Medical Centre, Trinidad and Tobago, W.I.

Harrison, P. 1994. The Impact of Oil on Trinidad and Tobago, 1966-1990. Working Paper Series No. 171. ISS, The Hague, the Netherlands.

Haslip-Viera, G., Ortiz de Montellano, B., Barbour, W. 1997. Robbing native American cultures: Van Sertima's Afrocentricity and the Olmecs. Current Anthropology 38 (3), 419 - 441.

Hasrat JA, Pieters L, Vlietinck AJ, 2004. Medicinal plants in Suriname: Hypotensive effect of *Gossypium barbadense*. J Pharm Pharmacol 56 (3): 381-7.

Hasrat, J.A., De Bruyne, T., De Backer, J.P., Vauquelin, G., Vlietinck, A.J. 1997a. Cirsimarin and cirsimaritin, flavonoids of *Microtea debilis* (Phytolaccaceae) with adenosine antagonistic properties in rats: leads for new therapeutics in acute renal failure. Journal of Pharmacy and Pharmacology 49 (11), 1150-6.

Hasrat, J.A., De Bruyne, T., De Backer, J.P., Vauquelin, G., Vlietinck, A.J.1997b. Isoquinoline derivatives isolated from the fruit of *Annona muricata* as 5-HTergic 5-HT1A receptor agonists in rats: unexploited antidepressive (lead) products. Journal of Pharmacy and Pharmacology 49 (11), 1145 - 9.

Hasrat, J.A., Pieters, L., Claeys, M., Vlietinck, A. 1997c. Adenosine-1 active ligands: cirsimarin, a flavone glycoside from *Microtea debilis*. Journal of Natural Products 60 (6), 638 - 641.

Hastrup, K., Elsass, P. 1990. Anthropological advocacy. Current Anthropology 31 (3), 301 - 311.

Hatten, R., Knapp, D. & Salonga, R. 2000. Action Research: Comparison with the Concepts of 'The Reflective Practitioner' and 'Quality Assurance'. Action Research E-Reports, 8. Available at: http://www.cchs.usyd.edu.au/arow/arer/008.htm. First published, 1997.

Hawkesworth, M. 1989. Knowers, knowing, known: Feminist theory and claims of truth. Signs 14 (3), 533 - 557.

Hayashi, K., Niwayama, S., Hayashi, T., Nago, R., Ochiai, H., Morita, N. 1988. *In vitro* and *in vivo* antiviral activity of scopadulcic acid B from *Scoparia dulcis*, Scrophulariaceae, against herpes simplex virus type 1. Antiviral Research 9 (6), 345 - 354.

Hayashi, T., Kawasaki, M., Miwa, Y., Taga, T., Morita, N. 1990. Antiviral agents of plant origin. III. Scopadulin, a novel tetracyclic diterpene from *Scoparia dulcis* L. Chemical and Pharmaceutical Bulletin 38 (4), 945 - 947.

Hayashi, T., Kawasaki, M., Okamura, K., Tamada, Y., Morita, N. 1992. Scoparic acid A, a α-glucuronidase inhibitor from *Scoparia dulcis*. Journal of Natural Products 55 (12), 1748 - 1755.

Hazlett, D.L. 1986. Ethnobotanical observations from Cabecar and Guaymí settlements in Central America. Economic Botany 40 (3), 339 - 352.

Hecht, S.S., Chung, F.L., Richie, J.P. Jr., Akerkar, S.A., Borukhova, A., Skowronski, L., Carmella, S.G. 1995. Effects of watercress consumption on metabolism of a tobacoo-specific lung carcinogen in smokers. Cancer Epidemiol Biomarkers Prev 4 (8), 877 - 884.

Heinen, H. Dieter and García-Castro, Alvarado. 2000. The multiethnic network of the Lower Orinoco in early Colonial times. Ethnohistory 47 (3-4): 561-579.

Heinrich, M., Rimpler, H., Antonio-Barrerra, N. 1992. Indigenous phytotherapy of gastrointestinal disorders in a lowland Mixe community (Oaxaca, Mexico): Ethnopharmacological evaluation. Journal of Ethnopharmacology 36 (1), 63 - 80.

Heinrich, M., Andrea Pieroni, Paul Bremner. 2005. Plants as medicines. In Prance,G. & M.Nesbitt (editors). Cultural history of plants. Routledge: Oxon and New York. Pp 205 – 238.

Hell, Bertrand. 1996. Enraged hunters: The domain of the wild in North-Western Europe. In Nature and Society: Anthropological Perspectives. Philippe Descola and Gísli Pálsson, eds. pp. 205 - 217. London: Routledge.

Hemlata, Kalidhar, S.B. 1993. Alatinone, an anthraquinone from *Cassia alata*. Phytochemistry 32 (6), 1616 - 1617.

Henry, John. 1998. Calls for a ceasefire in the Science wars. Book Review. Nature 395, 557 - 558.

Hernandez, T., Canales, M., Avila, J.G., Duran, A., Caballero, J., Romo de Vivar, A., Lira, R. 2003. Ethnobotany and antibacterial activity of some plants used in traditional medicine of Zapotitlan de las Salinas, Puebla (Mexico). J Ethnopharmacol. 88(2-3):181-8.

Hernández-Bermejo, J.E., García-Sánchez, E. 1998. Economic botany and ethnobotany in Al-Andalus (Iberian peninsula: tenth-fifteenth centuries), an unknown heritage of mankind. Economic Botany 52 (1), 15 - 26.

Herrera-Arellano A, Flores-Romero S, Chavez-Soto MA, Tortoriello J. 2004. Effectiveness and tolerability of a standardized extract from *Hibiscus sabdariffa* in patients with mild to moderate hypertension: a controlled and randomized clinical trial. Phytomedicine 11(5):375-82.

Herskovits, M. J., Herskovits, F.S. 1947 (1964). Trinidad village. New York: A. A. Knopf. Octagon Books Inc.

Higman, B.W. 1979. African and Creole Slave family Patterns in Trinidad. In: Crn, M.E. and Knight, F.W. (Eds.) 1979. Africa and the Caribbean: Legacies of a link. John Hopkins Press, Baltimore.

Hill, C.E. 1985. Local health knowledge and universal primary health care: A behavioral case from Costa Rica. Medical Anthropology 9 (1), 11 - 23.

Hilu, K.W., de Wet, J.M.J., Sergler, D. 1978. Flavonoid patterns and systematics in *Eleusine*. Biochemical Systematics and Ecology 6 (3), 247 - 249.

Hinrichsen, R.A. 2000. Are there scientific criteria for putting short-term conservation ahead of learning? No. Response to Kai N. Lee 1999: "Appraising adaptive management." Conservation Ecology 4 (1): r7. [online] URL: http://www.consecol.org/vol4/iss1/resp7.

Hirschhorn, H. 1981. Botanical remedies of South and Central America, and the Caribbean: An archival analysis. Part I. Journal of Ethnopharmacology 4 (2), 129 - 158.

Hirschhorn, H. 1982. Botanical remedies of South and Central America, and the Caribbean: An archival analysis. Part II. Conclusion. Journal of Ethnopharmacology 5 (2), 163 - 180.

Hirschhorn, H. 1983. Constructing a phytotherapeutic concordance based upon Tropical American and Indonesian examples. Journal of Ethnopharmacology 7 (2), 157 - 167.

Hirschmann, G.S., Rojas de Arias, A. 1990. A survey of medicinal plants of Minas Gerais, Brazil. Journal of Ethnopharmacology 29, 159 - 172.

Hiruma-Lima, C.A., Gracioso, J.S., Bighetti, E.J., Germonsén-Robineau, L., Souza Brito, A.R. 2000. The juice of fresh leaves of *Boerhaavia diffusa* L. (Nyctaginaceae) markedly reduces pain in mice. Journal of Ethnopharmacology 71 (1-2), 267-274.

Hodge, W. H., Taylor, D. 1957. The ethnobotany of the island Caribs of Dominica. Webbia 12 (2), 513 - 644.

Hoffman, B., Hölzl, J. 1987. New chalcones from *Bidens pilosa*. Planta Medica 54 (1), 52 - 54.

Hoffman, B., Hölzl, J. 1988. Further acylated chalcones from *Bidens pilosa*. Planta Medica 54 (5), 450 - 451.

Holland, J., Ramazanoglu, C. 1994. Coming to conclusions: power and interpretation in researching young women's sexuality. In: Maynard, M., Purvis, J. 1994. (Eds.) Researching women's lives from a feminist perspective. Taylor and Francis, London. Pp. 125 - 148.

Honychurch, P.N. 1986. Caribbean wild plants and their uses. Macmillan Education Ltd., London. 166 p.

Horigome, T., Sakaguchi, E., Kishimoto, C. 1992. Hypocholesterolaemic effect of banana (*Musa sapientum* L. var. Cavendishii) pulp in the rat fed on a cholesterol-containing diet. British Journal of Nutrition 68 (1), 231 - 44.

Hornborg, A. 1996. Ecology as semiotics: Outlines of a contxtualist paradigm for human ecology. In: Descola, P., Pálsson, G. 1996. (Eds.). Nature and society: anthropological perspectives. Routledge, London, pp. 45 - 62.

Horsten, S., van den Berg, A., Kettenes-van den Bosch, J., Leeflang, B., Labadie, R. 1996. Cyclogossine A: a novel cyclic heptapeptide isolated from the latex of *Jatropha gossypifolia*. Planta Medica 62 (1), 46 - 50.

Hosseinzadeh H, Nourbakhsh M: Effect of *Rosmarinus officinalis* L. aerial parts extract on morphine withdrawal syndrome in mice. *Phytother Res*. 2003, 17 (8): 938-41.

Hubbard, R. 1988. Some thoughts about the masculinity of the natural sciences. In: M.M. Gergen 1988 (Ed.). Feminist Thought and the Structure of Knowledge. New York University Press.

Hudson, J.B. 1990. Antiviral compounds from plants. CRC Press Inc., Boca Raton, Florida.

Hufford, C., Oguntimein, B. 1978. Non-polar constituents of *Jatropha curcas*. Lloydia 41 (2), 161 – 165.

Hulme, Peter. 2000. Remnants of Conquest: The Island Caribs and Their Visitors, 1877 - 1998. Oxford and New York: Oxford UP.

Hutter, J.A., Salman, M., Stavinoha, W.B., Satsangi, N., Williams, R.F., Streeper, B.T., Weintraub, S.T. 1996. Antiinflammatory C-glucosyl chromone from *Aloe barbadensis*. Journal of Natural Products 59 (5), 541 - 543.

IADB, 1995. Sixty-five million dollar loan to modernize agriculture in Trinidad and Tobago NR-190/95. Press release, September 21, 1995, Inter-American Development Bank.

Iauk, L., Galati, E.M., Kirjavainen, S., Forestieri, A.M., Trovato, A. 1993. Analgesic and antipyretic effects of *Mucuna pruriens*. International Journal of Pharmacognosy 31 (3), 213 - 216.

Ibrahim MA. 1996. Ethno-toxicology among Nigerian pastoralists. Pp. 54 - 59. In: *Ethnoveterinary research and development*, (Eds.). McCorkle CM, Mathias-Mundy E and Schillhorn van Veen T. 1996. London: IT Publications.

Ibrahim, D., Osman, H. 1995. Antimicrobial activity of *Cassia alata* from Malaysia. Journal of Ethnopharmacology 45 (3), 151 - 156.

Ibrahim, M.A. 1996. Ethno-toxicology among Nigerian pastoralists. In: McCorkle, C.M., Mathias-Mundy, E., Schillhorn van Veen, T. 1996. (Eds.) Ethnoveterinary research and development. IT Publications, London. Pp. 54 - 59.

IIRR, 1994. Ethnoveterinary medicine in Asia: An information kit on traditional animal health care practices. 4 Vols. International Institute of Rural Reconstruction, Silang, Cavite, Philippines.

Ikerd, J.E. 1993. The question of good science. American Journal of Alternative Agriculture 8 (2), 91 - 93.

Ilori, M., Sheteolu, A.O., Omonigbehin, E.A., Adeneye, A.A. 1996. Antidiarrhoeal activities of *Ocimum gratissimum* (Lamiaceae). J. Diarrhoeal Dis. Res. 14 (4), 283-5.

Im Thurn, E.F. (1883), 1967. Among the Indians of Guiana. Reprint. Dover Publications Inc, New York.

Indrayanto, G., Setiawan, B., Cholies, N. 1994. Differential diosgenin accumulation in *Costus speciosus* and its tissue cultures. Planta Medica 60 (5), 483-4.

Ingold, T. 1996. The optimal forager and economic man. In: Descola, P., Pálsson, G. 1996. (Eds.)). Nature and society: anthropological perspectives. Routledge, London, pp. 25 - 44.

Inniss, L.O. 1910. Trinidad and Trinidadians. A collection of papers, historical, social and descriptive about Trinidad and its people. Mirror Printing Works, Trinidad, B.W.I.

Inoue, K., Shimomura, K., Kobayashi, S., Sankawa, U., Ebizuka, Y. 1996. Conversion of furostanol glycoside to spirostanol glycoside by beta-glucosidase in *Costus speciosus*. Phytochemistry 41 (3), 725 - 727.

INRA-CARDI, 1991. Weeds of the lesser antilles, mauvais herbes des petites antilles. Institut National de la Recherche Agronomique, Paris.

IMA, 2006. Development of a National Programme of Action (NPA) for the Protection of the Marine Environment from Land-based Sources and Activities. Report on Tobago Stakeholders' Consultation 11 – 12 April 2006
http://www.ima.gov.tt/NPA%20Tobago%20Stakeholders'%20Consultation%20Final%20Report.pdf.

IMF, 2005. IMF Executive Board Concludes 2005 Article IV Consultation with Trinidad and Tobago Public Information Notice (PIN) No. 05/159 November 30, 2005.
http://www.imf.org/external/np/sec/pn/2005/pn05159.htm

Ioset, J.R., Marston, A., Gupta, M.P., Hostettmann, K. 2000. Antifungal and larvicidal cordiaquinones from the roots of *Cordia curassavica*. Phytochemistry 53 (5), 613-7.

Izzo, A.A., Sautebin, L., Borrelli, F., Longo, R., Capasso, F. 1999. The role of nitric oxide in aloe-induced diarrhoea in the rat. European Journal of Pharmacology 368, 43 - 48.

Jackson, Jean. 1989. Is there a way to talk about making culture without making enemies? Dialectical Anthropology 14, 127 - 143.

Jager, A.K., Hutchings, A., van Staden, J. 1996. Screening of Zulu medicinal plants for prostaglandin-synthesis inhibitors. Journal of Ethnopharmacology 52 (2), 95-100.

Jagtap AG, Shirke SS, Phadke AS. Effect of polyherbal formulation on experimental models of inflammatory bowel diseases. J Ethnopharmacol. 2004, 90(2-3):195-204.

Jain, S., Singh, S., Puri, H. 1994. Medicinal plants of Neterhat, Bihar, India. International Journal of Pharmacognosy 32 (1), 44 - 50.

Jainu M, Devi CS. Effect of *Cissus quadrangularis* on gastric mucosal defensive factors in experimentally induced gastric ulcer-a comparative study with sucralfate.J Med Food. 2004, 7(3):372-6.

Jakupovic, J., Baruah, R., Thi, T., Bohlmann, F., Msonthi, J., Schmeda-Hirschmann, G. 1985. New vernolepin derivatives from *Vernonia glabra* and glaucolides from *Vernonia scorpioides*. Plant. Med. J. Med. Plant. Res. 5, 378 - 380.

Janssen, A.M., Scheffer, J.J., Ntezurubanza, L., Baerheim Svendsen, A. 1989. Antimicrobial activities of some *Ocimum* species grown in Rwanda. Journal of Ethnopharmacology 26 (1), 57-63.

Jasanoff, S. 1999. Knowledge élites and class war. Millenium essay. Nature 401, 531.

Jayathirtha MG, Mishra SH: Preliminary immunomodulatory activities of methanol extracts of *Eclipta alba* and *Centella asiatica*. *Phytomedicine* 2004, 11(4):361-5.

Jedlickova, Z., Mottl, O., Sery, V. 1992. Antibacterial properties of the Vietnamese cajeput oil and ocimum oil in combination with antibacterial agents. J. Hyg. Epidemiol. Microbiol. Immunol. 36 (3), 303-9.

Jelager, L., Gurib-Fakim, A., Adersen, A. 1998. Antibacterial and antifungal activity of medicinal plants of Mauritius. Pharmaceutical Biology 36 (3), 153 - 161.

Jenett-Siems, K., Mockenhaupt, F.P., Bienzle, U., Gupta, M.P., Eich, E. 1999. *In vitro* antiplasmodial activity of Central American medicinal plants. Tropical Medicine and International Health 4 (9), 611 - 615.

Jeong, S-J., Miyamoto, T., Inagaki, M., Kim, Y-C., Higuchi, R. 2000. Rotundines A-C, three novel sesquiterpene alkaloids from *Cyperus rotundus*. Journal of Natural Products 63 (5), 673 - 675.

Jie, L. 1995. Pharmacology of oleanolic acid and ursolic acid. Review. Journal of Ethnopharmacology 49 (2), 57 - 68.

Jiggins, J., Gibbon, D. 1997. What does interdisciplinary mean? Experiences from SLU. Paper presented to the 13th European seminar on extension education. The Challenges for Extension Education in a Changing Rural World. Eds. A. Markey, J. Phelan, S. Wilson, University College Dublin, Ireland. Pp. 317 - 325.

Jiggins, J., Röling, N. 2000. Adaptive management: Potential and limitations for ecological governance. International Journal of Agricultural Resources, Governance and Ecology 1 (1), 28 - 42.

Jimenez Misas, C.A., Rojas Hernandez, N.M., Lopez Abraham, A.M. 1979. Biological evaluation of Cuban plants.II. [Article in Spanish] Rev. Cubana Med. Trop. 31 (1), 13 - 19.

Jimenez Misas, C.A., Rojas Hernandez, N.M., Lopez Abraham, A.M. 1979. Biological evaluation of Cuban plants.V. [Article in Spanish] Rev. Cubana Med. Trop. 31 (1), 37 - 43.

Jiu, J. 1966. A survey of some medicinal plants of Mexico for selected biological activities. Lloydia 29 (3), 250 - 259.

Johannsen, A.M. 1992. Applied anthropology and post-modern ethnography. Human Organization 51 (1), 71 - 81.

Johnson, P.B., Abdurahman, E.M., Tiam, E.A., Abdu-Aguye, I., Hussaini, I.M. 1999. *Euphorbia hirta* leaf extracts increase urine output and electrolytes in rats. Journal of Ethnopharmacology 65 (1), 63-9.

Joly, L., Guerra, S., Séptimo, R, Solís, P., Correa, M., Gupta, M., Levy, S., Sandberg, F. 1987. Ethnobotanical inventory of medicinal plants used by the Guaymi Indians in Western Panama. Part I. Journal of Ethnopharmacology 20 (2), 145 - 171.

Joly, L., Guerra, S., Séptimo, R, Solís, P., Correa, M., Gupta, M., Levy, S., Sandberg, F., Perera, P. 1990. Ethnobotanical inventory of medicinal plants used by the Guaymi Indians in Western Panama. Part II. Journal of Ethnopharmacology 28 (2), 191 - 206.

Joseph, E.L. 1837. History of Trinidad. Henry James Mills, London.

Joshi, A., Joshi, K. 2000. Indigenous knowledge and uses of medicinal plants by local communities of the Kali Gandaki Watershed area, Nepal. Journal of Ethnopharmacology 73 (1-2), 175 - 183.

Jovel, E.M., Cabanillas, J., Towers, G.H.N. 1996. An ethnobotanical study of the traditional medicine of the Mestizo people of Suni Miraño, Loreto, Peru. Journal of Ethnopharmacology 53 (3), 149 - 156.

Joyamma, V., Rao, S.G., Hrishikeshavan, H.J., Aroor, A.R., Kulkarni, D.R. 1990. Biochemical mechanisms and effects of *Mimosa pudica* (Linn) on experimental urolithiasis in rats. Indian J. Exp. Biol. 28(3), 237-40.

Joyeux, M., Mortier, F., Fleurentin, J. 1995. Screening of antiradical, antilipoperoxidant and hepatoprotective effects of nine plant extracts used in Caribbean folk medicine. Short Communication. Phytotherapy Research 9, 228 - 230.

Jukola, E., Hakkarainen, J., Saloniemi, H., Sankari, S. 1996. Blood selenium, vitamin E, vitamin A, and beta-carotene concentrations and udder health, fertility treatments, and fertility. J. Dairy Sci. 79 (5), 834- 45.

Juska, Arunas, Busch, Lawrence. 1994. The Production of Knowledge and the Production of Commodities: The Case of Rapeseed Technoscience. Rural Sociology 59, 581 - 597.

Kainer, K.A., Duryea, M.L. 1992. Tapping women's knowledge: plant resource use in extractive reserves, Acre, Brazil. Economic Botany 46 (4), 408 - 425.

Kaminjolo, J.S., Adesiyun, A.A. 1994. Rotavirus infection in calves, piglets, lambs and goat kids in Trinidad. British Veterinary Journal 150 (3), 293 - 299.

Kaminjolo, J.S., Adesiyun, A.A., Loregnard, R., Kitson-Piggott, W. 1993. Prevalence of *Cryptosporidium oocysts* in livestock in Trinidad and Tobago. Veterinary Parasitology 45 (3-4), 209-13.

Kamtchouing P, Mbongue GY, Dimo T, Watcho P, Jatsa HB, Sokeng SD: Effects of *Aframomum melegueta* and *Piper guineense* on sexual behaviour of male rats. *Behav Pharmacol*. 2002, 13 (3):243-7.

Kankofer, M., Wiercinsky, J., Kedzierski, W., Mierzynski, R. 1996a. The analysis of fatty acid content and phospholipase A_2 activity in placenta of cows with and without retained fetal membranes. Zentralblatt Fur Veterinarimedizin - Reihe A, 43 (8), 459 - 65.

Kankofer, M., Podolak, M., Fideckim M., Gondek, T. 1996b. Activity of placental glutathione peroxidase and superoxide dismutase in cows with and without retained fetal membranes. Placenta 17 (8), 591 - 4.

Kankofer, M., Maj, J.G. 1997. Enzyme activities in placental tissues from cows with and without retained fetal membranes. Deutsche Tierarztliche Wochenschrift 104 (1), 13 - 4.

Kapoor, L.D. 1990. Handbook of Ayurvedic medicinal plants. CRC Press Inc., Boca Raton, Florida, 416 pp.

Karimi G, Hosseinzadeh H, Ettehad N. 2004. Evaluation of the gastric antiulcerogenic effects of *Portulaca oleracea* L. extracts in mice. Phytother Res. 18(6):484-7.

Karpilovskaia, E.D., Gorban, G.P., Pliss, M.B., Zakharenko, L.N., Gulich, M.P. 1989. Inhibiting effect of the polyphenolic complex from *Plantago major* (plantastine) on the carcinogenic effect of endogenously synthesized nitrosodimethylamine. Farmakol Toksikol 52 (4), 64-7. [Article in Russian].

Kasonia, K.1995. Preliminary screening of plant extracts used in respiratory pathology in Kivu/Zaire on isolated guinea pigs rings trachea. Belgian Journal of Botany 128 (2), 165 - 175.

Kasture, V.S., Chopde, C.T., Deshmukh, V.K. 2000. Anticonvulsive activity of *Albizzia lebbeck*, *Hibiscus rosa sinensis* and *Butea monosperma* in experimental animals. Journal of Ethnopharmacology 71 (1-2), 65 - 75.

Katz, C. 1996. The expeditions of conjurers: Ethnography, power and pretense. In: Wolf, D.L 1996 (Ed.). Feminist dilemmas in fieldwork, West View Press, Boulder, Colorado, USA.

Kay, J.W. 1994. Politics without human nature? Reconstructing a common humanity. Hypatia 9 (1), 21 - 52.

Kay, M.A. 1996. Healing with plants in the American and Mexican West. University of Arizona Press, Tuscon, 315 pp.

Kelly, L., Regan, L., Burton, S. 1992. Defending the indefensible? Quantitative methods and feminist research. In: Hinds, H., Phoenix, A., Stacey, J. 1992. Working out: New directions for women's studies. The Falmer Press, London, Washington, DC. Pp. 149 - 160.

Kerr, E.A. 1998. Toward a feminist natural science: linking theory and practice. Women's Studies International Forum 21 (1), 95 - 109.

Khan, M.R., Omoloso, AD. 2002. Antibacterial activity of *Hygrophila stricta* and *Peperomia pellucida*. Fitoterapia 73(3):251-4.

Khobragade, V.R., Jangde, C.R. 1996. Antiinflammatory activity of bulb of *Allium sativum* Linn. Indian Veterinary Journal 73, 349 - 351.

Kielstra, N. 1979. Is useful action research possible? In: Huizer, G., Mannheim, B. 1979 (Eds.) The politics of anthropology: from colonialism and sexism toward a view from below. Mouton Publishers, the Hague, Paris. Pp. 281 -289.

Kim, G.S., Zeng, L., Alali, F., Rogers, L.L., Wu, F.E., McLaughlin, J.L., Sastrodihardjo, S. 1998. Two new mono-tetrahydrofuran ring acetogenins, annomuricin E and muricapentocin, from the leaves of *Annona muricata*. Journal of Natural Products 61(4), 432-6.

Kim, S.Y., Gao, J.J., Kang, H.K. 2000. Two flavonoids from the leaves of *Morus alba* induce differentiation of the human promyelocytic leukemia (HL-60) cell line. Biol. Pharm. Bull. 23(4), 451-5.

Kim, S.Y., Gao, J.J., Lee, W.C., Ryu, K.S., Lee, K.R., Kim, Y.C. 1999. Antioxidative flavonoids from the leaves of *Morus alba*. Arch. Pharm. Res. 22 (1), 81-5.

Kirszberg C, Esquenazi D, Alviano CS, Rumjanek VM: The effect of a catechin-rich extract of Cocos nucifera on lymphocytes proliferation. Phytother Res. 2003, 17(9):1054-8.

Kloppenburg, Jack, Jr. 1991. Social theory and the de/reconstruction of agricultural Science: Local Knowledge for an alternative agriculture. Rural Sociology 56 (4), 519 - 548.

Kloppenburg, Jack, Jr. 1992. Science in agriculture: A reply to Molnar, Duffy, Cummins and Van Santen and to Flora. Rural Sociology 57, 98 - 107.

Ko, F.N., Huang, T.F., Teng, C.M. 1991. Vasodilatory action mechanisms of apigenin isolated from *Apium graveolens* in rat thoracic aorta. Biochim Biophys Acta 115 (1), 69-74.

Koch, A. 1993. Investigations on the laxative action of aloin in the human colon. Planta Medica 59 (7) (Suppl), A689.

Konning GH, Agyare C, Ennison B. Antimicrobial activity of some medicinal plants from Ghana. Fitoterapia. 2004 75(1):65-7.

Koshimizu, K., Ohigashi, H., Huffman, M.A. 1994. Use of *Vernonia amygdalina* by wild chimpanzee: possible roles of its bitter and related constituents. Physiol. Behav. 56 (6), 1209-16.

Koshte, V.L., van Dijk, W., van der Stelt, M.E., Aalberse, R.C. 1990. Isolation and characterization of BanLec-1, a mannoside-binding lectin from *Musa paradisiac* (banana). Biochemical Journal 272 (3), 721 - 726.

Kreuger, R.A. 1988. Focus groups: a practical guide for applied research. Sage, London.

Kricher, John. 1989. A Neotropical Companion: An introduction to the Animals, Plants, and Ecosystems of the New World Tropics. Princeton: Princeton University Press.

Krimsky and Plough, 1988. In: Brown, P. and E.J. Mikkelson 1990 (Eds.). No Safe Place. Toxic Waste, Leukemia and Community Action. University of California Press, California.

Kubec R, Kim S, Musah RA, 2003. The lachrymatory principle of *Petiveria alliacea*. Phytochemistry 63 (1): 37-40.

Kubec R, Kim S, Musah RA: S-Substituted cysteine derivatives and thiosulfinate formation in *Petiveria alliacea* - part II. *Phytochemistry* 2002, 61(6): 675-80.

Kumar D, Mishra SK and Tripathi HC. 1991. Mechanism of anthelmintic action of benzylisothiocyanate. *Fitoterapia* 62: 403 - 410.

Kunz Thomas H and Diaz Carlos A. 1995. Folivory in fruit-eating bats, with new evidence from *Artibeus jamaicensis* (Chiroptera: Phyllostomidae). *Biotropica* 27: 106 - 120.

Kupchan, S.M., Doskotch, R.W., Bollinger, P., Mcphail, A.T., Sim, G.A., Renauld, J.A. 1965. The isolation and structural elucidation of a novel steroidal tumour inhibitor from *Acnistus arborescens*. Journal of the American Chemical Society 87 (24), 5805 - 5806.

Krumeich, A. 1994. The blessings of motherhood: Health, pregnancy and childcare in Dominica. Het Spinhuis, Amsterdam.

Labadie, R. P., Nat, J. M., van der, Simons, J. M., Kroes, B. H., Kosasi, S., Berg, A. J. J., van den, t'Hart, L. A., Sluis, W. G., van der, Abeysekera, A., Bamunuarachchi, A., De Silva, K. T. D. 1989. An Ethnopharmacognostic approach to the search for immunomodulators of plant origin. Planta Medica 55 (4), 339-348.

Lachman-White, D.A., Adams, C.D., Trotz, Ulric, O'D. 1992. A guide to the medicinal plants of coastal Guyana. Commonwealth Science Council, London, 350 pp.

Laferriere, J. 1994. Medicinal plants of the lowland Inga people of Colombia. International Journal of Pharmacognosy 32 (1), 90 - 94.

Lagreca L and Marotta E. 1985. Nutritional effect of pectin in swine during growth and before slaughter. *Arch. Latinoam. Nutr.* 35: 172-9. (in Spanish).

LaGuerre, J.G. (Ed.) 1984. Calcutta to Caroni: The East Indians of Trinidad. Longman Caribbean.

Laguerre, M. 1987. Afro-Caribbean folk medicine. Bergin and Garvey Publishers Inc. Massachusetts, USA.

Lakshmi Kumari P, Sumathi S: Effect of consumption of finger millet on hyperglycemia in non-insulin dependent diabetes mellitus (NIDDM) subjects. *Plant Foods Hum Nutr.* 2002, 57(3-4): 205-13.

Lal Jawahar, Chandra, S., Gupta, S., Tandan, S.K. 1990. Studies on anticonvulsant and anti-inflammatory actions of extracts of *Momordica charantia*. Indian Veterinary Journal 67, 82-83.

Lal, J., Gupta, P.C. 1973. Physcion and phytosterol from the roots of *Cassia occidentalis*. Phytochemistry 12, 1186.

Lal B, Kapoor AK, Agrawal PK, Asthana OP, Srimal RC. 2000. Role of curcumin in idiopathic inflammatory orbital pseudotumours. Phytother Res. 14 (6):443-7.

Lambie, N., Ngeleka, M., Brown, G., Ryan, J. 2000. Retrospective study on *Escherichia coli* infection in broilers subjected to postmortem examination and antibiotic resistance of isolates in Trinidad. Avian Diseases 44 (1), 155 - 160.

Landman, J., St. E. Hall, J. 1983. The dietary habits and knowledge of folklore of pregnant Jamaican women. Ecology of Food and Nutrition 12, 203 - 210.

Lanhers, M-C., Fleurentin, J., Cabalion, P., Rolland, A., Dorfman, P., Misslin, R., Pelt, J-M. 1990. Behavioural effects of *Euphorbia hirta* L.: sedative and anxiolytic properties. Journal of Ethnopharmacology 29 (2), 189 - 198.

Lanhers, M-C., Fleurentin, J., Dorfman, P., Mortier, F., Pelt, J-M. 1991. Analgesic, antipyretic and anti-inflammatory properties of *Euphorbia hirta*. Planta Medica 57 (3), 225-31.

Lans, C. 1996. Ethnoveterinary practices used by livestock keepers in Trinidad and Tobago. Unpublished M.Sc. thesis. Wageningen: Agricultural University, Dept. of Ecological Agriculture, the Netherlands.

Lans, C. unpublished. Research proposal for CNIRD. Medicinal Plant Research and Documentation in the wider Caribbean.

Lans, C. 2001. Creole remedies: case studies of ethnoveterinary medicine in Trinidad and Tobago, PhD dissertation, Wageningen University, the Netherlands.

Lans, C., Brown, G. 1998a. Observations on Ethnoveterinary medicines in Trinidad and Tobago. Preventive Veterinary Medicine 35 (2), 125 - 142.

Lans, C., Brown, G. 1998b. Ethnoveterinary medicines used for ruminants in Trinidad and Tobago. Preventive Veterinary Medicine 35 (3), 149 - 163.

Lans, C., Röling, N. 1998c. Feminist methods, women's traditional health knowledge and ethnoveterinary knowledge. Working Paper No.3. Centre for Gender and Development Studies, University of the West Indies, St. Augustine.

Lans, C., Harper, T., Georges, K., Bridgewater, E. 2000. Medicinal plants used for dogs in Trinidad and Tobago. Preventive Veterinary Medicine 45 (3-4), 201 - 220.

Lans, Cheryl, Harper, Tisha, Georges, Karla, and Bridgewater, Elmo. 2001. Medicinal and ethnoveterinary remedies of hunters in Trinidad. BMC Alternative and Complementary Medicine 1:10.

Lans, C. and Brown, G. 2004. The poultry surveillance unit in Trinidad and Tobago: A possible model for livestock-based extension. Journal of International Agricultural and Extension Education 11 (3): 5 – 12.

Lans, C., Brown, G., Borde, G., Offiah, V.N. 2004. Knowledge of traditional medicines and veterinary practices used for reproductive health problems in human and animal health. Journal of Ethnobiology 23 (2): 187 – 208.

Lastra AL, Ramirez TO, Salazar L, Martinez M, Trujillo-Ferrara J: The ambrosanolide cumanin inhibits macrophage nitric oxide synthesis: some structural considerations. *J Ethnopharmacol.* 2004, 95 (2-3): 221-7.

Latorre, D.L., Latorre, F.A. 1977. Plants used by the Mexican Kickapoo Indians. Economic Botany 31 (3), 340 - 357.

Latour, B. 1986. Visualization and cognition: thinking with eyes and hands; knowledge and society. studies in the sociology of culture past and present 1-40 In: Dewalt, B.R. Using Indigenous Knowledge to Improve Agriculture and Natural Resource Management. Human Organization 53 (2), 123-131.

Latour, B. 1988. The Pasteurization of France. Harvard University Press. Cambridge, Massachusetts.

Latour, B. 1993. Ethnography of a "High-Tech" Case. About Aramis. In: Lemonnier, P. 1993. Technological Choices. Transformation in material cultures since the Neolithic. Routledge, London.

Latour, Bruno. 1998. From the world of Science to the world of Research? Essays on Science and Society. Science 280, 208 - 209.

Latshaw JD. 1991. Nutrition - mechanisms of immunosuppression. Veterinary Immunonology Immunopathology 30:111 – 120.

Lave, J. 1996. The savagery of the domestic mind. In: Laura Nader 1996 (Ed.) Naked Science: Anthropological inquiry into boundaries, power, and knowledge. Routledge, New York and London. Pp. 87 - 101.

Laven, R.A., Peters, A.R. 1996. Bovine retained placenta: Aetiology, pathogenesis and economic loss. Review Article. Veterinary Record 139, 465 - 471.

Law, J. 1987. Technology and heterogeneous engineering: the case of Portuguese expansion. In: Bijker, W.E, Hughes, T.P., Pinch, T.J. 1987 (Eds.). The social construction of technological systems. New directions in the sociology and history of technology. Pp 111-134.

Law, J. 1991. Power, discretion and strategy. In: Law, J. 1991 (Ed.). A Sociology of Monsters. Essays on Power, Domination and Control. Sociological Review Monograph 38. Routledge, London.

Lawrence, E.A. 1998. Human and horse medicine among some Native American groups. Agriculture and Human Values 15 (2), 133 - 138.

Lawrence, P.A. 1999. The fashions and foibles of science. Nature 397, 487 - 488.

Leal, L.K.A.M., Ferreira, A.A.G., Bezerra, G.A., Matos, F.J.A., Viana, G.S.B. 2000. Antinociceptive, anti-inflammatory and bronchodilator activities of Brazilian medicinal plants containing coumarin: A comparative study. Journal of Ethnopharmacology 70 (2), 151 - 159.

Lee, Ik-Soo, Shamon, L.A., Chai, H-B., Chagwedera, T.E., Besterman, J.M., Farnsworth, N.R., Cordell, G.A., Pezzuto, J.M., Kinghorn, A.D. 1996. Cell-cycle specific cytotoxicity mediated by rearranged *ent-*

kaurene diterpenoids isolated from *Parinari curatellifolia*. Chemico-Biological Interactions 99 (1-3), 193 - 204.

Leite, J.R., de Seabra, M.L., Maluf, E., Assolant, K., Suchecki, D., Tufik, S., Klepacz, S., Calil, H,M., Carlini, E.A. 1986. Pharmacology of lemongrass (*Cymbopogon citratus* Stapf). III. Assessment of eventual toxic, hypnotic and anxiolytic effects on humans. Journal of Ethnopharmacology 17 (1), 75-83.

Lemos, T.L.G., Nogueira, P.C.L., Alençar, J.W., Craveiro, A.A. 1995. Composition of the leaf oils of four *Spondias* species from Brazil. Journal of Essential Oil Research 7 (5), 561 - 653.

Lemus, I., Garcia, R., Delvillar, E., Knop, G. 1999. Hypoglycaemic activity of four plants used in Chilean popular medicine. Phytotherapy Research 13 (2), 91-4.

Lentz, D.L., Clark, A.M., Hufford, C.D., Meurer-Grimes, B., Passreiter, C.M., Cordero, J., Ibrahimi, O., Okunade, A.L. 1998. Antimicrobial properties of Honduran medicinal plants. Short communication. Journal of Ethnopharmacology 63 (3), 253 - 263.

Lewis, D.A. 1989. Anti-inflammatory drugs from plant and marine sources. Birkhäuser Verlag, Basel, Switzerland.

Lewis, L. 1998. Masculinity and the dance of the dragon: reading Lovelace discursively. Feminist Review 59, 164 - 185.

Liaw CC, Chang FR, Lin CY, Chou CJ, Chiu HF, Wu MJ, Wu YC. 2002. New cytotoxic monotetrahydrofuran annonaceous acetogenins from *Annona muricata*.

Limmatvapirat C, Sirisopanaporn S, Kittakoop P., 2004. Antitubercular and antiplasmodial constituents of *Abrus precatorius*. Planta Med. 70 (3):276-8.

Lin, C., Shieh, W., Jong, T. 1992. A pyranodihydrobenzoxanthone epoxide from *Artocarpus communis*. Phytochemistry 31 (7), 2563 - 2564.

Littlewood, R. 1988. From vice to madness: The semantics of naturalistic and personalistic understandings in Trinidadian local medicine. Social Science and Medicine 27 (2), 129 - 148.

Littlewood, R. 1993. Pathology and identity: The work of Mother Earth in Trinidad. Cambridge University Press. Cambridge.

Liu, K.C.S., Lin, Mei-Tsu, Lee, Shoei-Sheng, L., Chiou, Jwo-Farn, Ren, S., Lien, E.J. 1999. Antiviral tannins from two *Phyllanthus* species. Planta Medica 65 (1), 43 - 46.

Liu, X.X., Alali, F.Q., Pilarinou, E., McLaughlin, J.L. 1998. Glacins A and B, two novel bioactive mono-tetrahydrofuran acetogenins from *Annona glabra*. Journal of Natural Products 61(5), 620-4.

Lizarralde, R., Beckerman, S., and Elsass P. 1987. Indigenous survival among the Barí and Arhuaco: Strategies and perspectives. IWGIA document no. 60. Copenhagen.

Lohezic-Le Devehat, F., Bakhtiar, A., Bezivin, C., Amoros, M., Boustie, J. 2002. Antiviral and cytotoxic activities of some Indonesian plants. Fitoterapia 73 (5): 400-5.

Lomniczi de Upton, I.M., de la Fuente, J.R., Esteve Romero, J.S., Garcia Alvarez Coque, M.C., Carda Broch, S. 1999. Chromatographic detection of sesquiterpene lactones in *Parthenium* plants from Northwest Argentina. Journal of Liquid Chromatography and Related Technologies 22 (6), 909-921.

Longanga Otshudi, A.L., Vercruysse, A., Foriers, A. 2000. Contribution to the ethnobotanical, phytochemical and pharmacological studies of traditionally used medicinal plants in the treatment of dysentery and diarrhoea in Lomela area, Democratic Republic of Congo (DRC). Journal of Ethnopharmacology 71 (3), 411 - 423.

Longino, Helen E. 1993. Feminist Standpoint Theory and the Problems of Knowledge. Review Essay. Signs 19, 201 - 212.

Longuefosse, J-L., Nossin, E. 1996. Medical ethnobotany survey in Martinique. Journal of Ethnopharmacology 53 (3), 117 - 142.

Lopes-Martins RA, Pegoraro DH, Woisky R, Penna SC, Sertie JA. The anti-inflammatory and analgesic effects of a crude extract of *Petiveria alliacea* L. (Phytolaccaceae). *Phytomedicine* 2002 9(3):245-8.

Lores, R.I., Cires Pujol, M. 1990. *Petiveria alleaceae* L. (anamu). Study of the hypoglycemic effect. Med. Interne 28 (4), 347-352.

Loro, J.F., del Rio, I., Pérez-Santana, L. 1999. Preliminary studies of analgesic and anti-inflammatory properties of *Opuntia dillenii* aqueous extract. Journal of Ethnopharmacology 67 (2), 213 - 218.

Loven, Sven. Origins of the Tainan Culture, West Indies Göteborg, Sweden: Elanders, 1935.

Lowe, H. 1972. Jamaican folk medicine. Jamaican Journal 6 (2), 20 - 24.

Lozoya, X., Meckes, M., Abou-Zaid, M., Tortoriello, J., Nozzolillo, C., Arnason, J. 1994. Quercetin glycosides in *Psidium guajava* L. leaves and determination of a spasmolytic principle. Archives of Medical Research 25 (1), 11 - 15.

Lubchenco, J. 1998. Entering the century of the environment: a new social contract for science. Science 279, 491 - 497.

Luis JG, Echeverri F, Garcia F, Rojas M. 1994, The structure of acnistin B and the immunosuppressive effects of acnistins A, B, and E. Planta Medica 60: 348–350.

Lutterodt, G.D. 1992. Inhibition of Microlax*-induced experimental diarrhoea with narcotic-like extracts of *Psidium guajava* leaf in rats. Journal of Ethnopharmacology 37 (2), 151 - 157.

Lynch-Brathwaite, B.A., Duncan, E.J., Seaforth, C.E. 1975. A survey of ferns of Trinidad for antibacterial activity. Planta Medica 27, 173 - 177.

MacDonald D, VanCrey K, Harrison P, Rangachari PK, Rosenfeld J, Warren C, Sorger G. 2004. Ascaridole-less infusions of *Chenopodium ambrosioides* contain a nematocide(s) that is(are) not toxic to mammalian smooth muscle. J Ethnopharmacol. 92(2-3):215-21.

MacGregor, F.B., Abernethy, V.E., Dahabra, S., Cobden, I., Hayes, P.C. 1989. Hepatotoxicity of herbal remedies. British Medical Journal 299 (4 November, 1989), 1156 -1157.

MacRae, W.D., Towers, G.H. 1984. *Justicia pectoralis*: a study of the basis for its use as a hallucinogenic snuff ingredient. Journal of Ethnopharmacology 12 (1), 93-111.

Mahabir, K. 1991. Medicinal and Edible Plants used by East Indians in Trinidad and Tobago. Chakra Publishing House, Trinidad and Tobago.

Mahato, S.B., Das, M.C., Sahu, N.P. 1981. Triterpenoids of *Scoparia dulcis*. Phytochemistry 20 (1), 171 - 173.

Mahiou, V., Roblot, F., Hocquemiller, R., Cavé, A., Rojas de Arias, A., Inchausti, A., Yaluff, G., Fournet, A. 1996. New prenylated quinones from *Peperomia galioides*. Journal of Natural Products 59 (7), 694 - 697.

Maiti R, Jana D, Das UK, Ghosh D. 2004. Antidiabetic effect of aqueous extract of seed of *Tamarindus indica* in streptozotocin-induced diabetic rats. J Ethnopharmacol. 92(1):85-91.

Malek F, Boskabady MH, Borushaki MT, Tohidi M. 2004. Bronchodilatory effect of *Portulaca oleracea* in airways of asthmatic patients. *J Ethnopharmacol.* 93(1):57-62.

Manabe M, Takenaka R, Nakasa T, Okinaka O. 2003. Induction of anti-inflammatory responses by dietary *Momordica charantia* L. (bitter gourd). *Biosci Biotechnol Biochem.* 67(12): 2512-7.

Mansingh, A., Williams, L.A.D. 1998. Pesticidal potential of tropical plants: II. Acaricidal activity of crude extracts of several Jamaican plants. Insect Science and Its Application 18 (2), 149 - 155.

Marcelle, G.B., Mootoo, B.S. 1975. Tetranotriterpenoids from the heartwood of *Carapa guianensis*. Phytochemistry 14 (12), 2717 - 2718.

Marcelle, G.B., Mootoo, B.S. 1981. 7alpha,11beta-diacetoxydihydronomilin, a new tetranortriterpenoid from *Cedrela mexicana* Trinidad. Tetrahedron Lett. 22 (6), 505 - 508.

Marglin, F.A. 1990b. Smallpox in two systems of knowledge. In: Marglin, F.A. and Marglin, S.A. (Eds.) 1990. Dominating Knowledge: Development, Culture and Resistance. Pp. 102 - 144.

Marglin, S.A. 1990a. Towards the decolonization of the mind. In: Marglin, F.A. and Marglin, S.A. (Eds.) 1990. Dominating Knowledge: Development, Culture and Resistance. Pp. 1 - 28.

Marglin, S.A. 1990c. Losing touch: the cultural conditions of worker accommodation and resistance. In: Marglin, F.A. and Marglin, S.A. (Eds.) 1990. Dominating Knowledge: Development, Culture and Resistance. Pp. 217 - 282.

Martin Calero, M., La Casa, C., Motilva, V., Lopez, A., Alarcon de la Lastra, C. 1996. Healing process induced by a flavonic fraction of *Bidens aurea* on chronic gastric lesion in rat. Role of angiogenesis and neutrophil inhibition. Z. Naturforsch. [C], 51(7-8), 570-7.

Martínez, M.J., Betancourt, J., Alonso-González, N., Jauregui, A. 1996a. Screening of some Cuban medicinal plants for antimicrobial activity (recent advances). Short communication. Journal of Ethnopharmacology 52 (3), 171 - 174.

Martínez, M.J., Betancourt, J., Alonso-González, N., Jauregui, A. 1996b. Screening of some Cuban medicinal plants for antimicrobial activity (recent advances). Pure and Applied Chemistry 62 (7), 1217 - 1222.

Martínez-Lirola, M.J., González-Tejero, M. R., Molero-Mesa, J. 1996a. Ethnobotanical resources in the province of Almería, Spain: Campos de Nijar. Economic Botany 50 (1) 40 - 56.

Martz, W. 1992. Plants with a reputation against snakebite. Review Article. Toxicon 30 (10), 1131 - 1142.

Mascia-Lees, F., Sharpe, P., Ballerino Cohen, C. 1989. The postmodernist turn in Anthropology: Cautions from a feminist perspective. Signs 5 (1), 7 - 33.

Masters, J. 1995. The History of Action Research, In: I. Hughes (Ed.) Action Research Electronic Reader, The University of Sydney, on-line http://www.behs.cchs.usyd.edu.au/arow/Reader/rmasters.htm (download date 10.10.2000).

Matadial, L., West, M.E., Gossell-Williams, M., The, T.L. 1999. The effect of *Bromelia pinguin* extract on the pregnant rat uterus. West Indian Medical Journal 48 (4), 198 - 199.

Matev, M., Angelova, I., Koichev, A., Leseva, M., Stefanov, G. 1982. Clinical trial of a *Plantago major* preparation in the treatment of chronic bronchitis. Vutr. Boles 21(2), 133-7. [Article in Bulgarian].

Mathias, E. 1998. Implications of the one-medicine concept for healthcare provision. Agriculture and Human Values 15 (2), 145 - 151.

Mathias, E., McCorkle, C.M. 1997. Animal health. In: Bunders, J., Haverkort, B., Hiemstra, W. 1996. (Eds.) Biotechnology: building on farmers' knowledge. MacMillan Education Publishing, Basingstoke UK. pp. 22 - 51.

Mathias, E., McCorkle, C.M., Schillhorn van Veen, T. 1996. Introduction: Ethnoveterinary research and development. In: McCorkle, C.M., Mathias-Mundy, E., Schillhorn van Veen, T. 1996. (Eds.). Ethnoveterinary Research and Development. IT Publications, London. Pp.1 - 23.

Mathias-Mundy, E. 1996. How can ethnoveterinary medicine be used in field projects? Indigenous Knowledge and Development Monitor 4 (2), 6 - 7.

Matsuse, I.T., Lim, Y.A., Hattori, M., Correa, M., Gupta, M.P. 1999. A search for anti-viral properties in Panamanian medicinal plants. The effects on HIV and its essential enzymes. Journal of Ethnopharmacology 64 (1), 15-22.

Matu EN, van Staden J. 2003. Antibacterial and anti-inflammatory activities of some plants used for medicinal purposes in Kenya. J Ethnopharmacol. 87(1):35-41.

Maturana, H., Varela, F. 1987. The tree of knowledge. In: Escobar, A. 1999. After nature: steps to an antiessentialist political ecology. Current Anthropology 40 (1), 1 - 30.

Maurice, P.D.L. Cream, J.J. 1989. The dangers of herbalism. British Medical Journal 299 (11 November, 1989), 1204.

Maxwell, A., Rampersad, D. 1991. A new dihydropiplartine and piplartine dimer from *Piper rugosum*. Journal of Natural Products (Lloydia) 54 (4), 1150-1152.

Maxwell, A., Seepersaud, M., Pingal, R., Mootoo, D.R., Reynolds, W.F. 1995. 3 beta-aminospirosolane steroidal alkaloids from *Solanum triste*. Journal of Natural Products 58 (4), 625 - 628.

Maynard, M. 1994. Methods, practice and epistemology: The debate about feminism and research. In: Maynard, M and Purvis, J. (Eds.) 1994. Researching Women's Lives from a Feminist Perspective. Taylor and Francis, London.

Mazumder UK, Gupta M, Pal D, Bhattacharya S. 2003. Chemical and toxicological evaluation of methanol extract of *Cuscuta reflexa* Roxb. stem and *Corchorus olitorius* Linn. seed on hematological parameters and hepatorenal functions in mice. Acta Pol Pharm. 60(4):317-23

McClure, S.A. 1982. Parallel Usage of Medicinal Plants by Africans and Their Caribbean Descendants. Economic Botany 36 (3), 291 - 301.

McCorkle, C.M, Green, E.C. 1998. Intersectoral healthcare delivery. Agriculture and Human Values 15 (2), 105 - 114.

McCorkle, C.M. 1989. Veterinary anthropology. Human Organisation 48 (2), 156 - 162.

McCorkle, C.M., Bazalar, H. 1996. Field trials in ethnoveterinary R&D: Lessons from the Andes. In: McCorkle, C.M., Mathias-Mundy, E., Schillhorn van Veen, T. 1996. (Eds.). Ethnoveterinary Research and Development. IT Publications, London. 338 pp. Pp. 265 - 282

McCorkle, C.M., Mathias-Mundy, E. 1992. Ethnoveterinary medicine in Africa. Africa 62 (1), 59 - 93.

McCorkle, C.M., Mathias-Mundy, E., Schillhorn van Veen, T. 1996. (Eds.). Ethnoveterinary Research and Development. IT Publications, London. 338 pp.

McElroy, J.L., de Albuquerque, K. 1990. Sustainable small-scale agriculture in small Caribbean islands. Society and Natural Resources 3, 109 - 129.

McManus OB, Harris GH, Giangiacomo KM, Feigenbaum P, Reuben JP, Addy ME, Burka JF, Kaczorowski GJ, Garcia ML. 1999. An activator of calcium-dependent potassium channels isolated from a medicinal herb. Biochemistry. 32(24):6128-33.

Melo, P., do Nascimento, M.C., Mors, W.B., Suarez-Kurtz, G. 1994. Inhibition of the myotoxic and hemorrhagic activities of crolatid venoms by *Eclipta prostrata* (Asteraceae) extracts and constituents. Toxicon 32 (5), 595 - 603.

Mercadante, A.Z., Steck, A., Rodriguez-Amaya, D., Pfander, H., Britton, G. 1996. Isolation of Methyl 9'Z-Apo-6'-Lycopenoate from *Bixa orellana*. Phytochemistry 41 (4), 1201 - 1203.

Merck, 1986. The Merck Veterinary Manual. 6th Edition. Merck and Co., Inc. Rahway, N.J., USA.

Messer, E. 1987. The hot and cold in Mesoamerican indigenous and Hispanicized thought. Social Science and Medicine 25 (4), 339 - 346.

Michal, J.J., Heirman, L.R., Wong, T.S., Chew, B.P., Frigg, M., Volker, L. 1994. Modulatory effects of dietary beta-carotene on blood and mammary leukocyte function in periparturient dairy cows. Journal of Dairy Science 77, 1408 - 1421.

Michie, C.A. 1992. The use of herbal remedies in Jamaica. Annals of Tropical Paediatrics 12, 31 - 36.

Middendorf, G., Busch, L. 1997. Inquiry for the public good: democratic participation in agricultural research. Agriculture and Human Values 14 (1), 45 - 57.

Mies, M. 1983. Towards a methodology for feminist research. In: Bowles, G. and Klein, R (Eds.) 1983. Theories of Women's studies. Routledge and Kegan Paul, London.

Miller, S.L., Tinto, W.F., McLean, S., Reynolds, W.F., Yu, M., and Carter, C.A.G. 1995. Isolation and characterisation of a new glabretal triterpene from *Quassia multiflora*. Journal of Natural Products (Lloydia) 58 (10), 1640-1642.

Milliken, W., Albert, B. 1996. The use of medicinal plants by the Yanomami Indians of Brazil. Economic Botany 50 (1), 10 - 25.

Mills, J., Pascoe, K.O., Chambers, J., Melville, G.N. 1986. Preliminary investigations of the wound-healing properties of a Jamaican folk medicinal plant (*Justicia pectoralis*). West Indian Medical Journal 35 (3), 190-193. University of the West Indies, Jamaica.

Milton, K. 1996. Environmentalism and cultural theory: exploring the role of anthropology in environmental discourse. Routledge, London, 266 pp.

Mimaki, Y., Inoue, T., Kuroda, M., Sashida, Y. 1996. Steroidal saponins from *Sansevieria trifasciata*. Phytochemistry 43 (6), 1325-31.

Mimaki, Y., Inoue, T., Kuroda, M., Sashida, Y. 1997. Pregnane glycosides from *Sansevieria trifasciata*. Phytochemistry 44 (1), 107-11.

Minguzzi S, Barata LE, Shin YG, Jonas PF, Chai HB, Park EJ, Pezzuto JM, Cordell GA, 2000. Cytotoxic withanolides from *Acnistus arborescens*. Phytochemistry 59(6): 635-41.

Ministry of Agriculture, Land and Marine Resources, 1990. Animal Health Sub-Division Field Service Report, Trinidad and Tobago.

Ministry of Agriculture, Land and Marine Resources, 1991. Animal Health Sub-Division Field Service Report, Trinidad and Tobago.

Ministry of Agriculture, Land and Marine Resources, Animal Health Subdivision. Annual Report 1994, Trinidad and Tobago.

Ministry of Agriculture, Land and Marine Resources. Veterinary Diagnostic Laboratory. Animal Health Sub-Division. Annual Report 1996, Trinidad and Tobago.

Ministry of Agriculture, Land and Marine Resources. Veterinary Diagnostic Laboratory. Animal Health Sub-Division, Annual Report 1998, Trinidad and Tobago.

Ministry of Food Production and Marine Exploitation, 1989. Division of Animal Production and Health. Poultry Surveillance Unit Annual Report, Trinidad and Tobago

Mintz, S.W. 1974. Caribbean transformations. Adline Publishing Co., Chicago.

Mintz, S.W. 1983. Reflections on Caribbean peasantries. Nieuwe West-Indische Gids 57 (1-2), 1 - 17.

Mirvish, S.S., Salmasi, S., Lawson, T.A., Pour, P., Sutherland, D. 1985. Test of catechol, tannic acid, *Bidens pilosa*, croton oil, and phorbol for cocarcinogenesis of esophageal tumors induced in rats by methyl-n-amylnitrosamine. J. Natl. Cancer Inst. 74 (6), 1283-90.

Mischel, F. 1959. Faith healing and medical pratice in the southern Caribbean. Southwestern Journal of Anthropology 15, 407 - 417.

Mitchell, M.F. 1983. Popular medical concepts in Jamaica and their impact on drug use. West. J. Med. 139 (6), 841-7.

Miyazawa, M., Okuno, Y., Nakamura, S., Kosaka, H. 2000. Antimutagenic activity of flavonoids from *Pogostemon cablin*. J. Agric Food Chem 48(3), 642-7.

Moerman DE. 1998. *Native American Ethnobotany*. Portland Timber Press.

Mohammed, P. 1995. Writing Gender into History: The negotiation of gender relations among Indian men and women in post-indenture Trinidad society, 1914 - 47. In: (Eds.) V. Shepherd, Bridget Brereton, Barbara Bailey. Engendering History: Caribbean women in historical perspective. Ian Randle Publishers, Jamaica. Pp. 20 - 47.

Mohammed, P. 1998. Towards indigenous feminist theorizing in the Caribbean. Feminist Review 59, 6 - 33.

Mohammed, P. 2000. 'But most of all mi love me browning': The emergence in eighteenth and nineteenth-century Jamaica of the mulatto woman as the desired. Feminist Review 65, 22 - 48.

Mohammed, S., Saka, S., El-Sharkawy, S.H., Manaf, A., Muid, S. 1996. Antimycotic screening of 58 Malaysian plants against plant pathogens. Pestic. Sci. 47 (3), 259 - 264.

Mole, R.R. 1924. The Trinidad snakes. Proceedings of the Zoological Society of London 1: 235 - 278.

Molnar, Joseph J., Duffy, Patricia A., Cummins, Keith A., Van Santen, Edzard. 1992. Agricultural science and agricultural counterculture: paradigms in search of a future. Rural Sociology 57, 83 - 91.

Monache, G.D., Botta, B., Vinciguerra, V., de Mello, J.F., Andrade Chiapetta de, A. 1996. Antimicrobial isoflavanones from *Desmodium canum*. Phytochemistry 41 (2), 537 - 544.

Mongelli, E., Romano, A., Desmarchelier, C., Coussio, J., Ciccia, G. 1999. Cytotoxic 4 Nerolidylcatechol from *Pothomorphe peltata* inhibits topoisomerase I activity. Planta Medica 65 (4), 376 - 378.

Monteiro, M.H., Gomes-Carneiro, M.R., Felzenszwalb, I., Chahoud, I., Paumgartten, F.J. 2001. Toxicological evaluation of a tea from leaves of *Vernonia condensata*. Journal of Ethnopharmacology 74 (2), 149-157.

Moodie, S. 1982. Some supersititions and beliefs of Hispano Trinidadians. In: Myth and superstition in Spanish-Caribbean literature. Conference Papers: Fifth Conference of Hispanists. University of the West Indies, Mona, Jamaica, 6 - 9 July, 1982. Pp 220 - 268.

Moodie-Kublalsingh, S. 1994. The cocoa panyols of Trinidad: An oral record. British Academic Press, London. 242 pp.

Moodie-Kublalsingh, unpublished. Fieldnotes.

Moore-Gilbert, B. 1997. Postcolonial theory: Contexts, practices, politics. Verso, London and New York, 243 pp.

Mootoo, B.S., Ali, A., Khan, A., Reynolds, W.F., McLean, S. 2000. Three novel monotetrahydrofuran annonaceous acetogenins from *Annona montana*. Journal of Natural Products 63 (6), 807-11.

Mootoo, B.S., Ali, A., Motilal, R., Pingal, R., Ramlal, A., Khan, A., Reynolds, W.F., McLean, S. 1999. Limonoids from *Swietenia macrophylla* and *S. aubrevilleana*. Journal of Natural Products 62 (11), 1514-7.

Mootoo, B.S., Jativa, C., Tinto, W., Reynolds, W.F., McLean, S. 1992. Ecuadorin, a novel tetranortriterpenoid of *Guarea kunthiana*. Structure elucidation by 2-D NMR spectroscopy. Canadian Journal of Chemistry 70 (5), 1260 - 1264.

Mootoo, B.S., Ramsewak, R., Khan, A., Tinto, W., Reynolds, W.F., McLean, S., Yu, M. 1996. Tetranortriterpenoids from *Ruagea glabra*. Journal of Natural Products 59 (5), 544 - 547.

Morales, M.A., Tortoriello, J., Meckes, M., Paz, D., Lozoya, X. 1994. Calcium-antagonist effect of quercetin and its relation with the spasmolytic properties of *Psidium guajava* L. Archives of Medical Research 25 (1), 17 - 21.

Morawski, J.G. 1988. Impasse in feminist thought? In: Gergen, M.M. 1988. Feminist thought and the Structure of knowledge. New York University Press, New York. 200pps.

Moreira, D.L., Kaplan, M.A.C., Guimaraes, E.F. 1997. 1-butyl-3,4-methylenedioxybenzene as the major constituent of essential oil from *Ottonia anisum* Sprengel (Piperaceae). Journal of Essential Oil Research 9 (5), 565 - 568.

Moreno Fraginals, M. 1976. The Sugar mill: The socio-economic complex of sugar in Cuba, 1769 - 1860. Monthly Review Press: New York and London.

Morgan, D.L. 1988. Focus groups as qualitative research. Sage, London.

Morison, S.E. 1963. Journals and other documents on the life and voyages of Christopher Columbus. New York: The Heritage Press.

Morrison, E.Y. St. A., Smith-Richardson, S., West, M., Brooks, S.E.H., Pascoe, K., Fletcher, C. 1987. Toxicity of the hyperglycaemic-inducing extract of the Annatto (*Bixa orellana*) in the dog. West Indian Medical Journal 36 (2), 99 - 103.

Morton, J.F. 1968a. The calabash (*Crescentia cujete*) in folk medicine. Economic Botany 22 (3), 273 - 280.

Morton, J.F. 1968b. A survey of medicinal plants of Curaçao. Economic Botany 22 (1), 87 - 102.

Morton, J.F. 1975. Current folk remedies of northern Venezuela. Quarterly Journal of Crude Drug Research 13, 97 - 121.

Morton, J.F. 1980. Caribbean and Latin American folk medicine and its influence in the United States. Quarterly Journal of Crude Drug Research 18 (2), 57 - 75.

Morton, J.F. 1981. Atlas of medicinal plants of middle America: Bahamas to Yucatan. Charles C. Thomas, Springfield, USA. 1420 pp.

Morton, Julia. 1990. Mucilaginous plants and their uses in medicine. Review Paper. Journal of Ethnopharmacology 29 (3), 245 - 266.

Muelas-Serrano, S., Nogal, J.J., Martínez-Díaz, R.A., Escario, J.A., Martínez-Fernández, A.R., Gómez-Barrio, A. 2000. *In vitro* screening of American plant extracts on *Trypanosoma cruzi* and *Trichomonas vaginalis*. Journal of Ethnopharmacology 71(1-2), 101-107.

Mukhopadhyay, S.K., Buddhadeb, D., Duary, B., Dasgupta, M.K. (Ed.)., Ghosh, D.C. (Ed.)., Gupta, D.D., (Ed.), Majumdar, D.K., (Ed.), Chattopadhyay, G.N. (Ed.), Ganguli, P.K. (Ed.), Munsi, P.S. (Ed.), Bhattacharya, D. 1995. Ethnobotany of some common crop field weeds in a sub-humid agricultural tract of West Bengal. Proceedings of the national symposium on sustainable agriculture in sub-humid zone, Sriniketan, West Bengal, India, 3 - 5 March 1995, pp. 272 - 277.

Müller, B.M., Franz, G. 1992.Chemical structure and biological activity of polysaccharides from *Hibiscus sabdariffa*. Planta Medica 58 (1), 60-7.

Munasinghe, V. 2001. Redefining the nation: the East Indian struggle for inclusion in Trinidad. JAAS, 4 (1), 1 - 34.

Munck, S.L., Croteau, R. 1990. Purification and characterization of the sesquiterpene cyclase patchoulol synthase from *Pogostemon cablin*. Arch. Biochem. Biophys. 282 (1), 58-64.

Muniappan M, Sundararaj T: Antiinflammatory and antiulcer activities of *Bambusa arundinacea*. J Ethnopharmacol. 2003, 88(2-3):161-7.

Muñoz, V., Sauvain, M., Bourdy, G., Arrázola, S., Callapa, J., Ruiz, G., Choque, J., Deharo, E. 2000b. A search for natural bioactive compounds in Bolivia through a multidisciplinary approach. Part III. Evaluation of the antimalarial activity of plants used by Alteños Indians. Journal of Ethnopharmacology 71 (1-2), 123 - 131.

Muñoz, V., Sauvain, M., Bourdy, G., Callapa, J., Rojas, I., Vargas, L., Tae, A., Deharo, E. 2000a. The search for natural bioactive compounds through a multidisciplinary approach in Bolivia. Part II. Antimalarial activity for some plants used by Mosetene indians. Journal of Ethnopharmacology 69 (1), 139 - 155.

Murakami A, Nakamura Y, Ohto Y, Yano M, Koshiba T, Koshimizu K, Tokuda H, Nishino H, Ohigashi H. 2000. Suppressive effects of citrus fruits on free radical generation and nobiletin, an anti-inflammatory polymethoxyflavonoid. Biofactors 12(1-4): 187-92.

Murdiati TB and Beriajaya Adiwinata G. 1997. Anthelmintic activity of papaya sap against *Haemonchus contortus* in sheep. *Parasitologi Indonesia* 10: 1 - 7. (in Indonesian).

Murdiati, T.B., Manurung, J. 1991. Study on the efficacy of ketepeng leaf (*Cassia alata* L.) against Psoroptic mange (*Psoroptes cuniculi*) in rabbits. (In Indonesian). Penyakit Hewan 23 (41), 50 - 52.

Murthy, D.R., Reddy, C.M., Patil, S.B. 1997. Effect of benzene extract of *Hibiscus rosa sinensis* on the estrous cycle and ovarian activity in albino mice. Biol. Pharm. Bull. 20 (7), 756-8.

Mustapha, Z. 1977. Folk medicine among the East Indians in Trinidad. Final Year Caribbean Studies Project. Faculty of Arts and General Science. University of the West Indies. St. Augustine, Trinidad and Tobago.

Nagaraju, N., Rao, K.N. 1990. A survey of plant crude drugs of Rayalaseema, Andhra Pradesh, India. Journal of Ethnopharmacology 29, 137 - 158.

Naipaul, V.S. 1962. The Middle Passage. Andre Deutsch, London.

Nakamura, C.V., Ueda-Nakamura, T., Bando, E., Melo, A.F., Cortez, D.A., Dias Filho, B.P. 1999. Antibacterial activity of *Ocimum gratissimum* L. essential oil. Memorias do Instituto Oswaldo Cruz 94 (5), 675-8.

Nakao, T., Gamal, A., Osawa, T., Nakada, K., Moriyoshi, M., Kawata, K. 1997. Postpartum plasma PGF metabolite profile in cows with dystocia and/or retained placenta, and effect of fenprostalene on uterine involution and reproductive performance. Journal of Veterinary Medical Science 59 (9), 791 - 4.

Nakashima, D., Guchteneire, P., de. 1999. 'Science and other systems of knowledge' : A new impetus for indigenous knowledge from the World Conference on Science. Indigenous Knowledge and Development Monitor 7 (3), 40.

Nakayama, T., Takeura, Y., Ueda, T. 1995. Visible spectrophotometric assay, purification, and molecular properties of a lipoxygenase from eggplant (*Solanum melongena* Linne) fruits. Biochem. Biophys. Res. Commun. 214 (3),1067-72.

Nalven, J. 1987. Measuring the unmeasurable: a microregional study of an undocumented population. In: Wulff, R.M., Fiske, S.J. 1987. (Eds.) Anthropological praxis: translating knowledge into action. Westview Press, USA. p. 34.

Nammi S, Boini MK, Lodagala SD, Behara RB: The juice of fresh leaves of *Catharanthus roseus* Linn. reduces blood glucose in normal and alloxan diabetic rabbits. BMC Complement Altern Med. 2003, 3(1):4.

Nandy, A., Visvanathan, S. 1990. Modern medicine and its non-modern critics: a study in discourse. In: Marglin, F.A. and Marglin, S.A. (Eds.) 1990. Dominating Knowledge: Development, Culture and Resistance. Pp. 145 - 184.

Nassis, C.Z., Haebisch, E., Giesbrecht, A. 1992. Antihistamine activity of *Bryophyllum calycinum*. Brazilian Journal of Medical and Biological Research 25 (9), 929 - 936.

Nations, M.K., Misago, C., Fonseca, W., Correia, L.L., Campbell, O.M.R. 1997. Women's hidden transcripts about abortion in Brazil. Social Science and Medicine 44 (12), 1833 - 1845.

Navarro, V., Villarreal, L. Ma., Rojas, G., Lozoya, X. 1996. Antimicrobial evaluation of some plants used in Mexican traditional medicine for the treatment of infectious diseases. Journal of Ethnopharmacology 53 (3), 143 - 147.

N'Dounga, M., Balansard, G., Babadjamian, A., David, P., Gasquet, M., Boudon, G. 1983. Contribution a l'étude de *Bidens pilosa* L. Identification et activite antiparasitaire de la phenyl-1 heptatriyne-1,3,5. Plantes Medicinales et Phytotherapie 17 (2), 64 - 75.

Nelkin, D. 1996. Controversy as a political challenge. In: Barnes, Barry, Edge, David (Eds.) Science in context: readings in the sociology of science. The Open University Press. Pp. 276 - 281.

Nelson, Lynn Hankinson. 1993. Epistemological Communities. In: Linda Alcoff and Elizabeth Potter (Eds.) Feminist Epistemologies, Routledge, New York and London. Pp. 121 - 159.

Nereu, F., Kock, J., McQueen, Robert J., Scott, John L. 1997. Can action research be made more rigorous in a positivist sense? The contribution of an iterative approach. Journal of Systems and Information Technology 1 (1), 1-24.

Newsom, Lee Ann. 1993. Native West Indian plant use. PhD dissertation, University of Florida.

Ngadjui, B., Kouam, S., Dongo, E., Kapche, G., Abegaz, B. 2000. Prenylated flavonoids from the aerial parts of *Dorstenia mannii*. Phytochemistry 55 (8), 915 - 919.

Ngassoum MB, Essia-Ngang JJ, Tatsadjieu LN, Jirovetz L, Buchbauer G, Adjoudji O. 2003. Antimicrobial study of essential oils of *Ocimum gratissimum* leaves and *Zanthoxylum xanthoxyloides* fruits from Cameroon. Fitoterapia 74(3):284-7.

Ngokwey, N. 1995. Home remedies and doctors' remedies in Feira (Brazil). Social Science and Medicine 40 (8), 1141 - 1153.

Nicholson, M.S., Arzeni, C.B. 1993. The market medicinal plants of Monterrey, Nuevo León, México. Economic Botany 47 (2), 184 - 192.

Niehoff, A., Niehoff, J. 1960. East Indians in the West Indies. Milwaukee Public Museum Publications in Anthropology 6. Milwaukee, Wisconsin.

Niehoff, J. 1959. Bush - the folk medicine of Trinidad. Shell Trinidad, 5 (6), 11 - 12.

Nigam, S., Saxena, V. 1975. Isolation and the study of the aurone glycoside leptosin from the leaves of *Flemengia strobilifera*. Planta Medica 27 (1), 98 - 100.

Nishino, H., Hayashi, T., Arisawa, M., Satomi, Y., Iwashima, A. 1993. Antitumor-promoting activity of scopadulcic acid B, isolated from the medicinal plant *Scoparia dulcis* L. Oncology 50 (2), 100 - 103.

Nitsch, U. 1991. Knowledge of agriculture. Paper presented at the 10th European Seminar on Extension Education: New focuses on European extension education: the issues. Vila Real, Portugal. Pp. 21 - 28.

Niwa, Y., Miyachi, Y., Ishimoto, K., Kanoh, T. 1991. Why are natural plant medicinal products effective in some patients and not in others with the same disease? Planta Medica 57 (4), 299 - 304.

Noda, Y., Kaneyuki, T., Igarashi, K., Mori, A., Packer, L. 1998. Antioxidant activity of nasunin, an anthocyanin in eggplant. Res. Commun. Mol. Pathol. Pharmacol. 102 (2), 175-87.

Novaretti, R., Lemordant, D. 1990. Plants in the traditional medicine of the Ubaye Valley. Journal of Ethnopharmacology 30 (1), 1 - 34.

Nunes, D.S. 1996. Chemical approaches to the study of ethnomedicines. In Medicinal Resources of the Tropical Resources of the Tropical Forest: Biodiversity and its Importance to Human Health. Michael Balick, Elaine Elisabetsky, and Sarah Laird, eds. pp. 41 - 47. New York: Columbia University Press.

Nwosu, M.O., Okafor, J.I. 1995. Preliminary studies of the antifungal activities of some medicinal plants against Basidiobolus and some other pathogenic fungi. Mycoses 38(5-6), 191-5.

Nyazema, N., Ndamba, J., Anderson, C., Makaza, N., Kaondera, K. 1994. The Doctrine of Signatures or Similitudes: A comparison of the efficacy of praziquantel and traditional herbal remedies used for the treatment of urinary schistosomiases in Zimbabwe. International Journal of Pharmacognosy 32 (2), 142 - 148.

Oakley, A. 1981. Interviewing women: A contradiction in terms. In: Helen Roberts (Ed.) 1981. Doing Feminist Research. Routledge and Kegan Paul, London.

Obikeze. D. S. 1997. Indigenous postpartum maternal and child health care practices among the Igbo of Nigeria. Indigenous Knowledge and Development Monitor 5 (2), 3-5.

O'Brien, W.E, Butler Flora, C. 1992. Selling appropriate development vs. selling-out rural communities: empowerment and control in Indigenous Knowledge discourse. Agriculture and Human Values 9 (2), 95 - 102.

Occhiuto, F., Sanogo, R., Germano, M.P., Keita, A., D'Angelo, V., De Pasquale, R. 1999. Effects of some Malian medicinal plants on the respiratory tract of guinea-pigs. Journal of Pharmacy and Pharmacology 51(11), 1299-303.

Offiah, V.N., Anyanwu, I.I. 1989. Abortifacient activity of an aqueous extract of *Spondias mombin* leaves. Journal of Ethnopharmacology 26 (3), 317 - 320.

Ohsaki, A., Kasetani, Y., Asaka, Y., Shibata, K., Tokoroyama, T., Kubota, T. 1995. A diterpenoid from *Portulaca pilosa*. Phytochemistry 40 (1), 205 - 207.

Ojala, T., Remes, S., Haansuu, P., Vuorela, H., Hiltunen, R., Haahtela, K., Vuorela, P. 2000. Antimicrobial activity of some coumarin containing herbal plants growing in Finland. Journal of Ethnopharmacology 73 (1-2), 299 - 305.

Oketch-Rabah, H.A., Lemmich, E., Dossaji, S.F., Theander, T.G., Olsen, C.E., Cornett, C., Kharazmi, A., Christensen, S.B. 1997. Two new antiprotozoal 5-methylcoumarins from *Vernonia brachycalyx*. Journal of Natural Products 60 (5), 458-61.

Olajide, O.A, Awe, S.O., Makinde, J.M. 1999. Pharmacological studies on the leaf of *Psidium guajava*. Fitoterapia 70 (1), 25 - 31.

Olajide, O.A. 1999. Investigation of the effects of selected medicinal plants on experimental thrombosis. Phytotherapy Research 13 (3), 231-2.

Oliver Bever, B.E.P. 1986. Medicinal plants in tropical West Africa. Cambridge University Press, Cambridge, 375 pp.

Oluwole, F.S., Bolarinwa, A.F. 1998. The uterine contractile effect of *Petiveria alliacea* seeds. Fitoterapia LXIX (1), 3-6.

Omisore NO, Adewunmi CO, Iwalewa EO, Ngadjui BT, Watchueng J, Abegaz BM, Ojewole JA. Antinociceptive and anti-inflammatory effects of *Dorstenia barteri* (Moraceae) leaf and twig extracts in mice. *J Ethnopharmacol.* 2004 95(1):7-12.

Onajobi, F.D. 1986. Smooth muscle contracting lipid-soluble principles in chromatographic fractions of *Ocimum gratissimum*. Journal of Ethnopharmacology 18 (1), 3-11.

Onawunmi, G.O., Yisak, W.A., Ogunlana, E.O. 1984. Antibacterial constituents in the essential oil of *Cymbopogon citratus* (DC.) Stapf. Journal of Ethnopharmacology 12 (3), 279-86.

Ong, H., Norzalina, J. 1999. Malay herbal medicine in Gemencheh, Negri Sembilan, Malaysia. Fitoterapia 70 (1), 10 - 14.

Opler, M.E. 1965. An Apache life-way. The economic, social, and religious institutions of the Chiricahua Indians. New York: Cooper Square Publishers.

Ortiz de Montellano, B. 1975. Empirical Aztec medicine. Science 188 (4185), 215 - 220.

Oryan, A., Zaker, S.R. 1998. Effects of topical application of honey on cutaneous wound healing in rabbits. Journal of Veterinary Medicine A 45 (3), 181 - 188.

Osim, E., Udia, P.M. 1993. Effects of consuming a kola nut (*Cola nitida*) diet on mean arterial pressure in rats. International Journal of Pharmacognosy 31 (3), 193 - 197.

Oubré, A.Y., Carlson, T.J., King, S.R., Reaven, G.M. 1997. From plant to patient: An ethnomedical approach to the identification of new drugs for the treatment of NIDDM. Diabetologia (1997) 40, 614 - 617.

PAHO, 1996. Biodiversity, biotechnology, and sustainable development in health and agriculture: emerging connections. Scientific publication No. 560. Washington, DC: Pan American Health Organization.

PAHO, 1997. Healthy people, healthy places. Annual Report of the Director 1995. Official Document 283, Washington, DC. 210 pp.

Pakrashi, A., Bhattacharya, K., Kabir, S.N., Pal, A.K. 1986. Flowers of *Hibiscus rosa-sinensis*, a potential source of contragestative agent. III: Interceptive effect of benzene extract in mouse. Contraception 34 (5), 523-36.

Pal, D., Panda, C., Sinhababu, S., Dutta, A., Bhattacharya, S. 2003. Evaluation of psychopharmacological effects of petroleum ether extract of *Cuscuta reflexa* Roxb. stem in mice. Acta Pol Pharm. 60(6):481-6.

Pal, A.K., Bhattacharya, K., Kabir, S.N., Pakrashi, A. 1985. Flowers of *Hibiscus rosa-sinensis*, a potential source of contragestative agent: II. Possible mode of action with reference to anti-implantation effect of the benzene extract. Contraception 32 (5), 517-29.

Pal, S., Nag Chaudhuri, A.K. 1989. Some pharmacological actions of *Bryophyllum pinnatum*. Planta Medica 55, 647-648.

Pal, S., Nag Chaudhuri, A.K. 1991. Studies on the anti-ulcer activity of a *Bryophyllum pinnatum* leaf extract in experimental animals. Journal of Ethnopharmacology 33 (1-2), 97-102.

Pal, S., Sen, T., Nag Chaudhuri, A.K. 1999. Neuropsychopharmacological profile of the methanolic fraction of *Bryophyllum pinnatum* leaf extract. Journal of Pharmacy and Pharmacology 51 (3), 313-318.

Palanichamy, S., Nagarajan, S. 1990. Antifungal activity of *Cassia alata* leaf extract. Journal of Ethnopharmacology 29 (3), 337 - 340.

Pálsson, G. 1996. Human-environmental relations. In: Descola, P., Pálsson, G. 1996. (Eds). Nature and society: anthropological perspectives. Routledge, London. Pp. 63 - 81.

Pannangpetch P, Vuttivirojana A, Kularbkaew C, Tesana S, Kongyingyoes B, Kukongviriyapan V. 2001. The antiulcerative effect of Thai *Musa* species in rats. Phytother Res. 15(5):407-10.

Pantin, R. 1999. An open letter to Peter Minshall. Sunday Express, September 19, 1999.

Pappas, G. 1990. Some implications for the study of the doctor-patient interaction: Power, structure, and agency in the works of Howard Waitzkin and Arthur Kleinman. Social Science and Medicine 30 (2), 199 - 204.

Paquette, Robert and Engerman, Stanley (eds.). 1996. The Lesser Antilles in the Age of European Expansion. University Press of Florida.

Pardo de Santayana M, Blanco E, Morales R. 2005. Plants known as te in Spain: An ethno-pharmaco-botanical review. J Ethnopharmacol. 98(1-2):1-19.

Park, E.J., Park, H.R., Lee, J.S., Kim, J. 1998. Licochalcone A: An inducer of cell differentiation and cytotoxic agent from *Pogostemon cablin*. Planta Medica 64 (5), 464-6.

Park, M.K., Park, J.H., Shin, G.Y., Kim, W.Y., Lee, J.H., Kim, K.H. 1996. Neoaloesin A: A new C-glucofuranosyl chromone from *Aloe barbadensis*. Planta Medica 62 (4), 363 - 365.

Passreiter, C.M., Medinilla Aldana, B.E. 1998. Variability of sesquiterpene lactones in *Neurolaena lobata* of different origin. Planta Medica 64 (5), 427 - 430.

Passreiter, C.M., Wendisch, D., Gondol, D. 1995. Sesquiterpene lactones from *Neurolaena lobata*. Phytochemistry 39 (1), 133 - 137.

Pathong, A., Kanjanapothi, D., Taesotikul, T., and Taylor, W.C. 1991. Ethnobotanical review of medicinal plants from Thai traditional books. Part II: Plants with antidiarrheal, laxative and carminative properties. Review paper. Journal of Ethnopharmacology 31 (2), 121 - 156.

Payne, C. 1974. Medicinal plants of Trinidad. Environmental Field program. Ohio: Antioch College.

Pemberton, C.A. 1990. Agricultural Diversification: Policies and Strategies. Proceedings of the 19th West Indian Agricultural Economic Conference, St. Augustine: University of the West Indies.

Peña, J. 1999. Pre-Columbian medicine and the kidney. Am. J. Nephrol. 19 (2), 148 - 154.

Pena, S.D. 1999. Origin of the Amerindians. Letter to the Editor. Science, 283 (5410), 2017.

Penissi AB, Rudolph MI, Piezzi RS. 2003. Role of mast cells in gastrointestinal mucosal defense. Biocell. 27(2):163-72.

Pereira, P.1969. Folk medicine as practised in Chaguanas, Trinidad. Caribbean Studies Thesis. University of the West Indies, St. Augustine, Trinidad.

Pereira, R.L., Ibrahim, T., Lucchetti, L., da Silva, A.J., Gonçalves de Moraes, V.L. 1999. Immunosuppressive and anti-inflammatory effects of methanolic extract and the polyacetylene isolated from *Bidens pilosa* L.. Immunopharmacology 43(1), 31-7.

Perez, C., Anesini, C. 1994. *In vitro* antibacterial activity of Argentine folk medicinal plants against *Salmonella typhi*. Journal of Ethnopharmacology 44 (1), 41 - 46.

Perez, G., Ocegueda, Z., Munoz, L., Avila, A., Morrow, W. 1984. A study of the hypoglucemic effect of some Mexican plants. Journal of Ethnopharmacology 12 (3), 253 - 262.

Perez-Guerrero C, Herrera MD, Ortiz R, Alvarez de Sotomayor M, Fernandez MA. 2001. A pharmacological study of *Cecropia obtusifolia* Bertol aqueous extract. J Ethnopharmacol. 76(3):279-84.

Pérotin-Dumon, Anne, 1996. Free coloureds and slaves in revolutionary Guadeloupe. Politics and political consciousness. In Paquette, Robert and Engerman, Stanley (eds.), The Lesser Antilles in the Age of European Expansion. University Press of Florida. Pp. 259 – 279.

Persad, K. 1999. Ministry of Black Culture and Gender Affairs. Sunday Express, August 29, 1999.

Perumal Samy, R., Ignacimuthu, S., Raja, D. P. 1999. Preliminary screening of ethnomedicinal plants from India. Short communication. Journal of Ethnopharmacology 66 (2), 235 - 240.

Peterson, J. 1988. Book review of John van Willigen's Applied Anthropology: An Introduction. American Anthropologist 90, 425 - 426.

Phan T.T., Hughes M.A., Cherry G.W., Le T.T., Pham H.M. 1996. An aqueous extract of the leaves of Chromolaena odorata (formerly Eupatorium odoratum) (Eupolin) inhibits hydrated collagen lattice contraction by normal human dermal fibroblasts. J. Altern. Complement. Med. 2 (3), 335-43.

Phan, T.T., Allen, J., Hughes, M.A., Cherry, G., Wojnarowska, F. 2000. Upregulation of adhesion complex proteins and fibronectin by human keratinocytes treated with an aqueous extract from the leaves of Chromolaena odorata. Eur. J. Dermatol. 10 (7), 522.

Phan, T.T., Hughes, M.A., Cherry, G.W. 2001. Effects of an aqueous extract from the leaves of Chromolaena odorata (Eupolin) on the proliferation of human keratinocytes and on their migration in an in vitro model of reepithelialization. Wound Repair Regen. 9 (4): 305-13.

Phillips, D. 1996. Medical professional dominance and client dissatisfaction. Social Science and Medicine 42 (10), 1419 - 1425.

Phuong, N.M., Van Sung, T., Ripperger, H., Adam, G. 1994. Sterol glucosides from Eleusine indica. Planta Medica 60 (5), 498.

Pickersgill, Barbara. 2005. In Prance,G. & M.Nesbitt (editors). Cultural history of plants. Routledge: Oxon and New York. Pp 153 – 172.

Pieroni, A. 2000. Medicinal plants and food medicines in the folk traditions of the upper Lucca Province, Italy. Journal of Ethnopharmacology 70 (3), 235 - 273.

Pieters, L., Bruyne, T., de, Claeys, M., Vlietinck, A., Calomme, M., vanden Berghe, D. 1993. Isolation of a dihydrobenzofuran lignan from South American Dragon's Blood (Croton spp.) as an inhibitor of cell proliferation. Journal of Natural Products 56 (6), 899 - 906.

Pillai MG, Thampi BS, Menon VP, Leelamma S: Influence of dietary fiber from coconut kernel (Cocos nucifera) on the 1,2-dimethylhydrazine-induced lipid peroxidation in rats. J Nutr Biochem. 1999, 10 (9): 555-60.

Pinch, T.J., Bijker, W.E. 1987. The social construction of facts and artifacts: or how sociology of science and the sociology of technology might benefit each other. In: Bijker, W.E, Hughes, T.P., Pinch, T.J. 1987 (Eds). The social construction of technological systems. new directions in the sociology and history of technology. Cambridge, MIT Press. Pp. 17-50.

Pino, J.A., Ortega, A., Rodriguez, M. 1999. Antimicrobial activity of the leaf oil of Lippia alba (Mill.) N.E. Brown from Cuba. Journal of Esssential Oil Bearing Plants 2 (1), 47 - 49.

Plowman, T. 1969. Folk uses of new world aroids. Economic Botany 23, 97 - 122.

Polanyi, M. 1967. The tacit dimension. New York.

Pöll, E. 1993. Medicinal plants from the Peten, Guatemala. Acta Horticulturae 330, 93 - 100.

Pomilio, A.B., Buschi, C.A., Tomes, C.N., Viale, A.A. 1992. Antimicrobial constituents of Gomphrena martiana and Gomphrena boliviana. Journal of Ethnopharmacology 36(2), 155-61.

Pomilio, A.B., Sola, G.A., Mayer, A.M., Rumi, L.S. 1994. Antitumor and cytotoxic screen of 5,6,7-trisubstituted flavones from Gomphrena martiana. Journal of Ethnopharmacology 44(1), 25-33.

Porac, J., Wade, J., Brown, J., de Vaughn, M. 2002. In: Bontis, N., Choo, C.W. (Eds.) 2002. The strategic management of intellectual capital and organisational knowledge: a collection of readings. Oxford University Press, New York.

Porta, E.A., Rappaport, A.M., Bras, G., Manning, C., Kawamura, T.M. 1972. Early sequential hepatic changes in fulvine-treated rats. West Indian Journal of Medicine 21, 186 - 200.

Porter, R.B., Reese, P.B., Williams, L.A., Williams, D.J. 1995. Acaricidal and insecticidal activities of cadina-4,10(15)-dien-3-one. Phytochemistry 40 (3), 735 - 738.

Posey, D.A. 1998. Changing fortunes: biodiversity and peasant livelihood in the Peruvian Andes. Journal of Latin American Studies 30 (3), 682 - 683.

Posey, Darrell A. and Plenderleith, Kristina. (eds.) 2002. Kayapó ethnoecology and culture New York: Routledge, 2002

Prakash, A.O., Mathur, A., Mehta, H., Mathur, R. 1990. Concentrations of Na+ and K+ in serum and uterine flushings of ovariectomized, pregnant and cyclic rats when treated with extracts of *Hibiscus rosa sinensis* flowers. Journal of Ethnopharmacology 28 (3), 337-47.

Prashar, R., Kumar, A., Hewer, A., Cole, K.J., Davis, W., Phillips, D.H. 1998. Inhibition by an extract of *Ocimum sanctum* of DNA-binding activity of 7,12-dimethylbenz[a]anthracene in rat hepatocytes *in vitro*. Cancer Letters 128 (2), 155 - 160.

Price, R., Price, S. 1997. Shadowboxing in the mangrove. Cultural Anthropology 12 (1), 3 - 36.

Pugliese, P.T., Jordan, K., Cederberg, H., Brohult, J. 1998. Some biological actions of alkylglycerols from shark liver oil. J. Altern. Complement. Med. 4(1), 87-99.

Purcell, T.W. 1983. Book Review of M. Lieber's Street Scenes: Afro-American culture in urban Trinidad. Nieuwe West-Indische Gids 57 (1-2), 119 - 122.

Puricelli L, Dell'Aica I, Sartor L, Garbisa S, Caniato R. 2003. Preliminary evaluation of inhibition of matrix-metalloprotease MMP-2 and MMP-9 by *Passiflora edulis* and *P. foetida* aqueous extracts. Fitoterapia 74 (3): 302-4.

Rabe, T., van Staden, J. 1997. Antibacterial activity of South African plants used for medicinal purposes. Journal of Ethnopharmacology 56(1), 81-7.

Raedeke, A.H., Rikoon, J.S. 1997. Temporal and spatial dimensions of knowledge: implications for sustainable agriculture. Agriculture and Human Values 14 (2), 145 - 158.

RAFI, 1995. Conserving Indigenous Knowledge. Integrating two Systems of Innovation. An independent study by the Rural Advancement Foundation International. Commissioned by the UNDP.

Rahman MM, Sarker SD, Byres M, Gray AL. 2004. New salicylic acid and isoflavone derivatives from *Flemingia paniculata*. J Nat Prod. 2004, 67(3):402-6.

Raja, D., Blanché, C., Xirau, J.V. 1997. Contribution to the knowledge of the pharmaceutical ethnobotany of La Segarra region (Catalonia, Iberian Peninsula). Journal of Ethnopharmacology 57 (3), 149 - 160.

Rajeshkumar, N.V., Kuttan, R. 2000. *Phyllanthus amarus* extract administration increases the life span of rats with hepatocellular carcinoma. Journal of Ethnopharmacology 73 (1-2), 215 - 219.

Randall, C., Randall, H., Dobbs, F., Hutton, C., Sanders, H. 2000. Randomized controlled trial of nettle sting for treatment of base-of-thumb pain. Journal of the Royal Society of Medicine 93 (6), 305 - 309.

Rao, M., Rao, M.N.A. 1998. Protective effects of cystone, a polyherbal ayurvedic preparation, on cisplatin-induced renal toxicity in rats. Journal of Ethnopharmacology 62 (1), 1 - 6.

Rao, V.S., Menezes, A.M., Viana, G.S. 1990. Effect of myrcene on nociception in mice. Journal of Pharmacy and Pharmacology 42 (12), 877-8.

Raphael KR, Sabu MC, Kuttan R. Hypoglycemic effect of methanol extract of *Phyllanthus amarus* Schum & Thonn on alloxan induced diabetes mellitus in rats and its relation with antioxidant potential. Indian J Exp Biol. 2002, 40 (8):905-9.

Rappaport, R.A. 1993. Distinguished lecture in general anthropology: the anthropology of trouble. American Anthropologist 95 (2), 295 - 303.

Rapport, N. 2001. Book Review of Clifford Geertz, 'Available light: anthropological reflections on philosophical tropics'. The Journal of the Royal Anthropological Institute 7 (1), 163 - 164.

Rapport, N., Overing, J. 2000. (Eds.). Social and cultural anthropology: the key concepts. Routledge, London and New York, 464 pp.

Rathi A, Rao ChV, Ravishankar B, De S, Mehrotra S. Anti-inflammatory and anti-nociceptive activity of the water decoction *Desmodium gangeticum*. J Ethnopharmacol. 2004, 95(2-3):259-63.

Ratnasooriya WD and Dharmasiri MG. 1999. Aqueous extract of Sri Lankan *Erythrina indica* leaves has sedative but not analgesic activity. *Fitoterapia* 70: 311 - 313.

Raudenbush B, Corley N, Eppich W: Enhancing athletic performance through the administration of peppermint odor. Journal of Sport and Exercise Pyschology 2001, 23 (2): 156 – 160.

Ravindranath N, Reddy MR, Mahender G, Ramu R, Kumar KR, Das B: Deoxypreussomerins from *Jatropha curcas*: are they also plant metabolites? *Phytochemistry* 2004, 65(16):2387-90.

Recio, M de Carmen, Giner, R.M., Máñez, S., Rios, J.L. 1995. Structural requirements for the anti-inflammatory activity of natural triterpenoids. Planta Medica 61 (2), 182 - 185.

Reddy, C.M., Murthy, D.R., Patil, S.B. 1997. Antispermatogenic and androgenic activities of various extracts of *Hibiscus rosa sinesis* in albino mice. Indian J. Exp. Biol. 35 (11), 1170-4.

Reeves, C. 1992. Egyptian medicine. Shire Egyptology Series No. 15. Shire Publications Ltd., Buckinghampshire.

Reyes, E. 1977. Roasted sour orange - the first spray deodorant. Trinidad Naturalist 1(8), 39 - 42.

Richards, P. 1989. Agriculture as a performance. In: R. Chambers, R. Pacey, and L.Thrupp (Eds.). Farmer first: farmer innovation and agricultural research. Intermediate Technology Publications. London.

Richards, P. 1993. Cultivation: knowledge or performance? In: M. Hobart 1993. (Ed.). An anthropological critique of development: the growth of ignorance. London, Routledge. Pp. 61 - 78.

Richards, P. 1996. Agrarian creolization: The ethnobiology, history, culture and politics of West African rice. In: R. Ellen, K. Fukui (Eds.). Redefining Nature: Ecology, culture and domestication. Berg, Oxford, Washington, D.C. pp. 291 - 318.

Richards, Paul and Ruivenkamp, Guido. 1996. New tools for conviviality: Social shaping of biotechnology. In: P. Descola & G. Pálsson (Eds.). Nature and society: Anthropological perspectives. London: Routledge.

Riddle, J.M. 1991. Oral contraceptives and early-term abortifacients during Classical Antiquity and the Middle Ages. Past and Present 132, 3 - 32.

Riley, Mary. 2003. Guayanese history, Makuski historicities, and Amerindian rights. In: Neil L. Whitehead (ed.) Histories and historicities in Amazonia. University of Nebraska Press, Lincoln and London. Pp. 141 – 159.

Rimbau V, Cerdan C, Vila R, Iglesias J: Antiinflammatory activity of some extracts from plants used in the traditional medicine of north-African countries (II). *Phytother Res.* 1999, 13(2):128-32.

Ringbom, T., Segura, L., Noreen, Y., Perera, P., Bohlin, L. 1998. Ursolic acid from *Plantago major*, a selective inhibitor of cyclooxygenase-2 catalyzed prostaglandin biosynthesis. Journal of Natural Products 61 (10), 1212 - 1215.

Ríos, J.L., Recio, M.C., Villar, A. 1987. Antimicrobial activity of selected plants employed in the Spanish Mediterranean area. Journal of Ethnopharmacology 21 (2), 139 - 152.

Rival, Laura M., Whitehead, Neil L. (eds.) 2001. Beyond the visible and the material: The Amerindianization of society in the work of Peter Rivière. New York: Oxford University Press.

Rivera, D., Obón, C. 1995. The ethnopharmacology of Madeira and Porto Santo Islands, a review. Journal of Ethnopharmacology 46 (2), 73 - 93.

Rivière, Peter. 1969. Marriage among the Trio. A principle of social organization. Oxford: Clarendon Press.

Robineau, L. (Editor), 1991. Towards a Caribbean ethnopharmacopoeia. TRAMIL 4 Workshop: Scientific Research and Popular Use of Medicinal plants in the Caribbean. UNAH, Enda-Caribe, Santo Domingo, DO.

Robinson, R.D., Williams, L.A., Lindo, J.F., Terry, S.I., Mansingh, A. 1990. Inactivation of *Strongyloides stercoralis* filariform larvae *in vitro* by six Jamaican plant extracts and three commercial anthelmintics. West Indian Medical Journal 39 (4), 213-217.

Robinson, M. 1998. Medical therapy of inflammatory bowel disease for the 21st century. *Eur J Surg Suppl.* (582): 90-8.

Rocha FF, Lapa AJ, De Lima TC: Evaluation of the anxiolytic-like effects of *Cecropia glazioui* Sneth in mice. *Pharmacol Biochem Behav.* 2002, 71(1-2):183-90.

Rocha, A.B., da Silva, J.B. 1969. Thin layer chromatographic analysis of coumarins and preliminary test for some active substance in the root of *Petiveria alliacea* L. In: Souza Brito, A.R.M. and Souza Brito, A.A. 1993. Forty years of Brazilian medicinal plant research. Journal of Ethnopharmacology 39, 53 - 67.

Rocheleau, D. 1994. Participatory research and the race to save the planet: questions, critique, and lessons from the field. Agriculture and Human Values 11 (2-3), 4 - 25.

Rohlehr, G. 1980. Talking about Naipaul. An interview with Selwyn Cudjoe. Carib No. 21981.

Rojas A, Bah M, Rojas JI, Serrano V, Pacheco S. 1999. Spasmolytic activity of some plants used by the Otomi Indians of Queretaro (Mexico) for the treatment of gastrointestinal disorders. Phytomedicine 6(5):367-71.

Rojas, G., Lévaro, J., Tortoriello, J., Navarro, V. 2001. Antimicrobial evaluation of certain plants used in Mexican traditional medicine for the treatment of respiratory diseases. Short communication. Journal of Ethnopharmacology 74 (1), 97 - 101.

Röling, N. 2000. Gateway to the global garden: Beta/Gamma Science for Dealing with Ecological Rationality. Eighth Annual Hopper Lecture, October 24, 2000,University of Guelph, Canada.

Röling, N., Jiggins, J., Coehoorn, C. 1999. The Santiago triangle: the cognitive systems as heuristic device for saving our souls. Paper for plenary session of 14th ESEE (Biannual European Seminar on Extension Education), Agricultural University of Krakow, Poland August 30 - September 4th, 1999.

Röling, N.G. 1988. Extension science, information systems in agricultural development. Cambridge University Press, 240 pp.

Rollocks, S.A. 1991. Folk medicine in Tobago: a study in cultural continuity. Caribbean Studies Thesis. University of the West Indies, St. Augustine, Trinidad.

Roper, N. 1987. Pocket Medical Dictionary. Churchill Livingstone & Longman Group UK, Ltd., Edinburgh, New York.

Rosello, M. 1995. Caribbean insularization of identities in Maryse Condé's work from *En attendant le bonheur* to *Les derniers rois mages*. Callaloo 18 (3), 565 - 578.

Rostlund, E. 1952. Freshwater fish and fishing in native North America. Berkeley: University of California Press.

Rotblat, Joseph, Sir. 1999. A hippocratic oath for scientists. Science 286, 1475.

Roth, G., Chandra, A., Nair, M. 1998. Novel bioactivities of *Curcuma longa* constituents. Notes. Journal of Natural Products 61 (4), 542 - 545.

Roth, Walter, E. 1915. An inquiry into the animism and folk-lore of the Guiana Indians. Annual Report of the Bureau of American Ethnology to the Secretary of the Smithsonian Institution 30 (1908 - 1909). Washington Government Printing Series, Washington, DC.

Rowland Atkinson and John Flint 2001. Accessing Hidden and Hard-to-Reach Populations: Snowball Research Strategies. Social Research Update 33.

Roy, B., Tandon, V. 1996. Effect of root-tuber extract of *Flemingia vestita*, a leguminous plant, on *Artyfechinostomum sufrartyfex* and *Fasciolopsis buski*: a scanning electron microscopy study. Parasitol Res 82(3), 248-52.

Ruffa MJ, Perusina M, Alfonso V, Wagner ML, Suriano M, Vicente C, Campos R, Cavallaro L.2002. Antiviral activity of *Petiveria alliacea* against the bovine viral diarrhea virus. Chemotherapy. 48 (3): 144-7.

Ruffa, M.J., Wagner, M.L., Suriano, M., Vicente, C., Nadinic, J., Pampuro, S., Salomon, H., Campos, R.H., Cavallaro, L. 2004. Inhibitory effect of medicinal herbs against RNA and DNA viruses. Antivir Chem Chemother. 15 (3): 153-9.

Russo, E.B. 1992. Headache treatments by native peoples of the Ecuadorian Amazon: A preliminary cross-disciplinary assessment. Review article. Journal of Ethnopharmacology 36 (3), 193 - 206.

Rutten T, Kruger C, Melzer M, Stephan UW, Hell R: Discovery of an extended bundle sheath in Ricinus communis L. and its role as a temporal storage compartment for the iron chelator nicotianamine. Planta 2003, 217 (3): 400-6.

Ryan, S. 1999. Independence battles. Sunday Express, August 29, 1999.

Ryan, S. 2001. Carnival and ethnicity. Sunday Express, March 4, 2001.

Ryu, S.B., Wang, X. 1998. Increase in free linolenic and linoleic acids associated with phospholipase D-mediated hydrolysis of phospholipids in wounded castor bean leaves. Biochim. Biophys. Acta 1393 (1),193-202.

Sachdewa, A., Khemani, L.D.1999. A preliminary investigation of the possible hypoglycemic activity of *Hibiscus rosa-sinensis*. Biomed. Environ. Sci. 12 (3), 222-6.

Sadekar, R.D., Pimprikar, N.M., Bhandarkar, A.G., Barmase, B.S. 1998. Immunopotentiating effect of *Ocimum sanctum* Linn. dry leaf powder on cell mediated immune (CMI) response in poultry, naturally infected with IBD virus. Indian Veterinary Journal 75, 168 - 169.

Saenz, M.T., Garcia, M.D., Quilez, A., Ahumada, M.C. 2000. Cytotoxic activity of *Agave intermixta* L. (Agavaceae) and *Cissus sicyoides* L. (Vitaceae). Phytotherapy Research 14 (7), 552-4.

Saidu, K., Onah, J., Orisadipe, A., Olusola, A., Wambebe, C., Gamaniel, K. 2000. Antiplasmodial, analgesic, and anti-inflammatory activities of the aqueous extract of the stem bark of *Erythrina senegalensis*. Journal of Ethnopharmacology 71 (1-2), 275 - 280.

Sakina, M.R., Dandiya, P.C., Hamdard, M.E., Hameed, A. 1990. Preliminary psychopharmacological evaluation of *Ocimum sanctum* leaf extract. Journal of Ethnopharmacology 28 (2), 143 - 150.

Salah, A.M., Dongmo, A.B., Kamanyi, A., Bopelet, M., Vierling, W., Wagner, H. 2000. *In vitro* purgative effect of *Ruellia praetermissa*. Scienf. ex. Lindau (Acanthaceae). Journal of Ethnopharmacology 72 (1-2), 269 - 272.

Samaroo, B. 1975. East Indian life and culture. In: Anthony, M and Carr, A 1975. (Eds.) David Frost introduces Trinidad and Tobago. Andre Deutsh Ltd, London.

Sampson, J.H., Phillipson, J.D., Bowery, N.G., O'Neill, M.J., Houston, J.G., Lewis, J.A. 2000. Ethnomedicinally selected plants as sources of potential analgesic compounds: Indication of *in vitro* biological activity in receptor binding assays. Phytotherapy Research 14(1), 24-9.

Samuelsen, A. 2000. The traditional uses, chemical constituents and biological activities of *Plantago major* L. A review. Journal of Ethnopharmacology 71 (1-2), 1 - 21.

Sanderson, Helen. 2005. Roots and tubers. In Prance,G. & M.Nesbitt (editors). Cultural history of plants. Routledge: Oxon and New York. Pp 61 – 76.

Sandhyakumary K, Boby RG, Indira M: Impact of feeding ethanolic extracts of *Achyranthes aspera* Linn. on reproductive functions in male rats. Indian J Exp Biol. 2002, 40(11):1307-9.

Santos, A.R.S., de Campos, R.O.P., Miguel, O.G, Filho, V.C., Siani, A.C., Yunes, R.A., Calixto, J.B. 2000. Antinociceptive properties of extracts of new species of plants of the genus *Phyllanthus* (Euphorbiaceae). Journal of Ethnopharmacology 72 (1-2), 229 - 238.

Sarg, T.M., Ateya, A.M., Farrag, N.M., Abbas, F.A. 1991. Constituents and biological activity of *Bidens pilosa* L. grown in Egypt. Acta Pharm. Hung. 61 (6), 317-23.

Sarin R: Insecticidal activity of callus culture of *Tagetes erecta*. Fitoterapia 2004, 75(1):62-4.

Sartori MR, Pretto JB, Cruz AB, Bresciani LF, Yunes RA, Sortino M, Zacchino SA, Cechinel VF. 2003. Antifungal activity of fractions and two pure compounds of flowers from *Wedelia paludosa* (*Acmela brasiliensis*) (Asteraceae). Pharmazie 58(8): 567-9.

Satrija F, Nansen P, Bjorn H, Murtini S and He S. 1994. Effect of papaya latex against *Ascaris suum* in naturally infected pigs. *Journal of Helminthology* 68: 343 - 346.

Satrija, F., Nansen, P., Murtini, S., He, S. 1995. Anthelmintic activity of papaya latex against patent *Heligmosomoides polygyrus* infections in mice. Journal of Ethnopharmacology 48 (2), 161 - 164.

Satyan, K.S., Prakash, A., Singh, R.P., Srivastava, R.S. 1995. Phthalic acid bis-ester and other phytoconstituents of *Phyllanthus urinaria*. Notes. Planta Medica 61 (3), 293-294.

Savickiene N, Dagilyte A, Lukosius A, Zitkevicius V. 2002. Importance of biologically active components and plants in the prevention of complications of diabetes mellitus. Medicina (Kaunas). 38(10):970-5. Article in Lithuanian.

Saxena, A.K., Singh, B., Anand, K.K. 1993. Hepatoprotective effects of *Eclipta alba* on subcellular levels in rats. Journal of Ethnopharmacology 40 (3), 155 - 161.

Saxena, V.K., Singhal, M. 1999. Novel prenylated flavonoid from stem of *Pithecellobium dulce*. Fitoterapia 70 (1), 98 - 100.

Scara, A., Guerci, A. 1982. Various uses of the castor oil plant (*Ricinus communis* L.): A review. Journal of Ethnopharmacology 5 (2), 117 - 137.

Scartezzini, P., Speroni, E. 2000. Review on some plants of Indian traditional medicine with antioxidant activity. Journal of Ethnopharmacology 71 (1), 23 - 43.

Schapoval, E.E.S., Winter de Vargas, M.R., Chaves, C.G., Bridi, R., Zuanazzi, J.A., Henriques, A.T. 1998. Antiinflammatory and antinociceptive activities of extracts and isolated compounds from *Stachytarpheta cayennensis*. Journal of Ethnopharmacology 60 (1), 53 - 59.

Scheper-Hughes, N. 1990. Three propositions for a critically applied medical anthropology. Social Science and Medicine 30 (2), 189 - 197.

Scheyvens, R., Leslie, H. 2000. Gender, ethics and empowerment: dilemmas of development fieldwork. Women's Studies International Forum 23 (1), 119 - 130.

Schillhorn van Veen, T.W. 1997. Sense or nonsense? Traditional methods of animal parasitic disease control. Veterinary Parasitology 71 (2-3), 177 - 194.

Schillhorn van Veen, T.W., de Haan, C. 1995. Trends in the organization and financing of livestock and animal health services. Preventive Veterinary Medicine 25, 225-240.

Schmeda-Hirschmann, G., Bordas, E. 1990. Paraguayan medicinal Compositae. Journal of Ethnopharmacology 28 (2), 163 - 171.

Scholz, E., Heinrich, M., Hunkler, D. 1994. Caffeoylquinic acids and some biological activities of *Pluchea symphytifolia*. Planta Medica 60 (4), 360-4.

Schon, D. 1991. The reflective practitioner: How professionals think in action. Ashgate Publishing Ltd, Avebury.

Scott, Julius, 1996. Crisscrossing empires. Ships, sailors, and Resistance in the Lesser Antilles in the Eighteenth Century In Paquette, Robert and Engerman, Stanley (eds.), The Lesser Antilles in the Age of European Expansion. University Press of Florida pp. 128 – 143.

Seaforth, C.E. 1991. A guide to the medicinal plants of Trinidad and Tobago. Commonwealth Secretariat, London.

Seeram, N.P., Jacobs, H., McLean, S., Reynolds, W. 1998. A prenylated benzopyran derivative from *Peperomia clusiifolia*. Phytochemistry 49 (5), 1389 - 1391.

Seeram, N.P., Jacobs, H., McLean, S., Reynolds, W.F. 1996a. Prenylated hydroxybenzoic acid derivatives from *Piper murrayanum*. Phytochemistry 43 (4), 863 - 865.

Seeram, N.P., Lewis, A.W., Jacobs, H., Nair, M.G., McLean, S., Reynolds, W.F. 2000. Proctoriones A-C: 2-acylcyclohexane-1,3-dione derivatives from *Peperomia proctorii*. Journal of Natural Products 63 (3), 399 - 402.

Seeram, N.P., Lewis, P.A., Jacobs, H., McLean, S., Reynolds, W.F., Tay, L.L., Yu, M. 1996b. 3,4-epoxy-8,9-dihydropiplartine. A new imide from *Piper verrucosum*. Phytochemistry 59 (4), 436 - 437.

Seiber, J.N., Nelson, C.J., Lee, S.M. 1982. Cardenolides in the latex and leaves of seven *Asclepias* species and *Calotropis procera*. Phytochemistry 21 (9), 2343 - 2348.

Selvam, R., Subramanian, L., Gayathri, R., Angayarkanni, N. 1995. The anti-oxidant activity of turmeric (*Curcuma longa*). Journal of Ethnopharmacology 47 (2), 59 - 67.

Sen, T., Nag Chaudhuri, A.K. 1989. Anti-inflammatory and antiulcer actions of *Pluchea indica*. Poster. Planta Medica 55, 647.

Serbin, A. 1981. In: E. Dew, 1982. Book Review of Nacionalismo, etnicidad y política en la República Cooperativa de Guyana. Nieuwe West-Indische Gids 56 (3-4), 184 - 185.

Sertié, J.A.A., Basile, A.C., Panizza, S., Matida, A.K., Zelnik, R. 1988. Pharmacological assay of *Cordia verbenacea*; Part 1. Anti-inflammatory activity and toxicity of the crude extracts of the leaves. Planta Medica 54 (1), 7 - 10.

Sethi, V., Koul, S., Taneja, S., Dhar, K. 1987. Minor sesquiterpenes of flowers of *Parthenium hysterophorus*. Phytochemistry 26 (12), 3359 - 3361.

Setzer, W., Green, T., Whitaker, K., Moriarity, D., Yancey, C., Lawton, R., Bates, R. 1995. A cytotoxic diacetylene from *Dendropanax arboreus*. Planta Medica 61 (5), 470 - 471.

Sezik, E., Yesilada, E., Tabata, M., Honda, G., Takaishi, Y., Fujita, T., Tanaka, T., Takeda, Y. 1997. Traditional medicine in Turkey VIII. Folk medicine in East Anatolia; Erzurum, Erzïncan, Agri, Kars, Igdir Provinces. Economic Botany 51 (3), 195 - 211.

Shah, R. 1999. Time for national heritage park. Sunday Express August 1, 1999.

Shannon, L.J. 1998. Book Review. Signs 23 (2), 543 - 546.

Sharma, G.L., Bhutani, K.K. 1988. Plant based antiamoebic drugs; part II. Amoebicidal activity of parthenin isolated from *Parthenium hysterophorus*. Planta Medica 54 (2), 120 - 122.

Sheridan, Richard, B. 1991. Slave medicine in Jamaica: Thomas Thistlewood's "Receipts for a Physick", 1750 - 1786. Jamaica Historical Review 17, 1 - 18.

Shimiz, K., Kondo, R., Sakai, K., Buabarn, S., Dilokkunanant, U. 2000. A geranylated chalcone with 5-alpha-reductase inhibitory properties from *Artocarpus incisus*. Phytochemistry 54 (8), 737-9.

Shinwari, M.I., Khan, M.A. 2000. Folk use of medicinal herbs of Margalla Hills National Park, Islamabad. Journal of Ethnopharmacology 69 (1), 45 - 56.

Shipochliev, T. 1981. Uterotonic action of extracts from a group of medicinal plants. Vet. Med. Nauki 18 (4), 94-8. [Article in Bulgarian].

Shirwaikar A, Rajendran K, Dinesh Kumar C, Bodla R: Antidiabetic activity of aqueous leaf extract of *Annona squamosa* in streptozotocin-nicotinamide type 2 diabetic rats. J Ethnopharmacol. 2004, 91(1):171-5.

Shiva, V. 1993. Monocultures of the mind. Perspectives on biodiversity and biotechnology. Zed Books, London and Malaysia.

Shore, C., Wright, S. 1996. British anthropology in policy and practice: a review of current work. Human Organisation 55 (4), 475 - 479.

Siddiqui, M.B., Mashkoor Alam, M., Husain, W. 1989. Traditional treatment of skin diseases in Uttar Pradesh, India. Economic Botany 43 (4), 480 - 486.

Siegel, P.E. 1991. On the Antilles as a potential corridor for cultigens into Eastern North America. Current Anthropology 32 (3), 332 - 334.

Sillitoe, P. 1998. The development of indigenous knowledge. Current Anthropology 39 (2), 223 - 252.

Silva, M.J., Capaz, F.R., Vale, M.R 2000. Effects of the water soluble fraction from leaves of *Ageratum conyzoides* on smooth muscle. Phytotherapy Research 14(2), 130-2.

Silva, S.A.G da, Costa, S.S., Mendonca, S.C.F., Silva, E.M., Moraes, V.L.G., Rossi-Bergmann, B. 1995. Therapeutic effect of oral *Kalanchoe pinnata* leaf extract in murine leishmaniasis. Acta Tropica 60 (3), 201 - 210.

Simko, S., Stanicova, J. 1990. Are lunar cycles related to sudden perishing of pigs in fattening? Pol'nohospodarstvo 36 (5), 470-476.

Simon, O.R., Singh, N. 1986. Demonstration of anticonvulsant properties of an aqueous extract of Spirit Weed (*Eryngium foetidum* L.). West Indian Journal of Medicine 35, 121 - 125.

Simpson, G.E. 1962. Folk medicine in Trinidad. Journal of American Folklore 75, 326 - 340.

Simpson, G.E. 1970. Religious cults of the Caribbean: Trinidad, Jamaica and Haiti. Institute of Caribbean Studies, University of Puerto Rico.

Singer, M. 1982. A rejoinder to Wiley's critique of critical medical anthropology. Medical Anthropology Quarterly 7 (2), 185 - 207.

Singer, M. 1990. Reinventing medical anthropology: toward a critical realignment. Social Science and Medicine 30 (2), 179 - 187.

Singer, M. 1994. Community - centered praxis: toward an alternative non-dominative applied Anthropology. Human Organization 53 (4), 336 - 344.

Singh K and Nagaich S. 1999. Efficacy of aqueous seed extract of *Carica papaya* against common poultry worms *Ascaridia galli* and *Heterakis gallinae*. *Journal of Parasitic Disease* 23: 113 - 116.

Singh KA. 1999. Nutrient contents in tree fodders and bamboo leaves of eastern Himalaya. *Indian Journal of Animal Nutrition* 16: 178 - 182.

Singh, K., Maheshwari, J. 1994. Traditional phytotherapy of some medicinal plants used by the Tharus of the Nainital district, Uttar Pradesh, India. International Journal of Pharmacognosy 32 (1), 51 - 58.

Singh, Y.N., Inman, W.D., Johnson, A., Linnell, E.J. 1993. Studies on the muscle-paralyzing components of the juice of the banana plant. Archives Internationales de Pharmacodynamie et de Therapie 324, 105 - 113.

Slikkerveer, L. Jan. 1990. Plural medical systems in the horn of Africa: The legacy of 'Sheikh' Hippocrates. Kegan Paul International, London and New York. 324 pp.

Slikkerveer, L. Jan. 1995. INDAKS: a bibliography and database on indigenous agricultural knowledge systems and sustainable development in the tropics. In: Warren, D.M., Slikkerveer, L.J., Brokensha D.W. (Eds.) (1995). The cultural dimension of development: indigenous knowledge systems. London: Intermediate Technology Publications. Pp. 512 - 516.

Smith, M.G. 1957. The African heritage in the Caribbean. In: V. Rubin 1960 (Ed.) Caribbean Studies: A Symposium. University of Washington Press, Seattle, Washington.

Sofowora, A. 1982. Medicinal plants and traditional medicine in Africa. John Wiley and Sons Ltd, Chichester, West Sussex.

Soon Kim, C. 1990. The role of the non-western anthropologist reconsidered: Illusion versus reality. Current Anthropology 31 (2), 196 - 201.

Sosa S, Balick MJ, Arvigo R, Esposito RG, Pizza C, Altinier G, Tubaro A, 2002. Screening of the topical anti-inflammatory activity of some Central American plants. J Ethnopharmacol. 81(2):211-5.

Sousa, Ivan de, Busch, L. 1998. Networks and Agricultural Development: The Case of soybean production and consumption in Brazil. Rural Sociology 63, 349 - 371.

Souza Brito, A.R.M. 1996. How to study the pharmacology of medicinal plants in underdeveloped countries. Journal of Ethnopharmacology 54 (2-3), 131 - 138.

Souza Formigoni, M.L., Lodder, H.M., Gianotti Filho, O., Ferreira, T.M., Carlini, E.A. 1986. Pharmacology of lemongrass (*Cymbopogon citratus* Stapf). II. Effects of daily two month administration in male and female rats and in offspring exposed "in utero." Journal of Ethnopharmacology 17(1), 65-74.

Spender, Dale. 1981. The gatekeepers: a feminist critique of academic publishing. In: Helen Roberts 1981 (Ed.). Doing feminist research, Routledge and Kegan Paul, London and New York. Pp. 186 - 202.

Sreejayan, Rao, M. 1997. Nitric oxide scavenging by curcuminoids. Journal of Pharmacy and Pharmacology 49 (1), 105 - 107.

Stanley L., Wise, S. 1990. Method, methodology and epistemology in feminist research processes. In: Stanley, Liz 1990 (Ed.). Feminist praxis: research, theory and epistemology in feminist sociology. Routledge, London. Pp. 20 - 47.

Stanley, L. 1990. Feminist praxis and the academic mode of production. An editorial introduction. In: Stanley L., Wise, S. 1990. Pp. 3 - 19.

Star, Susan Leigh. 1991. Power, technologies and the phenomenology of conventions: on being allergic to onions. In: John Law 1991 (Ed.) A Sociology of Monsters. Essays on Power, Technology and Domination. Routledge, London. Pp. 26 - 56.

Steggerda, M. 1929. Plants of Jamaica used by natives for medicinal purposes. American Anthropologist 31 (3), 431 - 434.

Steiner, 1924, Rudolf. Koberwitz Lecture 6. [on agriculture].

Stewart, C. 1999. Syncretism and its synonyms: reflections on cultural mixture. Diacritics 29 (3), 40 - 62.

Stokstad, E. 2000. Alternative medicine. Stephen Straus's impossible job. News Focus. Science 288 (5471), 1568 - 1570.

Strobel, M. Baj. 1985. Book review of Alice Peeters Représentations et pratiques populaires relatives à l'environment et a la santé aux Antilles Françaises, I: La Martiniques. Paris: CNRS. Nieuwe West-Indische Gids 59 (3-4), 244 - 247.

Suaeyun, R., Kinouchi, T., Arimochi, H., Vinitketkumnuen, U., Ohnishi, Y. 1997. Inhibitory effects of lemon grass (Cymbopogon citratus Stapf.) on formation of azoxymethane-induced DNA adducts and aberrant crypt foci in the rat colon. Carcinogenesis 18(5), 949-55.

Sudheesh, S., Presannakumar, G., Vijayakumar, S., Vijayalakshmi, N.R. 1997. Hypolipidemic effect of flavonoids from Solanum melongena. Plant Foods Hum. Nutrition 51(4), 321-30.

Sudheesh, S., Sandhya, C., Sarah Koshy, A., Vijayalakshmi, N.R. 1999. Antioxidant activity of flavonoids from Solanum melongena. Phytotherapy Research 13 (5), 393-6.

Suepaul, R. 1997. A survey of drugs resistance in seven (7) species of bacteria isolated from animals in Trinidad and Tobago from 1991 - 1995. Final Year Research project. School of Veterinary Medicine, Faculty of Medical Sciences, University of the West Indies, Trinidad and Tobago.

Sugimoto, K., Sakurai, N., Shirasawa, H., Fujise, Y., Shibata, K., Shimodo, K., Sakata, J. 1992. Bovine cases of urolithiasis treated with traditional herbal medicine, P-3. Journal of Veterinary Medical Science 54 (3), 579 - 582.

Suksamrarn, A., Chotipong, A., Suavansri, T., Boongird, S., Timsuksai, P., Vimuttipong, S., Chuaynugul, A. 2004. Antimycobacterial activity and cytotoxicity of flavonoids from the flowers of Chromolaena odorata. Arch Pharm Res. 27 (5): 507-11.

Sukumaran, K., Kuttan, R. 1991. Screening of 11 ferns for cytotoxic and antitumour potential with special reference to Pityrogramma calomelanos. Journal of Ethnopharmacology 34 (1), 93 - 96.

SunKee, K., Yeon, H.B., ShinJung, K., JungJoon, L., JaiSeup, R., KyongSoon, L., Kim, S., Hwang, B., Kang, S., Lee, J., Ro, J., Lee, K. 2000. Chemical components of Cyperus rotundus L. and inhibitory effects on nitric oxide. Korean Journal of Pharmacognosy 31 (1), 1 - 6.

Supratman, U., Fujita, T., Akiyama, K., Hayashi, H. 2000. New insecticidal bufadienolide, bryophyllin C, from Kalanchoe pinnata. Biosci. Biotechnol. Biochemistry 64 (6), 1310-2.

Sutton, J.A., Orr, B.D. 1991.The Use of the school essay as an RRA technique: A case study from Bong County, Liberia. RRA Notes. Participatory Methods for Learning and Analysis. No.14. IIED Sustainable Agriculture Program.

Taddei, A., Rosas-Romero, A.J. 1999. Antimicrobial activity of Wedelia trilobata crude extracts. Phytomedicine 6 (2), 133-4.

Tan, M.L. 1989. Traditional or transitional medical systems? Pharmacotherapy as a case for analysis. Social Science and Medicine, 29 (3), 301 - 307.

Tan, P.V., Dimo, T., Dongo, E. 2000. Effects of methanol, cyclohexane and methylene chloride extracts of Bidens pilosa on various gastric ulcer models in rats. Journal of Ethnopharmacology 73 (3), 415 - 421.

Tanaka, T., Nonaka, G-I., Nishioka, I. 1985. Punicafolin, an ellagitannin from the leaves of Punica granatum. Phytochemistry 24 (9), 2075 - 2078.

Tandon, V., Pal, P., Roy, B., Rao, H.S., Reddy, KS. 1997. In vitro anthelmintic activity of root-tuber extract of Flemingia vestita, an indigenous plant in Shillong, India. Parasitol. Research 83(5), 492-8.

Tarbes, M. G. González. 1989. On cross-cultural ethnomedical research. Current Anthropology 30 (1), 75 - 76.

Tavernier, E. M. 1999. Challenges to economic growth in Latin America and the Caribbean: A preliminary exploration. Paper presented to the Sixth International Conference of the Asociación Latinoamericana y del Caribe de Economía Agrícola, August 1999, UWI, St. Augustine, Trinidad and Tobago.

Taylor, D. 1950. The meaning of dietary and occupational restrictions among the island Carib. American Anthropologist 52, 343 - 349.

Taylor, Douglas. 1949. The interpretation of some documentary evidence on Carib culture. Southwestern Journal of Anthropology 5 (4): 379 - 392.

Terreaux, C., Maillard, M., Stoeckli-Evans, H., Gupta, M., Downum, K., Quirks, J., Hostettmann, K. 1995. Structure revision of a furanocoumarin from Dorstenia contrajerva. Phytochemistry 39 (3), 645 - 647.

Thebtaranonth, C., Thebtaranonth, Y., Wanauppathamkul, S., Yuthavong, Y. 1995. Antimalarial sesquiterpenes from tubers of Cyperus rotundus: structure of 10,12-peroxycalamenene, a sesquiterpene endoperoxide. Phytochemistry 40 (1), 125 - 128.

Thomas, Nadine. 2005. Trinidad and Tobago. WNV meeting. Oct 24 – 27 2005. Guadeloupe. www.caribvet.net/Informations/Documents/Downloads/WestNile102005/9-WN%20surveillance%20in%20Trinidad.pdf

Thompson, H., Morrison, E.Y. St. A., Pascoe, K., West, M., Fletcher, C. 1989. Isolation, purification and identification of the hyperglycaemic principle of the Annatto (*Bixa orellana*). West Indian Medical Journal 38 Suppl 1, 25.

Thrupp, L. 1989. Legitimatizing local knowledge: scientized packages or empowerment for third world people. In: Warren,D.M., Slikkerveer, J. and Titilola, S. (Eds.). Indigenous Knowledge Systems: Implications for Agriculture and International Development. Studies in Technology and Social Change. No. 11. Ames: Iowa State University, Technology and Social Change Program, pp. 138-153.

Tilly, Charles, 1998. *Durable Inequality*. Berkeley: University of California Press.

Tobago House of Assembly. Division of Agriculture, Forestry and Marine Affairs. 1992 Administrative Report.

Tobin, B.F. 1999. "And there raise yams": slaves' gardens in the writings of West Indian plantocrats. Eighteenth-Century Life 23 (2), 164 - 176.

Tona, L., Kambu, K., Mesia, K., Cimanga, K., Apers, S., De Bruyne, T., Pieters, L., Totte, J., Vlietinck, A.J. 1999. Biological screening of traditional preparations from some medicinal plants used as antidiarrhoeal in Kinshasa, Congo. Phytomedicine 6 (1), 59-66.

Tona, L., Kambu, K., Ngimbi, N., Mesia, K., Penge, O., Lusakibanza, M., Cimanga, K., De Bruyne, T., Apers, S., Totte, J., Pieters, L., Vlietinck, A.J. 2000. Antiamoebic and spasmolytic activities of extracts from some antidiarrhoeal traditional preparations used in Kinshasa, Congo. Phytomedicine 7(1), 31-8.

Tovar-Miranda, R., Cortés-García, R., Santos-Sánchez, N.F., Joseph-Nathan, P. 1998. Isolation, total synthesis, and relative stereochemistry of a dihydrofurocoumarin from *Dorstenia contrajerva*. Journal of Natural Products 61 (10), 1216-20.

Trinidad and Tobago Express Newspapers. Reeza consoles angry farmers. Sunday February 28, 1998. http://209.94.197.2/feb/feb28/politics.htm

2005-2006 Budget Speech. Trinidad and Tobago 2005-2006 Budget Statement, by Prime Minister Patrick Manning. http://www.knowprose.com/node/8716 as retrieved on 10 Jun 2006

Trollope, 1859. In: Naipaul, V.S. 1962. The Middle Passage. Andre Deutsch, London.

Tsi, D., Das, N.P., Tan, B.K. 1995. Effects of aqueous celery (*Apium graveolens*) extract on lipid parameters of rats fed a high fat diet. Planta Medica 61(1), 18-21.

TT Parliament, 2004. House of Representatives. House Debates. Friday October 1, 2004. http://www.ttparliament.org/hansard/house/2004/hh20041001.pdf.

Ubillas, R.P., Mendez, C.D., Jolad, S.D., Luo, J., King, S.R., Carlson, T.J., Fort, D.M. 2000. Antihyperglycemic acetylenic glucosides from *Bidens pilosa*. Planta Medica 66 (1), 82-3.

Uphof, J.C. Th. 1968. Dictionary of economic plants. 2nd ed. Verlag von J. Cramer.

Van den Berg, A.J.J., Horsten, S., Kettenes-van den Bosch, J.J., Beukelman, C., Kroes, B., Leeflang, B., Labadie, R. 1995b. Podacycline A and B, two cyclic peptides in the latex of *Jatropha podagrica*. Phytochemistry 42 (1), 129 - 133.

Van den Berg, A.J.J., Horsten, S., Kettenes-van den Bosch, J.J., Kroes, B., Beukelman, C., Leeflang, B., Labadie, R. 1995c. Curacycline A - a novel cyclic octapeptide isolated from the latex of *Jatropha curcas* L. FEBS Letters 358 (3), 215 - 218.

Van den Berg, M.E. 1984. Ver-o-Peso: the ethnobotany of an Amazonian market. Advances in Economic Botany 1, 140 - 149.

Van Harten, A.M. 1970. Melegueta pepper. Economic Botany 2, 208 - 216.

Vasconcelos, S.M., Macedo, D.S., de Melo, C.T., Paiva Monteiro, A., Rodrigues, A.C., Silveira, E.R,, Cunha, G.M., Sousa, F.C., Viana, G.S. 2004. Central activity of hydroalcoholic extracts from *Erythrina velutina* and *Erythrina mulungu* in mice. J Pharm Pharmacol. 56(3):389-93.

Vasquez, A.S. 1977. The philosophy of praxis. In: Warry, W. 1992. The eleventh thesis: applied anthropology as praxis. Human Organization 51 (2), 155 -163.

Vázquez, B., Avila, G., Segura, D., Escalente, B. 1996. Anti-inflammatory activity of extracts from *Aloe vera* gel. Journal of Ethnopharmacology 55 (2), 69 - 75.

Vázquez, F.M., Suarez, M.A., Pérez, A. 1997. Medicinal plants used in the Barros area, Badajoz Province (Spain). Journal of Ethnopharmacology 55 (1), 81 - 85.

Vedavathy, S., Rao, K. 1991. Antipyretic activity of six indigenous medicinal plants of Tirumala Hills, Andhra Pradesh, India. Journal of Ethnopharmacology 33 (1-2), 193 - 196.

Verpoorte, R., Dihal, P. 1987. Medicinal plants of Surinam IV. Antimicrobial activity of some medicinal plants. Short communication. Journal of Ethnopharmacology 21 (3), 315 - 318.

Vieira, R., Simon, J. 2000. Chemical characterization of Basil (*Ocimum* spp.) found in the markets and used in traditional medicine in Brazil. Economic Botany 54 (2), 207 - 216.

Vieira, C., Fetzer, S., Sauer, S.K., Evangelista, S., Averbeck, B., Kress, M., Reeh, P.W., Cirillo, R., Lippi, A., Maggi, C.A., Manzini, S. 2001. Pro- and anti-inflammatory actions of ricinoleic acid: similarities and differences with capsaicin. *Naunyn Schmiedebergs Arch Pharmacol*. 364 (2):87-95.

Vijaya, K., Ananthan, S. 1997. Microbiological screening of Indian medicinal plants with special reference to enteropathogens. J. Altern. Complement. Med. 3(1), 13-20.

Vijaya, K., Ananthan, S., Nalini, R. 1995. Antibacterial effect of theaflavin, polyphenon 60 (*Camellia sinensis*) and *Euphorbia hirta* on *Shigella* spp.--a cell culture study. Journal of Ethnopharmacology 49 (2), 115-8.

Vijayalakshmi, P., Vijayalakshmi, K.M., Nanda Kumar, N.V. 1999. Depolarizing neuromuscular junctional blocking action of *Parthenium hysterophorus* leaf extracts in rat. Phytotherapy Research 13(5), 367-70.

Vilayleck, E. 1996. The bles, a Caribbean creole disease. Bull. Soc. Pathol. Exot. 89(1), 57-67. [Article in French]

Voeks, R.A. 1996. Tropical forest healers and habitat preference. Economic Botany 50 (4), 381 - 400.

Von Poser, G.L., Moulis, C., Sobral, M., Henriques, A.T. 1995. Chemotaxonomic features of iridoids occurring in *Verbenoxylum reitzii* (Verbenaceae). Plant Systematics and Evolution 198 (3-4), 287 - 290.

Vyas, A.V., Mulchandani, N.B. 1986. Polyoxygenated flavones from *Ageratum conyzoides*. Phytochemistry 25 (11), 2625 - 2627.

Wagner, H. 1990. Search for plant derived natural products with immunostimulatory activity (recent advances). Pure and Applied Chemistry 62 (7), 1217 - 1222.

Waller, D.P. 1993. Methods in Ethnopharmacology. Journal of Ethnopharmacology 38 (2-3), 189 -195.

Walter, G. 1992. Communication and sustainable agriculture: building agendas for research and practice. Agriculture and Human Values 9 (2), 27-38.

Walter, G. 1993. Farmers' use of validity cues to evaluate reports of field-scale agricultural research. American Journal of Alternative Agriculture 8 (3), 107 - 117.

Warren, D.M., Slikkerveer, L.J., Brokensha, D.W. (Eds.) 1995. The cultural dimension of development: Indigenous knowledge systems. Intermediate Technology Publications, London.

Warry, W. 1992. The eleventh thesis: Applied Anthropology as praxis. Human Organization 51 (2), 155 - 163.

Waterton, Charles. 1973 [1893]. Wanderings in South America. London: Fellowes.

Watson-Verran, H., Turnbull, D. 1995. Science and other indigenous knowledge systems. In: S. Jasanoff, G. Markle, J. Petersen, T. Pinch (Eds.). Handbook of science and technology studies. Sage Publications, Inc. pp. 115 - 139.

Watt, J.M., Breyer-Brandwijk, M.G. 1962. The medicinal and poisonous plants of Southern and Eastern Africa, 2nd Edition. E & S Livingstone, Ltd., Edinburgh, UK, 1457 pp.

Weasel, Lisa. 1966. Dismantling the Self/Other Dichotomy in Science: Towards a Feminist Model of the Immune System. Hypatia 16 (1): 27-44.

Weaver, T. 1985. Anthropology as a policy science: part 1, a critique. Human Organisation 44 (2), 97 - 105.

Weenen, H., Nkunya, M., Bray, D., Mwasumbi, L., Kinabo, L., Kilimali, V. 1990. Antimalarial activity of Tanzanian medicinal plants. Planta Medica 56 (4), 368 - 370.

Weller, J.A. 1968. The East Indian Indenture in Trinidad. Caribbean Monograph Series 4, Institute of Caribbean Studies. University of Puerto Rico, Puerto Rico.

Weniger, B. 1991. Interest and limitation of a global ethnopharmacological survey. Journal of Ethnopharmacology 32 (1-3), 37 - 41.

Weniger, B., Haag-Berrurier, M., Anton, R. 1982. Plants of Haiti used as antifertility agents. Journal of Ethnopharmacology 6 (1), 67 - 84.

Werbner, P. 2001. The limits of cultural hybridity: On ritual monsters, poetic licence and contested postcolonial purifications. The Journal of the Royal Anthropological Institute 7 (1), 133 - 152.

Westkott, M. 1979. Feminist criticism of the social sciences. Harvard Educ Review 49 (4), 422 - 430.

Whitehead, 1997. The Discoverie of the Large, Rich and Bewtiful Empyre of Guiana. By Sir Walter Ralegh. Edited by Neil L. Whitehead. Norman: University of Oklahoma Press.

Wiese, J., McPherson, S., Odden, M,C., Shlipak, M.G. 2004. Effect of *Opuntia ficus indica* on symptoms of the alcohol hangover. *Arch Intern Med*. 164 (12):1334-40.

Wilbert, J. 1983a. *Warao* ethnopathology and exotic epidemic disease. Journal of Ethnopharmacology 8 (3), 357 - 361.

Wilbert, W. 1983b. The Pneumatic theory of female *Warao* herbalists. Soc Sci Med 25 (10), 1139 - 1146.

Wilbert, W. 1996. Environment, society and disease: the response of phytotherapy to disease among the *Warao* Indians of the Orinoco Delta. In: Balick, M.J., Elisabetsky, E., Laird, J.A. 1996. Medicinal Resources of the Tropical Resources of the Tropical Forest: Biodiversity and its importance to human health, Columbia University Press, New York, pp. 366 - 385.

Williams, A. 1997. The postcolonial *flaneur* and other fellow-travellers: Conceits for a narrative of redemption. Third World Quarterly 18 (5), 821 - 841.

Williams, B.F. 1989. A class act: Anthropology and the race to nation across ethnic terrain. Annual Review of Anthropology 18, 401 - 444.

Williams, L.A.D., Williams, L.C. 1998. Insecticidally active sesquiterpene furan from *Bontia daphnoides* L. Philippine Journal of Science 126 (2), 155 - 162.

Williams, R.O., Williams, R.O., Jnr. 1969. The useful and ornamental plants of Trinidad and Tobago. Government Printery, Trinidad and Tobago.

Wilson, P. 1969. Reputation and respectability: A suggestion for Caribbean ethnology. Man 4 (1), 70 - 84.

Wilson, P. 1973. Crab antics: the social anthropology of English-speaking Negro societies of the Caribbean. Yale University Press, New Haven.

Wilson, P.N. 1961. Agricultural Education in the West Indies. Society Paper. Agricultural Society of Trinidad and Tobago. No. 889. Journal of the Agricultural Society of Trinidad and Tobago. December.

Wittrock, B. 1985. Useful science and scientific openness: Baconian vision or Faustian bargain? In: Gibbons, M and Wittrock, B. 1985 (Eds.). Science as a commodity. threats to the open community of science. London, Longman, pp 156 - 167.

Wolf, D.L 1996. Feminist dilemmas in fieldwork. West View Press, USA.

Wong, W. 1976. Some folk medicinal plants from Trinidad. Economic Botany 30, 103-142.

Wood, D. 1968. Trinidad in transition: the years after slavery. Oxford University Press, London and New York, 318 pp.

Yadav NP, Dixit VK. 2003. Hepatoprotective activity of leaves of *Kalanchoe pinnata* Pers. J Ethnopharmacol. 86(2-3):197-202.

Yadava, R., Saini, V. 1990. *In vitro* antimicrobial efficacy of the essential oil of *Eupatorium triplinerve* leaves. Indian Perfumer 34 (1), 61 - 63.

Yamamoto, L.A., Soldera, J.C., Emim, J.A., Godinho, R.O., Souccar, C., Lapa, A.J. 1991. Pharmacological screening of *Ageratum conyzoides* L. (Mentrasto). Memorias do Instituto Oswaldo Cruz 86 Suppl 2, 145-7.

Yang, Y., Kinoshita, K., Koyama, K., Takahashi, K., Tai, T., Nunoura, Y., Watanabe, K. 1999. Anti-emetic principles of *Pogostemon cablin* (Blanco) Benth. Phytomedicine 6 (2), 89-93.

Yeşilada, E., Sezik, E., Honda, G., Takaishi, Y., Takeda, Y., Tanaka, T. 1999. Traditional medicine in Turkey IX: folk medicine in north-west Anatolia. Journal of Ethnopharmacology 64 (3), 195 - 210.

Yoosook, C., Panpisutchai, Y., Chaichana, S., Santisuk, T., Reutrakul, V. 1999. Evaluation of anti-HSV-2 activities of *Barleria lupulina* and *Clinacanthus nutans*. J Ethnopharmacology 67 (2), 179 - 187.

Youn JY, Park HY, Cho KH: Anti-hyperglycemic activity of *Commelina communis* L.: Inhibition of alpha-glucosidase. Diabetes Res Clin Pract. 2004, 66 Suppl 1:S149-55.

Young, R.E., Williams, L.A.D., Gardner, M.T., Fletcher, C.K. 1993. An extract of the leaves of the breadfruit *Artocarpus altilis* (Parkinson) fosberg exerts a negative inotropic effect on rat myocardium. Phytotherapy Research 7 (2), 190 - 193.

Yusuf, S., Agunu, A., Diana, M. 2004. The effect of *Aloe vera* A. Berger (Liliaceae) on gastric acid secretion and acute gastric mucosal injury in rats. *J. Ethnopharmacol.* 93 (1): 33-7.

Zamora-Martínez, M. C, Nieto de Pascual Pola, C. 1992. Medicinal plants used in some rural populations of Oaxaca, Puebla and Veracruz, Mexico. Journal of Ethnopharmacology 35 (3), 229 - 257.

Zeng, Y., Zhong, J.M., Ye, S.Q., Ni, Z.Y., Miao, X.Q., Mo, Y.K., Li, Z.L. 1994. Screening of Epstein-Barr virus early antigen expression inducers from Chinese medicinal herbs and plants. Biomed. Environ. Sci. 7 (1), 50-5.

Zimdahl, Robert, L. 1998. Rethinking agricultural research roles. Agriculture and Human Values 15 (1), 77 - 84.

Zulueta, M. Carmelita, A., Tada, M., Ragasa, C. 1995. A diterpene from *Bidens pilosa*. Phytochemistry 38 (6), 1449 - 1450.

Index

www.ingramcontent.com/pod-product-compliance
Lightning Source LLC
Chambersburg PA
CBHW051409200326
41520CB00023B/7171